PLANT ROOTS

PLANT

101 Reasons Why the Human Diet

ROOTS

Is Rooted Exclusively in Plants

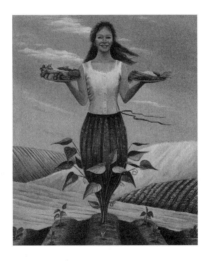

Rex Bowlby

OUTSIDE
THE BOX
publishing

Published by:
Outside the Box Publishing
P. O. Box 3402
Burbank, CA 91508-3402

Cover Design by Angie Underwood
Cover Illustration by Debby Fisher

Publisher's Cataloging-in-Publication
(Provided by Quality Books, Inc.)

Bowlby, Rex.
    Plant roots : 101 reasons why the human diet is
rooted exclusively in plants / Rex Bowlby. — 1st ed.
    p. cm.
    Includes bibliographical references and index.
    LCCN 2002116514
    ISBN 0-9672496-4-3

    1. Vegetarianism. 2. Diet. 3. Nutrition.
I. Title.

TX392.B69 2003   613.2'62
                          QBI03-200137

The information and ideas in this book are not intended as a substitute for the medical advice of your trained health professional. All matters regarding your health require medical supervision. Consult your physician before adopting the suggestions in this book, as well as about any condition that may require diagnosis or medical attention. The author and publisher disclaim any liability arising directly or indirectly from the use of this book.

Printed in the United States of America
First Edition
10 9 8 7 6 5 4 3 2 1

For

Ryan and Eric

May they live long and healthy lives

ACKNOWLEDGMENTS

To those that opened my eyes to the large chasm between the American perception and the reality.

To the individuals that directly contributed to this book: Debby Fisher for her talent, attitude, and portrayal of Olive, the veggie girl. Angie Underwood who believes you *can* judge a book by its cover. And Marilyn Weishaar for her sharp eyes and even sharper pencil.

To the hundreds of doctors, scientists, nutritionists, and educators whose wisdom, foresight, and compassion indirectly contributed to this book by way of their research and study, including: Keith Akers, Neal Barnard, Rynn Berry, William Harris, Frances Moore Lappé, Howard Lyman, John McDougall, Gary Null, John Robbins, Steven Rosen, and Joanne Stepaniak.

To the computer age and its products that have made writing, researching, and publishing so much more efficient: Microsoft® Word, Excel, and Bookshelf®, QuarkXPress™, Google.com™, and the World Wide Web.

To my family who, although they may not have always understood my quest, implicitly supported my efforts.

And to my dog, Gretchen, who I symbolically, but absurdly try to give the magnitude of love and affection sufficient to atone for all the animals that have been wronged by humans for the sake of food.

CONTENTS

"Although nature commences with reason and ends in experience it is necessary for us to do the opposite, that is to commence with experience and from this to proceed to investigate the reason."

(LEONARDO DA VINCI)

"A short saying often contains much wisdom."

(SOPHOCLES)

INTRODUCTION
THE DIET HAS CHOSEN US

When vegetarians are asked why they chose vegetarianism they give reasons such as, improving their health, saving the animals, protecting the environment, and increasing the global food supply.

They are all noble reasons, but are they really *reasons*? Might they instead be byproducts—beneficial consequences alerting us that humans were designed as natural herbivores? Therefore, it would be more correct to say that vegetarians didn't choose the diet—it chose them!

Plant Roots is based on the premise that the diet of humankind is rooted solely in plants—grains, legumes, vegetables, fruits, nuts, and seeds, to the exclusion of animals—meat, fish, dairy, and eggs. *Plant Roots* brings together evidence, inference, and common sense in a compelling whole to demonstrate this supposition—and just as importantly—to illuminate the reasons why we have strayed so far from our intended path.

Given that roughly 95 percent of Americans eat meat, the average citizen's initial reaction to the book might be to dismiss it as faddish, groundless, or extreme.[1] Their responses might be, "If we weren't meant to eat meat,

- wouldn't we see evidence that proves it?"

- wouldn't the revelation have made the news?"

- wouldn't a lot fewer people be eating meat?"

- wouldn't the nutritional information we get be less confusing?"

- wouldn't we have alternative sources for protein and iron?"

- wouldn't meat taste bad, instead of good?"

- wouldn't our life expectancy be getting shorter, not longer?"

- wouldn't *all* Americans that eat meat—95 percent—be suffering from a degenerative disease?"

They are all logical and rational responses—when they are viewed within the context of our culture. But our collective perception is greatly distorted. When we are able to break loose and step outside of our cultural reference—as 12 million American vegetarians have been able to do—these responses become flawed.[2]

In contrast to the meat-eater's reaction, a vegetarian's frame of reference might evoke these rebuttals: "If we *were* meant to eat meat,

- wouldn't our anatomy be designed the same as a carnivore's?"

- wouldn't our grand designer have made animals immobile, unable to run from us, to ensure the perpetuation of our species?"

- wouldn't we see far less breakdown of the incredible human body than we do—100 million Americans suffering from degenerative diseases and 50 percent of Americans overweight?"[3]

- wouldn't our human ancestors, who go back 8 million years, have evolved on a meat-based diet?"[4]

- wouldn't we see other countries and cultures suffering consequences rather than benefits from *not* eating meat?"

- wouldn't our environment be robust and stable, rather than what it is—damaged and deteriorating?"

- wouldn't we see a world well-fed and nourished, instead of a world where 2 billion people are malnourished—with a

curious equilibrium of 1 billion overfed and 1 billion underfed?"[5]

It's remarkable that people from the same country with so many
common experiences, could be so far apart in their perceptions on
such a fundamental and consequential issue as diet. But based on
the previous comparisons, American herbivores and omnivores are
just that.

Many cultural influences have shaped Americans' belief
that eating meat is a necessary and integral part of the human
dietary equation. These formidable factors are still at work distort-
ing the picture for the majority of Americans. Some of them are:

- ERRONEOUS INFORMATION: Some early nutritional data
  on protein has gone unchallenged and still assumed to be
  true.

- LEARNING AND CONDITIONING: Food habits are seen as
  needs and likes/dislikes, but they are really shaped by associations and rewards.

- ECONOMIC INTERESTS: The meat and dairy industries,
  and the healthcare industries, have a lot riding on our meat-
  eating habits.

- NEWS MEDIA AND ADVERTISING: This is where we
  obtain most of our nutritional information—sources that are
  not necessarily unbiased.

- HEALTHCARE: There is a misperception of what it is, and
  a gross underestimation of the influence of food on our
  health.

- ANIMALS: The fact that meat was once a living, breathing,
  sentient creature has become lost in our desensitization to
  nature.

- RELIGION: Given its underlying influence, the assumptions
  we might have made deserve a closer look.

- COMPLEXITY: The world, ever more complicated, has tended to foster conformity and diminish self-reliance.

These deeply ingrained elements are woven into the fabric of our lives. Unless we take the initiative to question the assumptions and seek out the readily available information, which these influences have masked, the factors will continue to stand as barriers to objectivity.

Plants Roots has done the legwork for the reader, assembling the relevant information, like pieces of a jigsaw puzzle, into a finished picture puzzle that is clear and unmistakable. Grouped into 11 chapters, each one of the book's 101 subjects represents a piece of the puzzle. The following brief chapter overviews provide a glimpse of what's ahead.

CHAPTER 1: There is more to EVIDENCE than test tubes, Bunsen burners, and technicians in white lab coats. If we relied solely on exact science to discover truths, we would surely miss a lot of them.

CHAPTER 2: They provide our fuel and manage our healthcare / immune system by pulling together minerals, vitamins, organic compounds, and phytochemicals into one efficient package—Nature's Nutrient Delivery System. Is there any reason *why* PLANTS couldn't be humankind's sole food source?

CHAPTER 3: Animal muscles designed to move body parts; the cows' lactating secretion and derivatives; the chicken embryo's gelatinous nourishment. These are the substances on which most Americans center their nutrition. MEAT AND DAIRY suggests that the foods we think we can't live without, are really the foods we can't *live* with.

CHAPTER 4: Is it possible something can do more damage than the inherent properties of animal-based foods such as fat and cholesterol? CONTAMINANTS advances two truths: Meat, a relatively inexpensive food, comes at a steep price. And there's more to meat than meets the eye.

CHAPTER 5: Rather than *what* we are eating, ANIMALS explores *who* we are eating, and also who we are. They are creatures with amazing character and a will to live, and we are supposedly humane and civilized. In the end we may change our opinion about which animal is the dumbest.

CHAPTER 6: What does THE ENVIRONMENT have to do with our food choices? Everything. Excluding meat from our diets would do more to benefit our natural resources than any other action. In essence our environment's health—like our health—is greatly dependent on what we choose to eat.

CHAPTER 7: Do DISEASE KILLERS indicate there are multiple design flaws in the human body? Are these diseases predominately due to heredity, aging, and bad luck as we perceive? Or are they Exhibit A in the evidence indicting animal-based foods of the crime: Food Impersonation.

CHAPTER 8: They generally won't end our lives, but DISEASE HARDSHIPS will have plenty to say about the quality of them. Britt Tilbones, Doctors Endd and Dometri, Colonel Otto M. Yune, and Sherlock Holmes help to explore this topic.

CHAPTER 9: Can theology provide direction or insight into the human diet? Given the fundamental importance to the success and survival of humankind, shouldn't it? RELIGION draws from both principles and the principals, and suggests that religion and vegetarianism might be a perfect marriage.

CHAPTER 10: Are there economic forces influencing our meat and dairy habits, and the perception of their effect on our health? MANIPULATION addresses protein, promotion, profits, politics, propaganda, and a pyramid in the quest for answers. Money talks— but do we have to listen?

CHAPTER 11: Sometimes seeing something in a way we have never seen it before can be the catalyst for INSIGHT and understanding.

Could one of the stories in the final chapter be the missing piece of the puzzle for the reader—the insight—to solidify the essence of *Plant Roots*?

Every decision we make impacts our lives. From simple everyday decisions that can have a minor effect, to a handful of decisions that are life-defining. The latter being decisions that affect the quality, and perhaps quantity—that is longevity—of our lives.

Every day, 140,000 times (3 meals/2 snacks) for the average lifespan, we place food into our bodies. What we choose as our food might be the most important decision we ever make. If we were to educate ourselves on only one issue in life, the subject of our diet should be the one we pick. We can't afford to be wrong.

Do we choose the Self-Induced Carnivorous Killer diet, hereafter referred to as the SICK diet, or do we choose the Wholly Eating Leaves to Live diet, hereafter referred to as the WELL diet?

If the premise of *Plant Roots* appears to be too unbelievable, consider this: Day in and day out for many centuries our ancestors watched the sun move across the sky. Who then, would have taken seriously the idea that it was the earth that revolved around the sun.

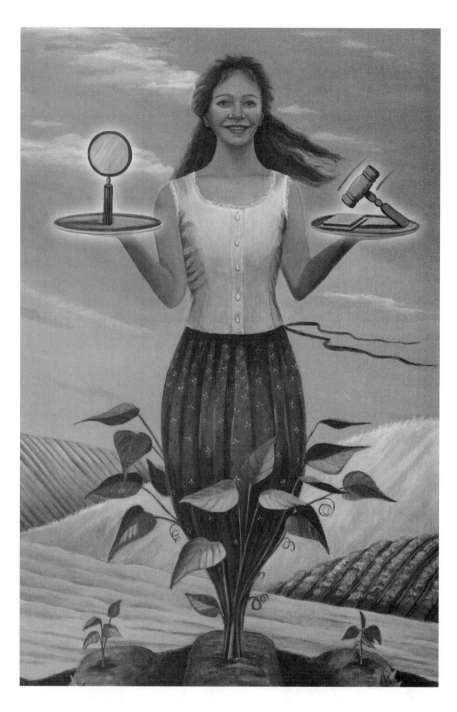

How Much Evidence Does It Take?

∾ 1 ∾
Evidence
BE PREPARED TO REACH A VERDICT

How much evidence does it take before one can conclude that the human diet should consist only of plant-based foods? Court is now in session. Become a jurist, absorb all the evidence, and be prepared to reach a verdict. Someone's life may depend on it.

Ahead in this chapter...

Is it possible there is more to SCIENTIFIC EVIDENCE than test tubes and Bunsen burners? If we relied on exact science to discover truths, we might miss a lot of them.

Can the EVOLUTION of humankind provide clues about the proper diet for our species?

Can we draw conclusions about our intended diet based on the human ANATOMY?

With 50 percent of Americans overweight, 1,800 diet books in print, and millions DIETING, can we conclude the human body has a major design flaw, or is there another problem?[1]

How many STUDIES will it take before we can reach a conclusion about the nature of the human diet? Do we recognize that studies can go on forever, but our lives don't?

A real-world experiment has been in progress for years, with millions of subjects in the pool, and no bias or manipulation. Can we learn anything from the diets of other COUNTRIES AND CULTURES?

Is there a difference between DEGENERATIVE AND INFECTIOUS DISEASE? If we have an 80 percent chance of dying from one, and a 2 percent chance of dying from the other, would we want to know more?[2]

How often does NATURE say one thing and wisdom another? Can Nature tell us anything about the natural diet of humankind?

1: Scientific Evidence

MORE THAN TEST TUBES AND BUNSEN BURNERS

HUMANS ARE HERBIVORES

Today it was announced on the lawns of the University of Utopia that humans were designed to subsist on a pure vegetarian diet to the exclusion of animals and their byproducts.

Dressed in white lab coats and holding test tubes and Bunsen burners, Doctor's Sy and Ince shared their results with media from all over the world. After 3 days of rigorously controlled experiments the good doctors exclaimed, "If our Bunsen burners hadn't kept going out we could have finished in 2 days."

Most probably, Americans, before accepting the idea that humans were designed as vegetarians and not meat-eaters, would want to see simple proof that came from an experiment. And then only after the news made front page headlines, came out of the mouths of network anchors, and been announced by the president in the Rose Garden, would they believe it. It's unlikely to happen.

The complexity of human physiology, the logistics of placing controlled settings in the real world, and the wide spectrum of variables involved, provide a scenario that is just the opposite of Americans' expectations and the fantasy press release. The scientific evidence will come in small pieces, in many forms, covering a long period of time.

Scientific evidence can be obtained from sources other than experiments done in a lab under controlled conditions with test tubes and Bunsen burners. The Encarta Desk Encyclopedia says this about scientific evidence:

"Science has tremendous scope, and its separate disciplines can differ greatly in terms of subject matter

and methods of observation. No single path to discovery exists in science, and no clear-cut description
can be given for all the ways in which scientific
truth is pursued."

In other words, if we are sincere about wanting to get at the truth of
what the natural human diet is, then we must broaden our thinking
to consider all the diverse data that comes under the umbrella of
scientific evidence.

To get us to start thinking outside the box—and under the
umbrella—here are 15 categories of evidence that are weaved into
the book. This is not an exact science, but if we relied on exact science to discover truths, we would surely miss a lot of them.

- EVOLUTION: Humans evolved over an 8 million year period.[1] What do we know about our diet during this span of
  time, and could our diet of the past influence our diet of the
  present?

- ANATOMY: Is our anatomy designed to eat and process
  meat? Can we learn anything by comparing our anatomy to
  the natural carnivores?

- CULTURES: The American diet is not the *world* diet.
  Beyond our shores are many diverse diets of many different
  countries. Can we learn anything about the relationship of
  disease and diet from other cultures?

- STUDIES: Studies often provide more "confusion than conclusion." Does the confusion mean that the picture is clouded, or do we only need to blow away the clouds to see a
  clear picture?

- SERENDIPITY: World War I and II provided unique circumstances, such as meat and dairy shortages for some
  countries. Did the apparent hardship turn out to be a definite
  blessing?

- POPULATIONS: Can subpopulations that have different diets, like Seventh-Day Adventists or poor Japanese women, provide insight into the nature of the human diet?

- GENETICS: Our perception is that genetics play an influential role in the determination of degenerative disease. Will we still think that way after looking at evidence provided by the observation of people of common races, who live in different parts of the world, with different diets?

- DISEASE: To what extent is disease, specifically degenerative disease, a byproduct of the foods we eat? This category might well be the most influential in our search for the truth.

- REVERSING DISEASE: Changing diets has been shown to stop and even reverse life-threatening degenerative diseases. What might it tell us about the source of disease when something as un-medical as food can have a medical-like solution?

- ANIMAL-BASED FOOD PROPERTIES: There are two compounds of animal-based foods that are as bad, if not worse, than fat and cholesterol. What are they, and why do we have the perception that we can't get enough of them?

- PLANT-BASED FOOD PROPERTIES: Plants pull the minerals from the earth, the energy from the sun, and manufacture a world of vitamins, chemicals, and compounds. What would make us think then that it couldn't be possible to be nourished exclusively by the plant kingdom?

- CHEMISTRY: Does animal protein cross-reaction cause autoimmune disease? Does animal fat cover insulin receptor sites promoting diabetes? Do chemoreceptors in the stomach that monitor nutrients have anything to do with overeating? The microscopic world can tell us a macroscopic bunch.

- ENVIRONMENTAL BYPRODUCTS: The sickness of our planet is manifested by the depletion and impairment of our natural resources. Can the diet that promotes human sickness be the same diet that promotes the earth's sickness?

- NATURE: Nature has a lot to tell us. We only need to stop, look around, and take note. After all, isn't observation the cornerstone of scientific evidence?

- RELIGION: True, religion is not scientific evidence. However, for those who are religious, might scripture and spiritual enlightenment carry equal weight?

Someday we may read the headlines, hear from the news anchors, and tune into the president in the Rose Garden, with all of them informing us that humans are indeed herbivores. But most likely it would come as confirmation, rather than revelation, meaning we should have made the diet change long ago.

Well, long ago is today. Let's have the revelation now.

2: Evolution

DO PLANTS LINE OUR EVOLUTIONARY PATH?

Would it help us to answer the question of whether humankind is a natural omnivore or herbivore (we can probably rule out carnivore), by looking at our evolutionary history? Certainly this is not the predominant issue facing us while waiting in the fast-food drive-through line trying to decide between a hamburger and a salad, but maybe it ought to cross our mind.

Most anthropologists would agree that for each species there is a natural, ideal type of food that leads to maximum vitality for that species. It is determined by the adaptation that each species has made to the available food during millions of years.[1] But there is not a consensus among anthropologists on what adaptation was made, and to which food, for humans. Anthropology is not an exact science. The archeological record does not give a clear linear story of human development.[2] Therefore, assumption, interpretation, and bias often drive opposing opinions. (Imagine the dilemma the meat-eating anthropologist is faced with if he or she should conclude humans are natural herbivores, and vice versa.)

Let's take a walk down our evolutionary path and see if it might be lined with plants.

- TIMELINE: Humankind and its ancestors evolved for 8 million years on a predominantly vegetarian diet until the ice age.[3]

- NUTRIENTS: Animals manufacture none of the nutrients essential to humans. Essential nutrients obtained from animal-based foods all originated in the plant kingdom.[4]

- DROUGHT: If nutrients from animals are redundant why did hominids eat meat? Climatic changes and drought during the Ice Age, 3.5 million years ago, rendered plants scarce. Consequently, in order to survive humans had to eat animals.[5]

- SPEED: Plants don't move but animals do. Humankind, because of its weight, could not chase down breakfast, lunch, or dinner. Meat consumption is inversely related to body weight; the smaller the primate, the more meat eaten. In a study of 21 primates observed, the smallest weighed less than 1 pound and ate 70 percent dietary animal matter. The largest, the gorilla, weighed 350 pounds and ate 1 to 2 percent animal matter.[6]

- INSTINCTS: What are we more likely to see: A human pouncing on a chicken, ripping it apart, salivating at the sight of its raw flesh, then sucking the warm blood from it? Or a human slicing an orange, inhaling the sweet fragrance, and salivating while sucking the flavorful juice?

- ANATOMY: A tangible result of evolution? Humans have a body structure (digestive system and hands/feet) designed to process plant-based foods, rather than meat. Our teeth, jaws, taste buds, intestines, saliva, hands/feet, vary significantly from the carnivores.[7]

- BIPEDAL: Some scientists have suggested that humans evolved initially into a two-legged primate for the purpose of reaching fruit growing in small trees. Fossilized remains indicate a very wide skeleton, which would have provided good support when standing upright to obtain the fruit, but would not have been very effective for walking.[8]

- DARWIN: If we believe the Darwinian version of evolution then we accept that we are primates descended from animals, and not separate from them. It then follows we should challenge the practical, religious, and philosophical justification for eating them.

- DISEASE: Another concrete product of evolution? The quantity and destruction of degenerative diseases tied to meat and dairy consumption might be trying to tell us something; maybe that we never adapted to eating animals and their byproducts.

Since we can do nothing about the past, we often think of it as being no longer relevant. School history class was often boring because of this perspective. And trying to relate to the millions of years of human evolution is like trying to imagine what exists on the other side of our universe. But to ignore what we know about our roots is to ignore an important piece of the puzzle. A piece that might make our next fast-food purchase decision an easy one.

3: Anatomy

NO CLAWS ON OUR HANDS OR FEET

If we look around the animal kingdom we might notice that mammals are built and constructed to get proper nourishment to ensure their survival. Anteaters have no teeth, but long snouts and sticky tongues to suck up ants and termites. Giraffes have long necks to reach into tall trees for their food. Lions have hooked claws and wide powerful jaws to catch and disassemble their meals.

The human mammal is no different. We, too, were built to get proper nourishment in order to thrive. How are we built then, and what does it tell us about which foods we were meant to survive on?

- CLAWS: We struggle to tear open letters or wrestle open jars with our supple pudgy fingers, but we can "pick and gather" with no problem. Chances are we wouldn't survive long catching, killing, and tearing prey with our hands. That is probably why carnivores come equipped with sharp claws.

- TEETH: When we look inside our mouths we see a majority of our teeth are short, with flat large surfaces. If we looked inside a carnivore's mouth—and please do so with caution—we would see long, sharp, canine teeth much the opposite of ours. One might conclude our teeth were designed to pulverize the cellulose walls of plants while the long, sharp teeth of the carnivore were meant to tear apart the flesh of animals.[1]

- JAW: The human jaw moves sideways in addition to moving up and down, while a carnivore jaw only moves up and down.[2] Their jaw is also double-hinged to open wider than we are capable of, presumably to make headway into a large animal. One might conclude the jaw moves sideways to work in concert with our flat teeth to grind down the starch-es of plants. We don't require quite the same opening to get our mouths around a stalk of celery or most other plant-based foods.

- SALIVA: If we analyzed human saliva (although it's proba-bly not something we care to do), it's alkaline, containing the chemical ptyalin. A carnivore's saliva is acidic, contain-ing the chemical hydrochloric acid. Ptyalin catalyzes the hydrolysis of starch from plants into maltose and dextrin. Hydrochloric acid is probably overkill for plants, but it works just fine for dissolving tissue, cartilage, and bone.[3]

- INTESTINE DESIGN: The human digestive system is com-posed of 25 feet of intestine. The many twists and turns makes the intestine look like a poorly designed racetrack. The insides are pocketed and pouched, and have an alkaline environment. The carnivore has a much shorter intestinal track with almost a straight shot from mouth to anus. The inside of the intestine is smooth and has an acidic environ-ment. Because the animal and human intestine designs are completely the opposite, might this be indicative that the foods they were each meant to manage could also be oppo-sites—not unlike plant-based and animal-based foods?[4]

- DIGESTION: The complex carbohydrates contained in plants, but not in animals, would logically require a com-plex intestinal system to break down their many compo-nents and nutrients. The short and compact acidic system of the carnivore might best be suited for the rapid breakdown and elimination of the carcinogen waste produced by meat. How do we know this? Unlike plants, meat has no fiber.[5] Therefore, meat has no inherent means to move itself quick-ly through our long, pouched, and winding intestine. The muscle, fat, and ligaments that make up meat can take 3 to 4 days to move sluggishly through our bowels causing some unpleasant consequences.[6]

After this brief analysis comparing the human digestive system with that of the natural carnivore, one of two possibilities emerges: Either Nature failed us in the engineering of our anatomy, or we failed when we selected animals as a food source. In either case, we appear to be left with just *one* possibility for our choice of diet: A Wholly Eating Leaves to Live (WELL) diet.

4: Dieting

DOES THE BODY HAVE A MAJOR DESIGN FLAW?

What do golf, the accordion, and diet books have in common? If our answer is: they exist for the continuing amusement of the Gods, we can go to the head of the class.

At the same time there are 1,800 diet books in print, Americans are fatter than they were in 1990, with 50 percent currently overweight, and 1 in 5 obese.[1] Doesn't it seem just a bit odd that after 8 million years of evolutionary refinement, the apparatus that regulates our food intake and impacts our very survival, is flawed for half the people in this country? Or is there another explanation. That maybe we are contributing to the mechanism's inefficiency. Let's look at the two fundamental ways we are doing this.

The first: Our digestive system monitors both calories and nutrients by way of chemoreceptors.[2] It wants us to get enough to eat as well as get us the proper nutrients. If we are eating the wrong foods and have met our caloric requirements, but not our nutrient requirements, our bodies will tell us to keep eating. Americans consuming the Self-Induced Carnivorous Killer (SICK) diet, are getting about 40 percent of their calories from fat, which is lacking nutrients, rather than the 10 to 15 percent they should be getting. So it is no surprise that the body will respond with a call to be fed more.[3] The result: overweight.

The second: A meat-based diet is made up of 40 percent carbohydrates in calories when the body should be receiving close to 80 percent carbohydrates, which it would receive on the WELL diet.[4] Carbohydrates are the body's primary fuel, converted to sugars more easily than protein or fat, and burned first by the body. Carbohydrates speed metabolism and are part of the cueing mechanism that alerts the body to fullness.[5] Carbohydrates are found mainly in plant-based foods, and complex carbohydrates and fiber are found *only* in plant-based foods. Fats found mainly in animal-based foods feed the body more than twice the calories for the same amount of food, as fat contains 9 calories per gram to 4 calories per gram of carbohydrate. The result: overweight.

Now we are overweight. Just look at us. We don't understand why, but since half of Americans are too, we don't feel so alone. We go to the bookstore, and then to the library, looking for just the right diet book. We're looking for one that is very scientific and precise because we figure since so many people are having such a hard time losing weight the secret must be very involved and complex. We also want a book that will give us the license to eat as many of the foods we like as possible. Given that the diet business is a $40 billion industry, most likely we are going to find exactly what we want.[6] But will our new diet work?

The human body has never heard of dieting, but it has heard of surviving. When we begin to diet and reduce our food intake the body assumes that we are running out of food, so logically it goes into conservation mode. This means it *conserves* fat and *slows* metabolism, completely contrary to weight loss.[7] Then when we come across an attractive hunk of food in a 5-gallon container the body is not sure if this is the only food it will see for some time. Before we know it we are scraping the bottom and licking the spoon. We think we are a failure for binging, but the body thinks it's a hero for saving our life.

It looks as if the best potential feature of diet books is the exercise one can get by stacking them on the floor for aerobic stair-stepping, or by walking them back to the library.

As it turns out the secret to weight loss and weight maintenance is a well-kept secret, possibly because there is no money—like $40 billion—to be made from it. It is a radical concept, quite different from any theory encountered in a diet book. The mechanism for losing weight and maintaining the correct weight is the same, and it is this: Eat a wide variety of whole, plant-based foods; the ones Nature put out for us—fruits, vegetables, whole grains, legumes, nuts, and seeds.

When we do, we naturally get the proper nutrients and ratio of carbohydrates, protein, and fat at roughly 80, 10, and 10 percent of calories, respectively.[8] We will lose weight, never feel hungry, maintain optimal health, and should never have a problem with our weight again. Pure vegetarians weigh 10 to 20 pounds less, have 30 percent less body fat, and 18 percent (20 to 2 percent) less obesity than those consuming an animal-based diet.[9]

The human body is an amazing, efficient machine. We only have to operate it properly and it will perform as it was meant to. Yes, it does sound too good to be true, so admittedly there are a few downsides.

We won't get to be part of the newest fad. We won't have interesting cocktail party talk. We won't have ready-made bedtime reading. We won't get the stimulating challenge of weighing food, counting calories, and calculating fat grams. And the worst part of the diet is: we only get to do it once. We will have to find other hobbies to take up our free time.

And as for the Gods? Sure, we want to keep them amused and happy. But even without diet books they are still left with golf and the accordion, assuring they will never be at a loss for a good laugh.

5: Studies

STUDIES CAN GO ON FOREVER BUT WE DON'T

The results of studies on nutrition come to us on almost a daily basis. For a number of reasons the collective data often provides us more "confusion than conclusion."

But studies, as part of a larger whole, can play an important role in furthering our knowledge. They can be narrowly designed to focus on a specific issue. They can corroborate data found in the real world. They can be manufactured to confirm or deny an opinion or theory. And although just one study is usually not conclusive—especially in the complex area of diet—it can move us closer to the truth.

Throughout the book results will be quoted from many scientific queries. The goal of "Studies" is to begin to peel the onion, posing some fundamental questions, and providing the results of studies that support the answers.

If we aren't familiar with some of the following information, it isn't because it's new. In fact, much of the data implicating animal-based foods in human disease has been around for some time. Like for instance, an article in *Scientific American* printed this observation: "Cancer is most frequent among those branches of the human race where carnivorous habits prevail." Was this observation made 5 years ago, 10 years ago, 20 or 30 years ago? No, it was made in 1892.[1]

Let's begin to peel the proverbial onion and explore the answers to the following questions.

Does meat give us strength? Does milk give us stronger bones? How much protein do humans require? Can disease caused by meat and dairy foods be reversed by avoiding them? Can avoiding meat extend our lives? Do cultural differences protect against disease? Can we fulfill our amino acid requirements with plant protein? Why is the risk of heart disease for women higher after menopause? Are the United States Department of Agriculture (USDA) food pyramid guidelines healthful?

- Does meat give us strength?

    In one Yale study, the score of vegetarians was double the score of meat-eaters in strength and endurance.[2] In another study in Paris, vegetarians averaged 2 to 3 times more stamina than meat-eaters and required only one-fifth the time to recover from exhaustion.[3]

- Does milk give us stronger bones?

    The Harvard Public School of Health tracked 75,000 nurses and found the women with the highest calcium consumption from dairy products had substantially more fractures than women who drank less milk.[4]

- How much protein do humans require?

    An adult male puts out 4.32 grams of urinary nitrogen per day. Each gram represents 6.25 grams of broken down protein. Thus, 27 grams of protein are required per day: 27 x 4 calories / gram = 108 calories / 2,400 calories = 4.5 percent protein / day.[5]

- Can disease caused by meat and dairy foods be reversed by avoiding them?

    Heart Disease: In a 12-year Esselstyn study, severe heart disease was reversed in 95 percent of those going on a pure vegetarian diet.[6] Diabetes: 75 percent of adult-onset diabetes patients stopped taking insulin soon after going on a pure vegetarian diet.[7] Arthritis: Six subjects going on a pure vegetarian diet had complete disappearance of symptoms after 7 weeks.[8]

- Can avoiding meat extend our lives?

    Vegetarian Seventh-day Adventist (SDA) men, on average, live 8.9 years longer than the typical North

American male, while SDA women, on average, live 7.5 years longer than the typical North American female.[9]

- Do cultural differences protect against disease?

  A National Cancer Institute study followed Japanese immigrants who moved to the United States and adopted the American SICK diet to see if they would maintain their low colon cancer rates. They did not. Their rates rose to the level of the typical American.[10]

- Can we fulfill our amino acid requirements with plant protein?

  Studies consistently show that the protein status of vegetarians is adequate. Vegetarians store amino acids in muscle tissue and have a constant supply of protein in the intestines. Vegetarians don't need to rely on protein combining to meet protein needs.[11]

- Why is the risk of heart disease for women higher after menopause?

  Iron makes atherosclerosis more likely to start. Women's iron levels are held down by the natural loss of iron through menstruation. Vegetarians are shown to have lower and safer amounts of iron stored in their bodies.[12]

- Are the USDA food pyramid guidelines healthful?

  The food pyramid includes 4 to 6 servings of meat/dairy foods per day. The 51,000 men who followed the pyramid guidelines for 8 years were only 11 percent less likely to develop cardiovascular disease, and no less likely to develop cancer.[13] In one study, 67,000 female nurses followed for 12 years were no less likely to develop any chronic disease by following the guidelines.[14]

The collective data pointing the accusatory finger at animal-based foods seems pretty convincing. Then one night while watching television we hear about another study and get confused again. A survey of 90,000 nurses found no relationship between fat consumption and breast cancer. How could one find fault with a study that has 90,000 data points? Here's how.

The study did not include a key population group—vegans. Therefore, all the subjects were consuming fat well above the 10 to 15 percent of calories recommended. The amount of fat the 90,000 nurses consumed then made little difference in their risk since they all exceeded the critical threshold.[15]

Studies are not the be all and end all. But when combined with other evidence, like data that emerges from the diets of other countries and cultures, the picture of humans as natural herbivores begins to come into focus.

Studies and evidence have implicated animal-based foods in human disease and other problems for more than 100 years, yet just 5 percent of Americans are vegetarians.[16] At what point do we say we have conducted enough studies, and have enough evidence, to decide we shouldn't be eating animal-based foods anymore?

Maybe we should keep in mind that studies can go on forever—but our lives don't.

6: Countries and Cultures

NO SLOPPY EXPERIMENTS OR BIAS

The result of yet another study about diet comes spilling out of the television onto the large pile of studies already on the floor. We're pretty sure it told us to eat something that we thought a previous study told us not to eat. Or was it the other way around? Oh well, we go back to eating our Salisbury steak confident we stand an even chance we've chosen the right food for dinner.

Studies and experiments often contradict themselves and each other. Maybe they were constructed with too few subjects. Maybe they didn't last long enough. Maybe those conducting the studies were incompetent. Maybe the designs were biased to ensure a predetermined result. Maybe the media is selective on what they report. Whatever the reason, we gave up long ago trying to sort through the morass of nutritional knowledge.

But don't despair. There is an ongoing experiment that provides some very clear results. It includes millions of subjects, over decades of time, and because nobody is running the experiment there are no incompetent technicians or bias. It's called "The Real-World Experiment of Countries' and Cultures' Diverse Diets." It may help to sort out the morass of nutritional information and illuminate the intelligence of our next dinner selection.

The following sampling of rankings is the result of plotting daily fat intake against disease for multiple countries. The rankings for cases or deaths are in parentheses.[1]

BREAST CANCER CASES (37 COUNTRIES):

- Cancer:
   Denmark (1)
   United States (7)
   Sri Lanka (37)
- Fat Intake:
   Denmark (1)
   United States (7)
   Sri Lanka (36)

INSULIN-DEPEND. DIABETES CASES (14 COUNTRIES):

- Diabetes:
  Denmark (1)
  United States (4)
  Japan (14)

- Fat Intake:
  Denmark (1)
  United States (5)
  Japan (14)

UTERINE CANCER DEATHS (8 COUNTRIES):

- Cancer:
  United States (1)
  Nigeria (7)

- Fat Intake:
  United States (1)
  Nigeria (8)

- Affluent women in Japan who eat meat have an 8.5 times greater risk of breast cancer than the poorer Japanese women who can't afford meat.[2]

- Residents of rural China subsist primarily on grains, legumes, fruits, and vegetables. As a result, coronary artery disease is virtually unknown. Cholesterol levels range from 90 to 150 milligrams per deciliter.[3]

- Coronary artery disease is 5 times lower for Greek men than American men—the Greek diet is plant-based.[4]

- The people of Nauru, who live on a small Polynesian island and subsist on vegetables, grains, and fruits, had no diabetes prior to World War II. After the war, their country fell into riches, people began to include meat in their diets, and one-third of the population developed diabetes.[5]

- The daily calcium intake for African Americans is more than 1,000 milligrams, and for black South Africans 196 milligrams. Which group has 9 times the hip fracture rate? Because of their animal-based, animal protein diets, African Americans do.[6]

- The four countries with the highest consumption of dairy products are the United States, Finland, Sweden, and England. The four countries with the highest rates of osteoporosis? The United States, Finland, Sweden, and England.[7]

- In the United States, 1 in 4 people suffers from osteoarthritis, a universal degenerative disease that strikes as we age. Except it's not so universal because it's a rare disease in China, Africa, and Japan where the diets contain little fat, cholesterol, and animal protein.[8]

- In the United States, 50 percent of the population older than 65 has hypertension with readings greater than 160 over 95.[9] Another universal degenerative disease due to aging? Like arthritis it is not so universal, because in New Guinea and several African countries, blood pressure *throughout life* remains at a constant 110 over 70.[10]

- Multiple sclerosis (MS) and Crohn's disease may not be thought of as diet-related diseases, but the facts are this: The nine countries with the highest rate of MS have a per capita fat consumption of 105 to 151 grams a day. The nine countries with the lowest incidence of MS have a per capita fat consumption of 24 to 60 grams a day.[11] In Japan, researchers found that the incidence of Crohn's disease is growing, and that animal protein is most closely linked with the disease.[12]

- The cultures with the highest animal-based food consumption, the Laplanders, Greenlanders, Eskimos, and Russian Kurgi, have a life expectancy of about 30 years. The cultures that eat little or no animal-based foods, the Yucatan Indians, Russian Caucasians, East Indian Todas, and Pakistan Hunzas, have a life expectancy of more than 90 years.[13]

No smoke and mirrors, slight of hand, or diversions went into the production of this data. It's simply data from the fallout of life. Life beyond our shores where Americans have little incentive to look, because after all, what could we learn from other countries and cultures who are nowhere near as technologically advanced, or as economically powerful as us? Apparently plenty.

7: Degenerative and Infectious Disease

TERMITES AND TORNADOES

Our perception of sickness is pretty basic. We get sick and then we go to the doctor. Then one of three things will happen. We get better, or we stay sick, or we die. Whether it is pneumonia or influenza, hypertension or diabetes, we aren't so concerned about how we became sick, we just want to get well. Sick is sick. Or is it?

If we said there was an 80 percent chance of dying from a degenerative disease, and a 2 percent chance of dying from an infectious disease, would we still be inclined to think, sick is sick?[1] In addition, if close to 70 percent of the time the cause of our death was due to what we ate, would we become a little more concerned about how we became sick?[2] The answer should be yes.

An infectious disease is an invasion by possibly contagious pathogenic microorganisms in a bodily part or tissue. Influenza, pneumonia, malaria, small pox, measles, and hepatitis are a few examples.

A degenerative disease is a gradual deterioration of specific tissues, cells, or organs with corresponding impairment or loss of function. Examples are heart disease, cancers, osteoporosis, arthritis, diabetes, and kidney disease. These are the sicknesses that have their roots in our meat-based diets. We call these diseases by different names because they take different courses and affect different organs. But it might be more informative to call them all by one name given their singular cause: maybe the SICK disease.

The infectious disease often hits hard and then goes away, much like a tornado hitting a building. The degenerative disease is more like termites that are ignored while they eat away in silence until one day the house collapses. An infectious disease is like being robbed at gunpoint; a degenerative disease is more like Uncle Harry coming to stay with us, and during the course of a few months embezzling all the funds in our bank account.

Although it is important to make a distinction between the causes of these two types of disease, it is just as important to differentiate them for how we perceive their remedies.

In the last 100 years, death from infectious disease in this country has dramatically decreased thanks to medical advances such as vaccines and antibiotics. Science has wiped out many diseases, and allows us to control and cure most others. Because of these events, our expectation is that science and medicine will perform the same magic on our new plague—degenerative diseases. Are they succeeding?

Medical advancements like bypass surgery, chemotherapy, cholesterol lowering drugs, insulin therapy, hypertension medicines, estrogen therapy, hip replacements, organ transplants, and what appears to be increased life expectancy, give most Americans the impression we are succeeding. But is that impression correct?

- According to *Nutrition Action* (June 1999), heart bypass surgery will extend life in 2 percent of cases.[3]

- According to the National Cancer Institute in Bethesda, Md. (2000), chemotherapy's success rate is 5.8 percent.[4]

- According to the *Journal of the American Medical Association* (1983), a study showed that for those with mild hypertension on drug therapy, the number of deaths was reduced by just 1 percent. Has this figure improved over the years? Given a person dies from a heart attack every minute in this country, probably not much.[5]

- According to the *New England Journal of Medicine* (1995), taking estrogen therapy for more than 5 years to reduce the risk of osteoporosis and heart disease will increase the risk of hormone-dependent ovarian and breast cancer by 30 to 40 percent.[6]

- According to the World Health Organization (WHO), the United States ranks 24th in the world in Healthy Life Expectancy (HALE).[7] And according to *The Growing*

Epidemic of Disease (David M. Homer), in 1900, a 55-year-old male could expect to live to age 72. In 1990, a 55-year-old male could expect to live to age 75. A modest 3-year improvement over 90 years.[8]

Yes, it's true we are going to die anyway. But wouldn't we rather live a long life by embracing the WELL diet and then die like Nature probably intended—peacefully in our sleep—rather than suffering the degeneration of our bodies, and reduction in quality of life?

The bathtub is overflowing and the medical profession is there to bail water from the tub to the sink, soak up the floor with towels, and build up the sides of the tub. Certainly these measures will help, but they will have nowhere near the impact of simply turning the water off.

8: Nature

SHE CAN'T SPEAK BUT SHE HAS MUCH TO TELL

Nature can't speak, but she has a lot to tell.

Did it ever occur to us that Nature provided cows' milk for baby cows, rather than a lifelong drink for humans?

Did it ever occur to us that Nature planned for plants to be our singular food source given that the ratio in calories of carbohydrates, proteins, and fats found in the plant kingdom match up with the ratio of human needs?[1]

Did it ever occur to us that Nature assumes that when we are dieting food is scarce, thus conserves fat and slows our metabolism?[2]

Did it ever occur to us that Nature, in placing 5 percent of calories as protein in breast milk at a critical stage of growth and development, wanted us to consume near that amount throughout life instead of the nearly 20 percent that we do consume?[3]

Did it ever occur to us that Nature gave us an anatomy that is optimal for consuming plant-based foods, and inefficient for eating animal-based foods?

Did it ever occur to us that Nature didn't give us the instinct to tear apart an animal, salivate, then enjoy the savory tissue and warm blood, because animals weren't intended to be on our menu?

Did it ever occur to us that if Nature wanted us to eat animals, unique nutrients would have been placed in them, when in fact no nutrients exist in meat that aren't already present in plants?[4]

Did it ever occur to us that Nature built into our design a complex regulatory apparatus to ensure we maintain the proper weight, so given that 50 percent of Americans are overweight, what might that tell us about the foods we are eating?[5]

Did it ever occur to us that Nature, to ensure our survival, intended our food source to be stationary rather than mobile?

Did it ever occur to us that Nature, after placing our ancestors on a plant-based diet for most of 8 million years, would have any particular reason to change things?[6]

Did it ever occur to us that Nature would have provided enough food to feed the planet, so the fact that 1.2 billion people are *underfed* and malnourished, and 1.2 billion people are *overfed* and malnourished is not coincidental, but indicative we have chosen the wrong foods to eat?[7]

Did it ever occur to us that Nature created our forests as earth's air filter, rather than as an obstacle to be cleared to graze cattle and grow their food?[8]

Did it ever occur to us that Nature built us a body free of defects, with the intent of us dying in our sleep of old age?[9]

Did it ever occur to us that Nature, given that vegetarians have shown in studies to have more strength, greater stamina, and higher IQs than those consuming a meat-based diet, intended us to select our food from the plant kingdom?[10]

Did it ever occur to us that Nature spent millions of years designing our foods motivated by the assurance of our survival, while commercial enterprise has spent a few years designing genetically engineered foods motivated by financial gain?

Did it ever occur to us that Nature gave us a signaling system, including pain, to tell us to STOP an activity rather than starting an activity to mask the problem, like taking prescribed drugs and medicines?[11]

Did it ever occur to us that Nature has given us a cancer-fighting immune system that chemotherapy defeats?[12]

Did it ever occur to us that Nature didn't intend for girls to bear children at 12.5 years of age, that 175 years ago puberty was reached at age 17 when meat consumption and fat intake were significantly lower?[13]

Did it ever occur to us that Nature intended menopause to be a natural and problem-free event—which it is for vegetarians—in the continuum of a woman's life, rather than as a disease to be treated with drugs?[14]

Did it ever occur to us that Nature provided the sun, wind, and water to be used as safe, renewable power sources, with no dangers, pollutants, or hazardous byproducts?

Did it ever occur to us that Nature might suggest that we belong to the earth, instead of the earth belonging to us?[15]

Did it ever occur to us that Nature would think us more humble and less arrogant if we acknowledged that we live on a small planet in a galaxy tucked away in the corner of the universe in which there are far more galaxies than people?[16]

Did it ever occur to us that Nature never says one thing and wisdom another?[17]

It has occurred to some that it's time for humankind to give back the reins to Nature.

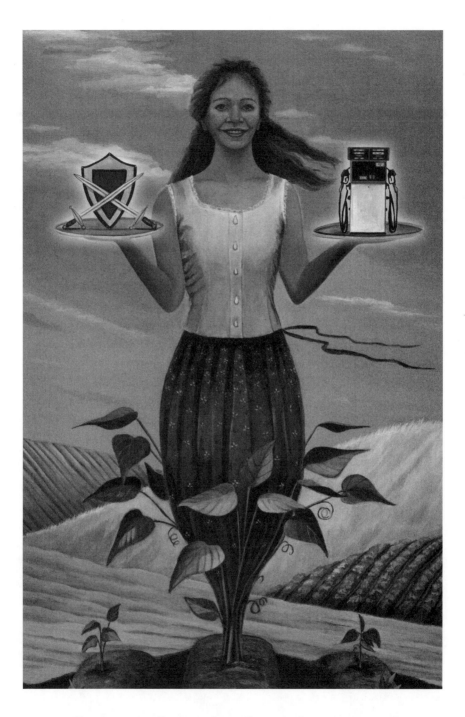

They Fuel, Defend, and Do Battle

~ 2 ~
Plants
NATURE'S NUTRIENT DELIVERY SYSTEM

Given that food is necessary for human survival would Nature have placed our nourishment in a system that could run from us, or one that was stationary? Is there any reason why plants couldn't be our sole food source?

Ahead in this chapter...

The critical command and control systems of the body are regulated by complex CARBOHYDRATES. The percentage of these compounds in meat? Virtually zero.[1]

VITAMINS necessary for man's survival, chiefly originate from plant sources. True, meat also contains vitamins—because animals require vitamins for survival, too.[2]

CALCIUM does not originate from a cow's udder, nor IRON from a 16-ounce sirloin. All minerals essential to humankind were baked into the earth upon its formation.

Every defense system must be armed with the proper weapons to operate effectively. What might those weapons be if a vegetarian's IMMUNE SYSTEM has shown the ability to destroy cancer cells by more than double?[3]

ANTIOXIDANTS AND PHYTOCHEMICALS fight disease, bolster the immune system, and retard aging. We don't know fully how they do it, but we do know where they almost entirely originate: plants.[4]

If vegetarians have been shown in tests to have twice the stamina of meat-eaters and 70 percent of 12-year-olds have significant artery plaque, what does this say about the often-heard view that ATHLETES and CHILDREN are short-changed by a vegetarian diet?[5]

Can the VITAMIN B_{12} be used to defend a meat-based diet or is this issue another test of faith for the vegetarian?

Thought plant-based foods were boring? Get out a score-card and be ready to compare them against animal-based foods in VARIETIES AND FLAVORS, colors, textures, and aromas.

9: Carbohydrates

PHILLIP ONCARBS

As much as we hear about protein and fat, one would think they are the predominant players in the nutritional game—the performers that require the most attention. As it turns out these two nutrients, although they play major roles, see way too much playing time, and as a result we continue to lose. Big time. Meanwhile our star players, carbohydrates, sit on the bench wondering why no one has figured out they are the key to victory and our long-term success.

The optimal ratio of carbohydrates, fat, and protein should be roughly 80, 10, and 10 percent of calories, respectively.[1] A Wholly Eating Leaves to Live (WELL) diet would provide that ratio. The current Self-Induced Carnivorous Killer (SICK) diet runs a ratio close to 40, 40, and 20 percent.[2] Given that our main energy source is carbohydrates, why aren't they in the spotlight? When protein and fat in excess are troublemakers, why do they garner most of the attention?

Maybe this phenomenon parallels life. Who gets the most attention in the classroom? The naughty kids or the good students who go quietly about their work? Who do we highlight in the sports world? The star that strikes for another million or the star that gives a million to build a community center? Who makes the evening news? Top teachers, exceptional parents, and sacrificing social workers, or killers, rapists, and swindlers? Is this the way it should be?

Oh sure, carbohydrate rich foods such as potatoes, pasta, and bread were in the spotlight at one time. Do we remember why? They were being accused of contributing to the obesity of America. As it turns out they just happen to be innocent bystanders in the vicinity where the bad guys—butter, cheese, sour cream, bacon, meat sauce, and the like—were hanging out. Guilt by association. Now it's time to redeem their reputation. Now it's time to trumpet the credentials of the good guys for a change.

Those frenzied and in-your-face television commercials

hawking miracle cleaning products and do-everything tools seem to be successful. Maybe that approach could also work for carbohydrates.

The commercial might go something like this:

*****

"Hi Friends. Phillip Oncarbs here. Do you want to BOOST your metabolism, INCREASE your serotonin, and REDUCE your risk of cancer and heart disease?[3] Do you want to LOSE weight easily, LOWER your cholesterol, and REDUCE your risk of diabetes and high blood pressure?[4]

"Of course you do! Now you can have all of these benefits in one simple product. Just one. Carbohydrates. The most abundant organic compounds in nature. Simple and complex. Glucose and fructose. Starch and fiber. They are powered by the sun and they will power YOU.

"Carbohydrates burn clean with fewer byproducts and are more easily converted into energy.[5] Carbohydrates stimulate the thyroid gland hormones, stimulate the hormone norepinephrine, all to increase your metabolism to make you a lean, mean, efficient machine![6] And don't forget that carbohydrates naturally increase the production of serotonin in your brain, AND without a prescription and the side effects of antidepressants.[7]

"Carbohydrates travel with an enforcer called fiber that will protect you from the ravages of many degenerative diseases. Fiber binds with carcinogens, fats, and cholesterol and eliminates them from your body to reduce the risk of colon cancer, heart disease, and diverticulitis.[8] Complex carbohydrates cause insulin resistance to decrease, slowing absorption of sugars into the bloodstream, reducing the risk of diabetes.[9]

"I know you've heard this before: *Do you want to lose weight and keep it off, without always feeling hun-*

gry? The problem is you continue to hear it because— it never happens! And it won't until you start filling your stomach with COMPLEX CARBOHYDRATES. Their properties cue your brain to let you know you've had enough to eat.[10] The fiber with its bulk fills up your gas tank, making the needle reach the "full" indicator quicker. The fact is you will lose weight and maintain the loss without even trying. It's not magic. It's CARBOHYDRATES!

"Carbohydrates are to you as gasoline is to your car. Fat is to you as the oils are to your car. Protein is to you as the maintenance fluids: radiator water, antifreeze, windshield cleaner, and battery water are to your car. Now repeat after me:

> While fat has a place in you
> But not too much you know
>
> And protein mends your tissues
> And also helps them grow
>
> Don't forget carbs are Nature's gas
> That makes your engine go!

"So where do you fill up? That's the best part because complex carbohydrates are abundant, inexpensive, AND legal. They are designed by Nature and manufactured by the earth and sun. You can find them at the grocery store, whole foods store, farmers' market, roadside stand, and even in your backyard if you so desire! Whole grains contain 85 percent complex carbohydrates in calories. Fruits 80 percent. Vegetables 65 percent. Legumes 65 percent.[11] And meat? Virtually ZERO percent! None, zip, nada.[12]

"Now that you know what carbohydrates can do. Now that you know where you can find them. Now that you know you can't live without them, this is Phillip Oncarbs saying, my name says it all: FILL UP ON CARBS!"

10: Vitamins

THE ANIMALS NEED THEM FOR SURVIVAL, TOO

Vitamins are mysterious creatures. We can't see them, smell them, or taste them. But we know we need them because, well, that's what our mothers always told us. Most of us aren't exactly sure where vitamins come from or what happens when they get inside of us. We just know if we don't get them, and in sufficient quantities, we will suffer poor health.

Vitamins find their way into breakfast cereals (fortified), breads (enriched), and small plastic containers (compressed into pills). All done to make sure we don't come up short—maybe literally. So what are vitamins? Where do they come from? Why do we need them? And are these the ways Nature intended for us to get them?

Vitamins are organic molecules required for normal metabolism, but cannot be made in adequate amounts by humans and animals.[1] Many of them work as catalysts to facilitate chemical reactions. Others are coenzymes requiring the presence of other vitamins, minerals, or proteins to accomplish the reaction.[2] The body needs 13 vitamins, which are divided into two types: fat-soluble (vitamins A, D, E, and K), and water-soluble (B_1, B_2, B_3, B_6, B_{12}, pantothenic acid, folate, biotin, and vitamin C). Water-soluble vitamins are required in our diet daily. Fat-soluble vitamins are stored in fat and called upon as needed.[3]

Where do these vitamins originate? Is it from animals? From the soil? Certainly not from breakfast cereals, bread, or from thin air in the laboratory.

Vitamins originate almost entirely from plants. Vitamins are present in animal tissue only if the animal consumes foods containing them or harbors microorganisms capable of synthesizing them—animals, like humans, need vitamins for their own survival. In essence, animals contain no vitamins that don't already exist in plants or microorganisms (required for vitamin synthesis), therefore obtaining our vitamins from animals is an added layer on the food chain. Why not go to the source: plants?[4]

Vitamin C *is* synthesized by animals, but the plant kingdom can more than meet our needs.[5] Vitamin A (retinol), Vitamin B_3 (Niacin), Vitamin D (Calciferol) are argued to be hormones, synthesized by humans, therefore should not be classified as vitamins. Vitamin B_{12} is made neither by plants or animals, but by bacteria.[6]

If Nature wrote a simple instructional booklet on vitamins it might go like this:

*****

Not all nutrients for humans and animals could be baked into the earth upon its formation like minerals, or synthesized by the body like hormones, therefore vitamins were engineered into the plant kingdom.

Plants use the sun's energy to grow and make vitamins so they can live, then the vitamins are turned over to humans *and* animals so they can live.

The vitamins are contained in all six parts of the plant: flower, fruit, leaf, stem, seed, and root.[7] Examples of foods from these six parts are:

FLOWER: broccoli, artichoke, and cauliflower.
FRUIT: strawberry, apple, and orange.
LEAF: lettuce, spinach, and cabbage.
STEM: celery, asparagus, and leek.
SEED: bean, nut, and wheat.
ROOT: carrot, turnip, and radish.

*****

Unfortunately, we've chosen to disregard Nature's simple and safe Vitamin Delivery System in favor of a manmade chaotic hybrid that includes:

- Choosing to get our vitamins second-hand from animals after they have eaten plants, because like us they can't make vitamins either. This might be compared to chewing someone else's already-chewed gum.[8]

- Adding vitamin D to cows' milk when humans manufacture all they require with exposure to sunlight. As an additive it can be harmful and toxic; as a hormone that humans make, it is regulated by the body and is safe.[9]

- Turning whole grain flour into white flour by stripping away the bran, meal, and millings that contain roughly 75 percent of the six B vitamins, and 95 percent of vitamin E, then chemically replacing some of the vitamins and calling a food "enriched." The bran, meal, and millings are then fed to the animals we eat, and the American SICK diet is left with only 1 percent of its food accounted for by whole grains.[10]

- Over sterilizing our ecosystem by chlorinating our drinking water, chemically treating our soil, and sanitizing our foods to the extent of destroying many of the microorganisms that produce vitamin B_{12}.[11]

- Getting vitamins from questionable sources (coal tar, petroleum chemicals, and animal byproducts) to manufacture supplements. Supplements that contain vitamins far removed from nature, that is from organic plants. This results in the potential for reduced efficiency, synergy, missing catalysts, and toxicity.[12]

Unfortunately, there is no booklet to explain things to us. Nature probably never imagined we would get ourselves into a predicament like this, and then continue to make matters worse.

But like young children who think they can stay one step ahead of a lie, we apparently think we can do the same. The only difference being is that children aren't punished until *after* they have been found out.

11: Calcium

SANTA CLAUS, THE TOOTH FAIRY, AND CALCIUM

Santa Claus, the Easter Bunny, the Tooth Fairy, and calcium. Which is the misfit? The correct response is the Tooth Fairy—the other three can't fly. If we thought calcium was the correct response because there is no myth or fantasy attached to it, think again.

As children we believed in Santa Claus, the Easter Bunny, and the Tooth Fairy. As adults we believe if we don't consume enough dairy products it will lead to a calcium deficiency, and if we don't get enough calcium it will lead to osteoporosis. Either the childhood beliefs, or the adulthood beliefs, are harmless fantasies that do no long-term damage. Want to hazard a guess as to which is which?

If the answer isn't clear maybe taking the following 10 question, true/false quiz, will help to discern it. Remember, no talking. No looking at your neighbor's paper. Place your pencils down when finished. Please begin.

1. A study found that women drinking three glasses of milk per day, and consuming 1,500 milligrams of calcium (the Recommended Daily Allowance is 1,000 milligrams) for 1 year, had a negative calcium balance.[1]

    TRUE. Corroborating the study, Eskimos routinely ingest 2,500 milligrams of calcium daily and maintain a negative calcium balance, and also have one of the highest number of osteoporosis cases in the world.[2]

2. In a 12-year Harvard study of 78,000 women, those who got the most calcium from dairy products broke more bones than women who rarely drank milk.[3]

    TRUE. And not because those who got the most calcium were also acrobatic skiers or circus performers. This study is corroborated by the fact that the four countries with the highest intake of dairy products, Finland, Sweden, the United States, and England, are also the four countries with the highest rates of osteoporosis and hip fractures.[4]

3. A calcium deficiency is rare in vegans and vegetarians.

TRUE. One study showed that when animal protein was replaced with plant protein subjects maintained a positive calcium balance on 457 milligrams a day.[5] Another study indicated similar results with subjects on a low-protein plant-based diet, maintaining a positive balance on 500 milligrams a day.[6] The average daily vegan intake for calcium is 637 milligrams.[7]

4. Those subsisting on the WELL diet, have less incidence of osteoporosis than those subsisting on the SICK diet.

TRUE. For example, the Bantu women of Africa consume 240 to 450 milligrams of calcium on a predominately vegan diet. The demand on their calcium needs reaches into the red as many of the women bear 10 children and then nurse them for longer than 1 year. Are they ravaged with osteoporosis? They can't even spell it—not because they're illiterate—because the disease is almost unknown amongst them.[8]

5. The sulfur containing amino acids of animal protein are responsible for the mass exodus of calcium from the bones.[9]

TRUE. Although we might think the top priority of calcium is our bones, it's not. Its most important job is the work it does in our bloodstreams: Regulating nerve and muscle function, clotting, and balancing the pH which becomes acidic from animal protein.[10] What do we think are in those antacids we take to neutralize excess stomach acid?

6. No matter how much calcium we consume by way of dairy products or supplements, even if we latched our mouths onto the udder of a cow 3 hours each day, if we are eating an animal-based diet (which contributes 70 percent of its protein in animal protein) we will have a calcium deficit.

> TRUE. One study showed that women who consumed a high ratio of animal to vegetable protein suffered 3 times the rate of bone loss, and 4 times the rate of hip fractures.[11] Another study showed that subjects ingesting 1,400 milligrams of calcium daily on a high-protein diet still could not reach a positive balance.[12]

7. Kidney stones are a byproduct of a meat-based diet.

> TRUE. Where do we think all that calcium spilled into the bloodstream to neutralize the pH ends up. It ends up in the urine in high concentrations causing stones to form. Twelve percent of the population will get them. Twelve percent of the population may require no other incentive to change its diet.[13]

8. The genes of a race, or population of people, are not factors in determining the risk of osteoporosis.

> TRUE. African Americans in this country, who ingest 1,000 milligrams of calcium a day, have 9 times the hip fracture rate of South African blacks who ingest 196 milligrams of calcium a day.[14]

9. The U.S. RDA for calcium is set twice as high to compensate for the American meat-based diet.

> TRUE. The U.S. RDA is 1,000 milligrams a day. The World Health Organization (WHO) sets the RDA at 500 milligrams a day.[15]

10. Calcium is a mineral that comes from the soil by virtue of being baked into the planet during its formation, and makes up 3 percent of the earth's crust.[16]

> TRUE. Calcium isn't made in a cow's udder, an animal's tissue, or a pharmaceutical lab. Most foods from the plant kingdom including vegetables, grains, legumes, fruits, nuts, and seeds have all pulled up calcium from the earth's soil in ample amounts to easily cover our daily calcium requirements.[17]

All done? Put your pencils down. Did the quiz clarify the issue as to which are the harmless fantasies causing no long-term damage—the childhood or the adult?

If your answer was that the three childhood mythical figures created long-term damage far worse than any foods ever could, then please take as much time as you need to address the issue. When that's taken care of, we will get back to discussing diet.

12: Iron

LIKE A FIRE, IT CAN WARM OR IT CAN BURN

The mineral iron may be a microcosm of Nature's plan for us to acquire our food exclusively from plants.

Let's suspend reality for a moment. A theatrical producer has dropped off a short one-act science fiction play involving space travel that is currently without a star. Would you like to try out? Don't worry if you have never acted before, all you have to do, is to do what you are doing now—read.

Here is the set-up. You are an alien that lives on the planet, Monotonous. You have been granted one wish. Your wish is to become a human being and live on earth. You are dropped to earth, and after getting up and dusting yourself off, you realize you're hungry, but you don't know what humans eat. Fortunately for you a car drives by, stops, and hands you a leaflet. After reading the leaflet entitled *Iron*, you head off looking for food, assured of what the human diet is. This is the leaflet you will read:

*****

Welcome to earth. We hope it is all that you imagined. I know you must be hungry, so allow me to provide you some insight into our diet. You may find this hard to believe, but even after 8 million years of evolution, we on earth are not all eating the same diets. There are two distinct camps. Rather than bog you down with the mountains of knowledge available, and make your first day a hardship, I think I can sum it up by telling you about the nutrient, iron.

Humans require iron to produce hemoglobin that carries oxygen through the blood. Without iron we would eventually get sick and die. However, too much iron can be every bit as deadly. Like a fire, it can warm or it can burn.

Our bodies store iron, thus the more iron ingested and absorbed, the more we have in us. Iron acts with oxygen to encourage free radical damage. Outside the body the result is corrosion and rust, inside the body the result is atherosclerosis and heart disease.[1] The risk was demonstrated in a study of 2,000 subjects.[2]

Excess iron also encourages DNA damage, which can lead to cancer. Restricting iron to the cancer cell slows division of the cell. A study of 10,000 subjects has proven this.[3] Finally, overall tissue damage because of too much iron can accelerate the aging process.[4]

Iron is found in a variety of foods. It is found in many vegetables, legumes, grains, nuts, seeds, and fruits.[5] It is also found in red meat. Because calorie for calorie foods from the plant kingdom contain more iron than red meat—for instance spinach contains 14 times more iron than does the typical sirloin steak—vegetarians take in more iron than omnivores.[6] However, vegetarians typically have *lower* iron stores than do meat-eaters.[7] The omnivore male has 1,000 to 2,000 milligrams of stored iron, while the vegetarian male has 480 milligrams.[8] (The RDA is 18 milligrams.) Why such a contradiction?

Plants contain a predominately different kind of iron than does meat. Meat contains non-heme and heme iron; plants contain only non-heme iron. Generally non-heme iron is less absorbable, thus it keeps the body's stores lower.[9] However, when the body is deficient in iron, non-heme iron in plant-based foods has the capability to increase its absorption rate 10 times, while the combination irons in red meat can only manage a two-fold increase. Additionally, when a meal has a small amount of iron, the non-heme iron will increase its absorption 3 times while the heme iron will not change its uptake at all.[10]

Nature mirrors the body's sophisticated balancing routine by placing both enhancers of iron absorption, like vitamin C, and inhibitors of iron absorption, like phytates, in the plant kingdom.[11] The iron and iron helpers in plant-based foods have far greater flexibility in maintaining the correct balance of iron in the body, while much of the iron from meat continually adds to the omnivore's iron stores with potentially grave consequences.

Women provide us additional insights into the effects of iron. During the childbearing years, women's iron stores are depleted monthly due to menstruation. During childbearing years women's risk of heart disease is significantly less than men's, and after menopause becomes the same as theirs.[12] Coincidence? The flip side shows that during child bearing years 10 to 20 percent of women are deficient in iron.[13] Why might this be?

Women are often worried about getting sufficient protein and calcium, and errantly increase their dairy consumption to compensate. Dairy is not only deficient in iron, it also inhibits its absorption.[14] Both these factors may be significant contributors to women's iron deficit.

Iron may well be a microcosm of Nature's plan for us to acquire our food from the plant kingdom. Certainly our knowledge and insight of this nutrient provides a persuasive argument.

We hope you enjoy your life on earth as a human being. If you don't mind when you have finished reading this please pass it on to the nearest omnivore. They'll be the ones rusting.

*****

Not bad for a first reading. I believe the part is yours. Congratulations! Now all you have to do is practice it for the play—and memorize it for life.

13: Immune System

WE BETTER ARM OUR DEFENSES

Let's do a word association.

> AUTHOR: Immune system.

> READER: Colds. More rest. Infection. Vaccinations.

Let's switch roles.

> READER: Immune system.

> AUTHOR: Cancer. Autoimmune disease. Plants. Defense.

Given the sharp contrast in associations is it possible there is more than one immune system? Or is it more likely we greatly underrate and misunderstand the immune system?

The immune system is to us as the military defense system is to the United States—protecting, fighting, and sacrificing to ensure our preservation. If we fail to properly arm our military soldiers, our country risks great peril. If we fail to arm the immune system, *we* risk great peril.

Today, the American SICK diet includes 33 percent more dairy products, 50 percent more beef, and 280 percent more poultry than our diet did in 1900.[1] Today, cancer is the 2nd leading cause of death; 100 years ago it was the 10th leading cause of death.[2] Today, cancer is the second leading cause of death in children under 15; in 1950 it was a medical rarity.[3] Today, according to the National Cancer Institute, 80 percent of cancers are due to factors that we control.[4]

Apparently we have chosen the wrong weapons for our battle. That's unfortunate given the powerful array of potent deterrents that have already been designed, manufactured, and are ready for deployment. Let's visit the weapons depot.

PHYTOCHEMICALS: Found only in plant-based foods—fruits, vegetables, whole grains, and legumes. More than 1,000 have been identified and their secrets are just beginning to be understood.[5] They have been shown to support immune function combating tumors, viruses, heart disease, and diabetes. They aren't involved with normal maintenance processes as vitamins and minerals, but they are an integral part of the body's military industrial complex.

VITAMINS: Manufactured chiefly by, and found predominately in, plants. Meats also contain vitamins, as animals eat plants and require vitamins, like we do.

- Vitamin C is probably the most important vitamin for the health of the immune system.[6] It works together with vitamin E in improving oxygen utilization and stimulating the immune system.

- Beta-carotene (converted to vitamin A in the body) significantly increases the percentage of cells in the body acting as natural killer cells, and increases T-helper cells which are white blood cells that act as generals directing the battle plan.[7]

- Vitamin A has potent anti-virus properties.[8]

- Vitamin B_6 enhances the ability of the body's white blood cells to combat offending pathogens.[9]

MINERALS: Originating beneath our feet, they were born with the earth. Because we are unable to absorb them through our feet, plants have been assigned the role as middlemen to bring them to us. Animals can do the same, but the minerals in meat come with some unwanted baggage.

- Calcium is a vital mineral that plays many roles in the immune system. It is involved in the synthesis of the enzymes that T-cells use to defeat pathogenic invaders.[10]

- Selenium is an essential trace mineral involved in antibody synthesis.[11]

- Iron plays an essential role in the production of all white blood cells, and it is involved in the synthesis of antibodies.[12]

- The thymus gland requires zinc to manufacture the T-cells that fight pathogens entering the body.[13]

- Manganese is necessary for normal antibody production.[14]

OTHER IMMUNE BOOSTERS: Another branch of our military, coming to us by way of the plant kingdom, might be called Special Forces.

- Soybean isoflavins stimulate natural killer cell activity.[15]

- Echinacea has profound immune-enhancing effects and antiviral activities.[16]

- Astragalus appears to help restore normal immune function for cancer patients.[17]

- Garlic and ginger boost the immune system.[18]

- Goldenseal, panax ginseng, and licorice exhibit immuno-stimulatory properties.[19]

Our enemies appear to stand little chance when we defend our bodies with plant-based foods. Their properties hold our attackers at bay, or destroy them if they infiltrate us.

One study conducted in the laboratory took white blood cells from vegetarians, and from non-vegetarians, and compared their capacity to kill cancer cells. The result? Vegetarians had more than double the ability to destroy cancer cells.[20] Pure vegetarians have been shown to have a very low incidence of viral, bacterial, and fungal infections owing to a highly functional immune system response. They also have been shown to have significantly fewer tooth caries, cavities, and plaque buildup than their omnivore counterparts.[21]

Meat and dairy contain some of the vitamins and minerals that maintain and strengthen the immune system. But they are more than offset by enemies of our defenses resident in these foods, such as:

- Animal protein has shown to be implicated in autoimmune disease, as amino acid sequences similar to ours confuse the immune system, resulting in its attack on us.[22] Rheumatoid arthritis, insulin-dependent diabetes, lupus, and multiple sclerosis are a few of the consequences of this phenomenon.[23]

- Animal fat has shown to greatly decrease natural killer cell activity, and impact the clearing system that removes antigen-antibodies implicated in autoimmune disorders.[24]

- Iron, especially the heme iron resident in meat, creates excess iron storage, which promotes free radical damage implicated in atherosclerosis, cancer, and aging.[25]

Supplements have their place in specific situations and in limited use. But as supplements the nutrients are no longer in their natural environment, where they work together to do the most good; not unlike having all the soldiers and weapons but without coordination, leadership, and training.[26] And if one is using supplements to crutch and compensate for the SICK diet, it will have an impact— an impact on par with putting out a three-alarm fire with a water pistol.

Our ever-increasingly complex world brings with it ever-increasing threats to our country. From time to time our enemies attempt to penetrate our defenses and endanger our way of life. To date we have been ready.

Our ever-increasingly complex world brings with it ever-increasing environmental threats to our bodies. From time to time our microscopic enemies attempt to penetrate our defenses and endanger our lives. Will *we* be ready?

14: Antioxidants and Phytochemicals

DISCOVERIES OR EXPLANATIONS?

Scientists are discovering thousands of biologically active compounds that promote longevity and safeguard against disease. They are called antioxidants and phytochemicals. Some are so new that computer spell checkers fail to recognize them. Carotenoids, glucarates, tocotrienols, saponins, flavonoids, phytates, and lignans are but a few. They have demonstrated the potential to slow or reverse cancer, reduce the risk of heart disease and stroke, lower cholesterol, bolster the immune system, reduce blood pressure, and protect against cataracts, arthritis, and overall aging.[1] The list of benefits go on.

If we think it will be years before these compounds will be perfected, then difficult to find due to the demand, and price prohibitive so only the wealthy can afford them, think again. Because they are available now, in abundant quantity, at our local grocery store, for $1.00 to $3.00 a pound.

Unbeknown to us, these compounds have been inherent in fruits, vegetables, whole grains, and legumes for 350 million years. Recently identified were 40 of these compounds in broccoli, 50 in onions and garlic, 70 in tarragon, and 170 in oranges.[2] Although one might refer to these as *discoveries*, vegetarians and many in the scientific and nutritional communities, are more likely to refer to them as *explanations*. Further confirmation of what they already know: The plant kingdom was designed to fuel, guard, and do battle for the human body.

These compounds do their job by neutralizing free radicals. (Not the ones from the sixties; they were far less destructive.) Free radicals are unstable oxygen molecules caused by environmental influences such as stress, injury, pollution, and fat-laden and iron-rich foods that bounce around the body looking for trouble.[3] They attack and damage the cell membrane, and sometimes the DNA, with little remorse. The result is disease.

Antioxidants found predominately in plants, and phytochemicals found only in plants, do battle by standing guard outside our cells and then sacrificing themselves for the good of the cell—not unlike a secret service agent taking a bullet for the president.[4] It should come as no surprise then that herbivores have twice the natural cell-protecting capabilities that omnivores do.[5]

Vitamin C, vitamin E, and beta-carotene are antioxidants, compounds we probably have heard of. These particular antioxidants have proven disease-fighting prowess in addition to their nutritive value for normal physiologic function. Vitamin C patrols the bloodstream for free radicals and knocks them out. Vitamin E works within the cell to protect it if a free radical gets through. Beta-carotene, prevalent in carrots, has substantial anticancer and anti-aging properties.[6] (Ever see a sick or aging Bugs Bunny?)

When we go to the grocery store, it might be a temptation to head to the supplement section rather than the produce section. After all, it would seem more efficient to ingest the star nutrients without all the riffraff. However, we would be making a mistake, because each plant contains a world of individual, yet interacting compounds. Although so much is yet to be uncovered about the power of plants, it's clear that the stars must work together with other nutrients for them to do their magic and shine.[7] Take Abbot away from Costello, or Laurel away from Hardy, and we might be left with four guys looking for work. The smart money has to be on Nature's altruistic design rather than the supplement industries' profit motive.

The synchronicity of plants and humans goes back 8 million years. The human body has evolved into a finely tuned and flawless mechanism that is interwoven and allied with the plant kingdom. Plants nourish it, defend it, and do battle for it, and as the years go by the chemistry of foods will be better understood.

In the meantime have a carrot, and sit down and enjoy a good Laurel and Hardy movie.

15: Athletes

GENTLEMEN, START YOUR ENGINES!

If the average human being is a Ford Taurus, then the world-class athlete is a high performance Indy racecar. If the fuel formula that powers that racecar doesn't match up with the engine specifications for which the fuel was designed, the engine's optimum perform-ance won't be achieved. The same goes for the athlete's engine.

The question then becomes: Were athletic engines designed to run on New York strips or Idaho potatoes? Since there are no engine specs available to answer that, we will have to find the way to the finish line all by ourselves.

A word association response to "athlete" in the category of foods and nutrients might elicit words such as protein, iron, steak, eggs, liver, chops, and so on. Without these foods and nutrients how else could the athlete reach peak performance by transforming into a carnivorous predator, blood thirsty for victory, and primed for the kill? The scientific and dietary communities have some ideas on how else:

- Athletes who are winning are loading up on carbohydrates, not protein.[1]

- Carbohydrates should make up the largest portion of the athlete's diet; high-carbohydrate diets optimize muscle and liver glycogen stores, and have been shown to optimize per-formance during prolonged and moderate intensity exer-cise.[2]

- The quantity of protein in the athletes' diet is rarely a con-cern.[3]

- It is surprising to note that most meats are only average sources of iron when compared to many grains and legumes.[4]

- Vegetarians have shown no negative performance effects due to decreased iron stores.[5]

- Vegetarian diets can meet the needs of competitive athletes.[6]

Experiments in the laboratory bear these declarations out.

- Tests in strength and endurance at Yale University showed vegetarians had twice the stamina of meat-eaters. Comparable tests by a doctor in Paris brought similar results: Vegetarians had 2 to 3 times greater stamina than meat-eaters, and required just one-fifth the time to recover.[7]

- In another test, immediately after subjects were fed a vegetarian diet they pedaled stationary bicycles almost 3 times longer than subjects who were fed a meat and dairy diet.[8]

- A test conducted with grip meters resulted in vegetarians having double the score of meat-eaters, with the vegetarians coming back from fatigue far more rapidly than did meat-eaters.[9]

We might be inclined to question how nerdy white-coat-wearing, clipboard-toting, pocket-protecting scientists working in a laboratory a few thousand light years away from the competitive arena of world-class athletic competition could have a clue about the sports world. It's a fair question. So let's leave the lab and enter the stadium.

If the scientists and dieticians are all wrong, and the conventional perception that protein, iron, and meat are necessary for peak performance is correct, then we shouldn't be able to find too many vegetarian world-class athletes.

A brief data search returned more than 100 world-class vegetarian athletes, in 25 different sports, with two-thirds of the athletes reaching the pinnacle of their sport. The sports covered the range of endurance, strength, agility, and coordination.

They included baseball, basketball, bodybuilding, boxing,

cycling, distance swimming, distance walking, fitness building, football, gymnastics, hang gliding, ice skating, karate, marathon running, rowing, sailing, skiing, snowboarding, soccer, tennis, track and field, triathlons, weightlifting, windsurfing, and wrestling.

These athletes fueled by the plant kingdom have achieved such titles as world champion, Olympic gold medallist, world record holder, Heisman trophy winner, Most Valuable Player, tournament winner, grand slam winner, Ironman, national champion, Mr. Universe, Mr. America, and World Cup champion.

A sampling of the 100 athletes and their accomplishments include:[10]

- Paavo Nurmi: Distance runner and one-time holder of 20 world records, and holder of 9 Olympic medals.

- Gilman Low: Body builder and holder of 9 world records.

- Peter Hussing: European heavyweight boxing champion.

- Edwin Moses: Olympic Gold Medallist who went undefeated for 8 years.

- Carl Lewis: 9-time Olympic gold medallist in track and field.

- Dave Scott: 6-time ironman triathlon winner.

- Alan Jones: Marine captain and polio victim, who set records with 17,003 continuous sit-ups, and 43,000 consecutive jump ropes.

- Nicky Cole: First woman to walk to the North Pole.

- Johnny Weissmuller: Holder of 6 world swimming records in his time.

- Art Still: Professional football player and defensive end MVP.

- Billy Jean King, Chris Evert, Martina Navratilova, and Serena Williams: Winners of enough combined championship tennis trophies to fill a swimming pool.

- Bill Pearl: Bodybuilder and 4-time Mr. Universe.

- Ridgly Abele: Karate world champion and 8-time national champion.

- Cheryl Marek and Estelle Gray: World champion cross-country tandem cyclists.

- Ruth Heidrich: Winner of over 800 triathlons and running races.

- A Japanese baseball team: Went from last place to champions after every member was required to switch to a vegetarian diet.

Whether we are an athlete going out for the sixth grade track team, or closing in on a world record, this list of athletes and their accomplishments would have to make us think twice about the contents of our next meal—and every meal after that.

Does this mean that these athletes wouldn't have amassed these impressive records if they ate a meat-based diet? We will never know.

Does this mean that becoming a world-class athlete is impossible if we don't become a vegetarian? Of course not.

What it might tell us, however, is that the fuel we put in our bodies will have a measurable impact on our performance. Maybe making the difference between achieving a world record or making the sixth grade track team.

And who knows, it's entirely possible there are many athletes who have not divulged they are vegetarians. Why do anything to jeopardize a competitive edge, might be their thinking. After all, they want to be in the driver's seat when the starter calls out, "Gentlemen, start your engines!"

16: Children

THEY ARE NOT A UNIQUE SPECIES

Children are not a unique species—although sometimes the way they act leaves room for doubt. They are mammals, Homo sapiens, human beings, just like adults. The biochemical processes, and the foods that drive those processes, should be common for both children and adults. So why when most people accept the idea of adults embracing a vegetarian diet, do we—even adult vegetarians—balk at the notion of the same diet for children?

All humans need proper nutrition and while children are growing it is even more critical they receive a balanced diet. Iron, calcium, vitamin D, and protein are four of the more important nutrients necessary for proper development. What is the best way to ensure that these nutrients are received?

- IRON: The best sources of iron are dark green vegetables.[1] The vitamin C in fruits and vegetables enhances iron absorption.[2] Dairy products are low in iron, and they can cause a mild chronic blood loss from the digestive tract further decreasing iron stores.[3]

- CALCIUM: Calcium is found in almost all plant-based foods. Excluding animal protein from the diet helps the body retain calcium.[4] The Recommended Daily Allowance (RDA) is set 2 times higher for calcium, to compensate for a high-protein animal-based diet.[5] The high sodium content of many processed foods inhibits the absorption of calcium.[6]

- VITAMIN D: This vitamin is really a hormone and is satisfied, except on rare occasions, by exposure to sunlight.[7]

- PROTEIN: A good variety of plant sources easily meets the protein needs of all humans, including children.[8]

So if all four nutrients are easily obtained from plants, and in sufficient quantities, where is the controversy over whether children's nutritional needs are being met on a vegetarian or vegan diet?

The common feeding experience of the American family with children probably goes something like this:

- Parents, to save time at the grocery store and in the kitchen, purchase highly processed convenience foods that often lack the nutritional punch of unprocessed whole foods.

- Parents further sacrifice nutrition for time by making use of fast food restaurants found at most corners and highway off-ramps.

- Parents encourage three big meals a day and discourage snacking, when children with their smaller stomachs and need for calories should be eating smaller meals throughout the day.

- Parents reward children with empty calorie sweets. Parents serve pizza, hot dogs, cake, soda, and ice cream at parties. These not so nutritional foods come to be associated with fun times, and thus come to be in high demand on a regular basis.

That's when parents step up to the child-rearing plate and proclaim, "It would be irresponsible of us to put our children at risk by not providing them with the nutrients they need. We'll give them meat and dairy foods to ensure this doesn't happen."

Ironically, the adage our parents taught us, "Two wrongs don't make a right" might well apply here.

OK, so parents are bent on compensating for their questionable family food habits by serving their children meat and dairy foods. What could be the harm so early in their lives?

- In one study 70 percent of 12-year-olds had a significant amount of atherosclerotic plaque in their arteries.[9]

- In 1996, the Centers for Disease Control and Prevention announced that 25 percent of children from 6 to 17 years old were overweight.[10]

- It has been reported that 17 percent of 6th-to-8th graders have cholesterol levels higher than 180 milligrams per deciliter.[11]

- Plaque has been found in children 2 years old.[12]

- Milk is suspected of triggering juvenile diabetes.[13]

- The highest rates of leukemia are found in children ages 3 to 13, who consume the most dairy products.[14]

- Children are more susceptible to food poisoning, like E. coli, due to their underdeveloped immune systems.[15]

- The concentration of pesticides in animal-based foods increases long-term cancer risk, and antibiotics increase resistance to disease.[16]

Bigger is better, faster is better, more is better. These are the presumptions to which Americans usually subscribe. In many cases embracing the proverbs takes us to higher heights, but in the area of nutrition they don't apply. Instead, they take us to lower lows.

BIGGER IS BETTER: We praise the mother whose baby is putting on the most weight, yet breast-fed babies and herbivore children stay slimmer and healthier than their omnivore counterparts throughout their lives.[17]

FASTER IS BETTER: The WELL diet may encourage a later menarche, which has been shown to be associated with reduced risk of breast cancer in epidemiological studies.[18] Does anyone ever question how Nature could have made such a blunder in giving a 12-year-old girl the capability of having a baby long before she has the maturity to take care of it? It may well be that Nature designed the human body to grow up more gradually, to reach puberty later, and to last longer. Much the opposite of what occurs for those raised on an omnivore diet.

MORE IS BETTER: Too much protein and too much iron can lead to a whole host of potentially adverse consequences, from heart disease, to osteoporosis, to cancer.[19]

Populations the world over have been raising healthy vegetarian children for hundreds of years. Even so, the typical response from the average American is, "If you insist on taking up the vegetarian fad, go ahead, but don't subject your children to it."

On the other hand here are some typical responses from some not-so-average Americans:

- The American Dietetic Association (ADA) approves a vegetarian diet for all ages, including infants and toddlers who are in a high-growth stage of life.[20]

- The Physicians Committee for Responsible Medicine (PCRM) recommends a vegetarian diet for everyone.[21]

- The director of pediatrics at Johns Hopkins University, Dr. Frank Oski, says, "Children do not need dairy products to grow up strong and healthy."[22]

- The late Dr. Benjamin Spock recommended a vegan diet for children.[23]

- Well-informed dietitians, doctors, and other health professionals now accept that vegetarianism is a healthy option for infants and children of all ages.[24]

Every parent *wants* their children to be healthy, and every parent *wants* their children to eat properly. Some slight changes in our habits, perceptions, and awareness, when it comes to children and nutrition, will go a long way toward satisfying these wants.

Children are not an alien life form or made from unique ingredients. They are a smaller version of us. One day they will be our size though, and that's the day when we can look them in the eye. And when we do, we want to be able to tell them that we did our very best.

17: Vitamin B$_{12}$

ANOTHER TEST OF FAITH

Mother Nature is not as easy going as we might expect. First, she makes matters difficult for vegetarians by clouding the protein issue, resulting in the most frequently asked question of vegetarians by non-vegetarians: "How do you get enough protein?" Now that we have a better understanding of protein, sufficient to answer the question, Mother Nature has created a new challenge for the vegetarian.

The B$_{12}$ vitamin, cobalamin, is not made by, or found in, plants, but can be found in meat, poultry, dairy products, and eggs.

Consequently, moving up fast to become the new most frequently asked question of vegetarians by non-vegetarians is, "How do you get your B$_{12}$?" The implication being, if we were designed to be herbivores how could this important nutrient be left out of the vegetarian diet equation. The question seems to be a valid one given that an omnivore diet apparently supplies adequate amounts of B$_{12}$.

Let's examine what we know—and what we don't know—and see if we can begin to unravel the mystery.

Mother Nature has started the ball rolling with a number of clues, contradictions, and facts. However, for now, all that it adds up to is another test of faith for the vegetarian.

- Where can we find vitamin B$_{12}$?

  The vitamin B$_{12,}$ cobalamin, helps make red blood cells and aids in the proper functioning of the nervous system.[1] Our bodies need one-tenth of a microgram per day, which means humans only need one-fiftieth of an ounce *for life.*[2]

  Although it is the only vitamin not made by plants, it is not made by animals either. It is made by bacteria. The bacteria is found in the soil and stream water. It is also found in animals presumably by way of the soil and stream water. And it grows in the colons and mouths of humans.[3]

- How do we get B_{12}?

One theory suggests that before we over-sanitized our food supply with modern day hygienic methods, we got the bacteria-producing B_{12} indirectly from our food by way of the soil and natural water.[4] We may or may not get any from these sources now.

There is a B_{12}-like substance in fermented foods. However, it appears to be an analog and actually inhibits the absorption of the real thing.[5]

The bacteria grows in humans' mouths and colons, but evidently it can only be absorbed in the small intestine, where some but not much B_{12} has been detected.[6]

Some research shows organically grown plants can uptake some B_{12} from the soil into their roots, but even though we don't need very much, apparently the amount is not enough.[7]

It might also be obtained second-hand from the meat of animals that presumably get it from soil and water. But research suggests that when meat is cooked B_{12} is less available for absorption.[8]

And if the mystery wasn't already complicated enough, B_{12} can be found in sea vegetables like Japanese raw nori.[9]

- Can we *get* B_{12}, once we *got* B_{12}?

Even after we have enough B_{12} in the body, we can't absorb or utilize it in the small intestine without a protein called *intrinsic factor* that is produced in the stomach.[10] A test can be done to determine the presence of this protein, but the results of this test can be ambiguous.[11] Other nutrient deficiencies such as iron, B_6, and folic acid can reduce the effectiveness of B_{12}.[12] The answer to the question, then, is an emphatic maybe.

- How much B_{12} do we need?

  Some authorities say we need blood levels of 200 pg/ml; some say 350 pg/ml.[13] Some research shows too much can cause cancer and too little can cause heart disease.[14] Some suggest we can store 3 to 5 years worth of B_{12} and recycle it through the body for a period of 10 to 30 years, while others suggest we should take in some every 2 to 3 days.[15]

  Some say vegetarians may not be getting enough; some say meat and dairy eaters may not be getting enough; some say *no one* is getting enough.[16]

  And the first sign of trouble? Any agreement on this one? Of course not. Some say anemia and some say nerve damage.[17]

- Are vegetarians at risk for a B_{12} deficit?

  They don't appear to be since 95 percent of cases of B_{12} deficiency have occurred in *non-vegetarians*. This has been as a result of poor absorption.[18] A B_{12} deficiency is so uncommon in vegans that the medical press still records the cases.[19] Comprehensive studies in England showed no deficiencies in vegans.[20] And one study showed even vegans without B_{12} supplementation have adequate levels of the vitamin.[21]

Certainly the answer to this last question might have us scratching our heads wondering if the controversy over B_{12} should be a controversy. If vegetarians and vegans are getting sufficient amounts why is this an issue?

Since it is the only nutrient that humans need that doesn't appear to come from plants, it is conspicuous. And because we don't really know how vegetarians are obtaining B_{12} it makes everyone a little nervous and feeling vulnerable.

So it comes as no surprise that the logical, and perhaps politically safe, advice from the nutritional community is for vegetarians to supplement their diet with B_{12} until more is known. This is like waving a red flag to non-vegetarians. Omnivores can use this controversy to question the herbivore's conviction, and defend their diet all in one breath, leaving the vegetarian with not much more than an anemic retort.

However it is a long way from, "We don't know a lot about B_{12} right now," to "Because of what we know about B_{12}, humans were meant to eat meat." Even the most ardent steak lovers would have to pause, if even for a moment, and ask themselves why Mother Nature would have planned for humans to get their B_{12} micronutrients from half-ton cattle.

Someday the B_{12} mystery will be solved. Most likely the answer won't require vegetarians to have to reassess the intelligence of their diet choice. And just as likely vegetarians won't be able to rest. Why? Because given Mother Nature's track record they can expect another test of faith.

18: Varieties and Flavors

The young man had made it to the final group competing for first prize in the annual World's Championship Chili Cook-off. He called his chili, "Hot Bottom Revenge." He waited patiently as the judges deliberated. They broke up and began to head his way. He won! He couldn't believe it. Well actually he could.

With not a lick of meat in his chili—just a grain and soy combination meat analog—he really had an unfair advantage over his competition. He considered returning the first prize for not using meat. But then thought better of it figuring they would never believe him anyway.

Something like this could happen, maybe already has. Certainly its impact would be immeasurable in underscoring the idea that foods from the plant kingdom, and foods made from them like meat analogs, run circles around animal-based foods in variety, color, texture, flavor, and aroma.

- VARIETY: There are 115 commonly eaten varieties of vegetables, fruits, legumes, nuts, and grains, compared to four commonly eaten varieties of meats—beef, chicken, pork, and fish.

- COLOR: Plant-based foods cover a wide spectrum of vibrant colors, from the intense red of a bell pepper to the bright green of cooked broccoli, compared to three meat colors—muddy brown, dirty red, and dingy white.

- TEXTURE: The crisp crunch of an apple and the snap of a carrot, compared to the sponginess of muscle and the greasiness of fat.

- FLAVOR: The sweetness of a cashew and the tartness of a tangerine, compared to, ahhhh, compared to—the taste of gravy, marinade, or breading—butter, steak sauce, barbecue sauce, secret sauce, or tartar sauce—mustard, ketchup, mayonnaise, or relish—salt, pepper, spices, or seasonings—cranberry jelly, horse radish, mint jelly, or sweet and sour sauce. Can we blame the meat-eater for covering up a flavor that's probably not very savory given what it really is—cooked, dead flesh?

- AROMA: Stir-fried vegetables with tofu and couscous, and tomato and rosemary soup, compared to: see *Flavor*.

At first glance the meat analog (meat substitute) is a strange food. Plant-based foods such as tofu, soybeans, grains, and vegetables are made to look and taste like familiar animal-based foods: hamburgers, hot dogs, bacon, sausage, lunch meat, ground beef, turkey, chicken, ham, pepperoni, ice cream, and cheese. Although it might appear as if these analogs are recognizing meat and dairy as legitimate foods, many people see them as the food version of the nicotine patch—a way to break a bad habit and transition to a better place—a place filled with whole foods and good health.

If we currently place meat at the center of our meals then it's probably hard to imagine how those obligatory soups, salads, grains, vegetables, and the like, imposing on the fringes of our plates could possibly make a real meal. Maybe that perception comes from past experience.

Let's contrast our previous experiences with how a future experience *could be*:

- SALAD: Iceberg lettuce in a tiny bowl smothered in thick red, white, or orange dressing with bacon bits, in contrast to: A Creole spinach and hot pepper salad with rice noodles, in an olive oil and rice vinegar dressing.

- SOUP: Heavily salted broth with strands of noodles, some shriveled peas, and three or four small bloated pieces of, possibly meat, in contrast to: A black bean soup garnished with diced scallions and soy cream.

- GRAINS: Sticky, starchy, and tasteless white rice, in contrast to: a bulgur and pine nut pilaf with red pepper and parsley.

- VEGETABLES: A vegetable medley of limp pale carrots, mealy beans, and unrecognizable yellow bits, in contrast to: Millet with roasted eggplant, zucchini, and yellow pepper, mixed with lemon juice and mint.

Maybe the contrasts were exaggerated some, but probably not all that much. Having a hard time visualizing the possibilities? It's understandable. Let's remedy that and take a drive together to the local farmers' market, and then to the whole foods store. Seatbelts on? Here we go.

FIRST STOP: THE FARMERS' MARKET. Take a look. This is what fruits and vegetables were meant to look like. All the colors of the rainbow and more. Organically grown, freshly picked, touched only by Nature, with hundreds of life-affirming nutrients, all in one place, costing but dimes and quarters an item. The shopping and picking is exciting, the meal preparation and cooking is soothing, and the dining and consumption is sensual. A complete sensory experience all in one. On to the next stop.

SECOND STOP: THE WHOLE FOODS STORE. Over there are rows of bins filled with dried beans, whole grains, lentils, peas, nuts, and seeds. Unprocessed and direct from the earth. We can fill up seven or eight bags with whatever quantity we want, and center our meals on these foods for dollars a week.

Well, we're back at home base. One hopes that our little excursion was educational and that it will begin to change the way we shop for, think about, and prepare our foods. The local grocery conglomerate may play less of a role in our future food procurement as we choose One-Ingredient Whole Foods from sources closer to Nature.

It's human nature to balk at trying new things, to change, be different, and acquire new habits. Ironically, *this* is what being human is all about. To exercise our free will, to grow, learn, and experience all that life has to offer. To deny this gift makes us little different than the animals that we eat.

Next time a chili cook-off comes to town, maybe we should enter. After all, we now have the beginnings of a recipe that just might make us a winner. And if we do win, and they want to know our secret, we should go right ahead and tell them the truth: It's in the hours of stirring.

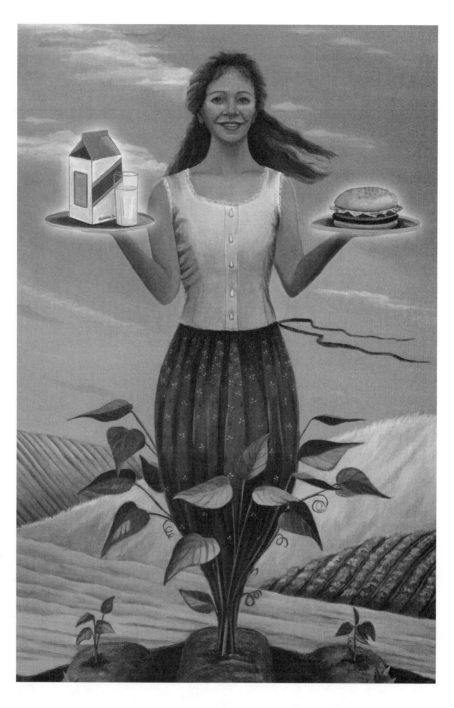

The Elements of a SICK Diet

≈ 3 ≈
Meat and Dairy
CAN'T LIVE WITHOUT OR CAN'T LIVE WITH?

The American Self-Induced Carnivorous Killer (SICK) diet is centered on the following: Animal muscles designed to move body parts, the cows' lactating secretion and products made from it, and the chicken embryo's gelatinous nourishment. Also known as meat, milk, dairy, and eggs, these so-called foods we think we can't live without, are foods we can't *live* with.

Ahead in this chapter...

Is BEEF a proud American icon, backbone of the American economy, a symbol of status, and deliverer of strength, virility, and quality nutrition? Or is beef an American distortion, backbreaker of the economy, symbol of environmental destruction and global hunger, and deliverer of illness and chronic disease?

Turning a pig into food is like turning gold into tin. Pigs have a lot of heart, and the so-called foods we make from them called PORK products, may well have an impact on ours.

If CHICKEN AND FISH are healthy replacements for red meat, then it makes good sense to jump out of the frying pan and into the fire.

Consider what a MILK that is formulated to turn a 90-pound calf into a 450-pound cow in 1 year might do to the human body.

Is it possible to spin-off foods from milk? Take a test matching up DAIRY PRODUCTS with their descriptions to find out.

Is it remotely possible that Nature did in fact formulate the perfect food, place it in chicken EGGS, and hide it under hens?

Since a picture is worth a thousand words, a mural of CHOLESTEROL AND FAT is portrayed, with symbolic color combinations, in five unique mini-paintings.

19: Beef

The American Heritage Dictionary's definition of beef is:

> "The flesh of a slaughtered full-grown steer, bull, ox, or cow."

That's it. Quite a stark contrast to what we might expect given that there is so much more information about beef not in the definition.

Whether we subscribe to the Wholly Eating Leaves to Live (WELL) diet as a vegetarian, or the Self-Induced Carnivorous Killer (SICK) diet as a beef lover, this definition leaves a lot to be desired. It needs to be expanded to complete the beef picture. Let's attempt to do so from the vegetarian's perspective, and the meat-eater's point of view.

Those that eat beef might provide a version like this:

> "Meat from a slaughtered full-grown steer, bull, ox, or cow. A food necessary for human health due to its nutrients of protein, iron, and B vitamins, providing among other things, strength and virility. Beef is an icon of Americana and the backbone of the U.S. economy."

Those that abstain from beef might pen a version like this:

> "Meat from a slaughtered, sentient, full-grown steer, bull, ox, or cow. A food unnecessary and injurious to human health due to its many properties, among them fat, cholesterol, and excessive protein and iron. In addition to the promotion of degenerative diseases such as heart disease and cancer, beef is implicated in impotence and reduced stamina. The

production of beef impairs the environment and contributes to global hunger. Its early production infringed on the land of Native Americans, and today the cost drain makes it a backbreaker of the U.S. economy."

Maybe this is why the dictionary definition is so sparse; the diverse perceptions made a consensus impossible. Which version is the truth?

Americans have been nursed on the first definition, and apparently the suckling hasn't ceased, because 95 percent of Americans currently populate their plates with meat. If contrary information was brought forth in line with the second definition, would a weaning begin? Let's find out by briefly touching on some of the issues surrounding beef such as properties, health, environment, global hunger, economics, and image.

PROPERTIES: The food that we call beef is in essence muscles and ligaments designed to move the body parts of the steer. The elements inherent in these parts are cholesterol, saturated fat, animal protein, and heme iron.

The first property, cholesterol, the human body makes. The second one, saturated fat, we don't need at all. The third and fourth, animal protein and heme iron, we need, but not in the type or the quantity that beef or any other animal provides.

Not inherent, but as potentially damaging are the antibiotics, hormones, and pesticides used to fatten, speed growth, and minimize disease in the cattle and their food. These contents have a slightly different effect on us.

Rounding out the cast of infamous properties are *live* pathogens (like E. coli), that prey on *dead* flesh (like beef).

HEALTH: Given the properties of beef, the potential for adverse health consequences shouldn't be too surprising. The implication of beef, and other meat and dairy products, in some degenerative diseases is well-known: heart disease, atherosclerosis, stroke, and hypertension for instance. Some a little less known: kidney disease, diabetes, and cancer. And then some possibly not known at all: osteoporosis, autoimmune disease, impotence, and Alzheimer's disease. The human body was not designed and built by a bunch of amateurs. It was not meant to fall apart at *any* age.

ENVIRONMENT: Although more subtle, and less known, the production of beef has virtually the same impact on our earth as it does on the human body. Recycling, car-pooling, and low-flow toilets are nice gestures, but they have nowhere near the impact that giving up beef would have. Included in beef's impact on our natural resources are the depletion of water, soil, energy, forests, and the animal waste pollution of inland waterways and oceans. Remember, it's not THE environment, it's OUR environment.

GLOBAL HUNGER: Out of sight out of mind, yes—a reality to ignore, no. The inefficiency of producing beef is no better symbolized, and no more profound, than its impact on the world food supply, and those affected by it. It takes 16 pounds of grain to produce 1 pound of feedlot beef—grain that produces 15 times the calories and 8 times the protein of beef.[1] Feed the grain to humans, rather than the animals, and we have all but alleviated global hunger.[2] Instead, 1 billion people on the planet are underfed and malnourished, and conservatively 40 to 60 million people a year die of starvation.[3]

ECONOMICS: A conservative estimate places the cost of healthcare for beef and meat consumption at $123 billion a year. Industry receipts for beef and meat are roughly $100 billion a year.[4] That's a $23 billion deficit. Add to this, government subsidies, tax breaks, and the cost for ecological repairs. Thus beef, along with other meats, are quantifiably the backbreaker rather than the backbone, of the American Economy.

IMAGE: We have already discovered that beef is the backbreaker rather than backbone of our economy. Are there any other misperceptions lurking about?

Does beef endow virility? If we can use impotence as the barometer then it appears to do the opposite. One in three middle-aged men suffer from impotence,[5] which in 85 percent of cases is caused by artery damage due to fat and cholesterol.[6] Why would this be surprising. A clogged artery to the heart can cause heart failure, a clogged artery to the brain can cause stroke, so why couldn't a clogged artery to any other organ in the body cause equal devastation.

Does beef give us strength? According to studies vegetarians exhibit greater strength and stamina than do omnivores.[7]

And what about beef being a part of Americana? If we define Americana as a proud part of our culture and history, then probably not. The grazing of cattle requires huge amounts of land. Much of the land happened to be already occupied by Native Americans. The cattle wiped out vegetation and other animals that the Indians had built their cultures around.[8] Cowboys and Indians probably wasn't the same game then, that youngsters play now.

Given what we have learned maybe it's time to update the dictionary definition of "beef." Then again, maybe the most appropriate update would be to delete the word all together.

20: Pork

Turning a pig into food is like turning gold into tin. Pigs as animals have much to add to the lives of humans. They are fun loving and friendly. They have an intelligence level on par with chimpanzees. And they have rescued humans to save their lives. Overall, they are sensible, clean, and social. Many people keep them as pets as they would a dog.[1]

Conversely, pigs as food have nothing to add to the lives of humans. In reality, as a food, they are more apt to take away the lives of humans.

Ninety million pigs are slaughtered every year in the United States.[2] The foods made from pigs, like the pigs themselves, contain variety, flexibility, and companionship.

VARIETY: Ham, bacon, sausage, pork chops, wieners, pork rinds, cured meats, chitlins, ham hocks, and hog maws. Names that help us forget about what it is we are really consuming.

FLEXIBILITY: Bacon for breakfast, ham sandwich for lunch, pork chops for dinner, and pork rinds for snacks.

COMPANIONSHIP: Ham and cheese, bacon and eggs, pork and beans. The byproducts of these foods provide yet another kind of versatility. Contained in these foods are a wide array of elements not quite as friendly as the pigs themselves: saturated fat, cholesterol, sodium, nitrites, pesticides, parasites, and hostile viral pathogens are contained in the 23 pigs the average American will consume in his or her lifetime.[3]

FAT CHANCE: The fatter the pig farmer can make the pig, the more money the pig will bring at market. However, fatter translates into fat when it comes to the foods made from the pig. Pork sausage contains 83 percent fat, bacon 82 percent fat, and ham 70 percent fat.[4] Additionally, a 3.5-ounce serving of the average pork product contains 70 milligrams of cholesterol, the same as beef.[5] And the usable protein we receive from pork runs at 19 percent of calories, 3 to 4 times too much.[6] But this is only the beginning in the pig's attempt to get even.

WE'VE BEEN CURED: Potassium nitrite and sodium nitrite are added to cured meats like bacon, Vienna sausage, and spiced ham to give these foods their blood color, tanginess to the palate, and ability to retard the growth of botulism. What could be wrong with that? These nitrites combine with the natural stomach and food chemicals (secondary amines) to create nitrosamines, among the most powerful cancer causing agents known.[7] That's what could be wrong with that.

GOING UP? Ham and bacon have high levels of sodium, that can make for high levels of blood pressure, that can make for high levels of sickness and sorrow.[8]

GRAY AREA: Pork wieners would be gray, and probably less marketable, if it weren't for the red blood cells from slaughtered animals added for color. However, it may not be worth the trade-off as the coloring additive has been shown to be carcinogenic.[9]

NONDISCRIMINATION: Pesticides are used to kill pests in the pig's food and environment. Plant-based foods require nowhere near the pesticide use. Thus it is no surprise that pork contains the accumulation of pesticides up to 14 times more concentrated than those in plant-based foods.[10] Unfortunately, pesticides continue to kill after they are finished with the pests as they can cause birth defects, tumors, and more in humans.[11]

TRICKY WORM: Eating undercooked pork can lead to trichinosis, a pesky worm that's right at home reproducing in our intestines. At only 300 cases a year, and a 5 percent fatality rate, it's hardly something to worry about, unless we are one of the 300 cases or 15 who die.[12]

CHILD ABUSE? Another hazard of undercooked pork is toxoplasmosis. Approximately 30 percent of all pork products are contaminated with this pathogen.[13] For most adults it's nothing more than a bout with the flu, however for pregnant women it's a slight bit more—the potential of serious consequences to their unborn child.

A LONG PASS: A virus called Nipah can lead to deadly encephalitis in humans. It can be passed from pigs to humans. An outbreak in Borneo in the year 2000 caused more than 100 deaths and required the slaughter of more than 1 million pigs. Sure, Borneo is far away, then again viruses have no problem with travel.[14]

SHARING: Hepatitis E virus (HEV) can also be passed from swine to humans. Pork may be the reservoir responsible for sporadic acquired cases of acute hepatitis reported in regions with relatively mild climates. Apparently sharing is another trait we can attribute to pigs.[15]

Even if the additives, parasites, and viruses were not players in the game of pork roulette, the saturated fat and cholesterol, eternal enemies of our heart, should be reason enough to walk briskly in the opposite direction if presented a plate of pork or other pork product. But if our plan is to not do so, our ever-resourceful species has developed a work-around scheme. Pig hearts are being considered as organ transplants because of their anatomical similarity to the human heart.

If the absurdity of replacing our heart, with the heart of the animal we consumed that ruined our heart isn't evident, then we should fear for the future of our species.

21: Chicken and Fish

IT MAY SOUND LIKE PROGRESS

"I have really cut back on eating red meat. I try to eat only chicken and fish," we like to tell our critical doctor, healthy friends, and vegetarian acquaintances.

In essence, we are attempting to improve our health by replacing red meat with chicken and fish so we can get the protein we need without all the fat. It sounds like progress, but then so does getting a stay of execution for 24 hours.

We should be getting 10 to 15 percent of our calories from fat.[1] Even if we bake it, pull off the skin, and consume only the white meat, chicken still contains 23 percent fat in calories. A roasted chicken contains 51 percent fat.[2] When it comes to fish, salmon contains 52 percent fat, trout 32 percent, and even halibut has 19 percent fat.[3] By replacing red meat with fish and chicken to reduce our fat intake, we may be doing our consciences some good, but not our bodies.

In their next campaign those creating ads for beef should tout, "Calorie for calorie, chicken and fish contain twice as much cholesterol as beef." Because per 100 calories fish contains 50 milligrams, chicken 44 milligrams, beef 29 milligrams, and pork 24 milligrams of cholesterol.[4] Then again, maybe that wouldn't be such a good idea given the RDA for cholesterol—since the body makes all that it needs—is zero milligrams.[5]

Our perception of protein is this: "We have to make sure we get enough. We can never get too much." The human body's requirement for protein is 5 to 10 percent of total calories.[6] This is easily satisfied with the WELL diet both in quantity and quality.[7] Chicken and fish contain roughly 23 percent and 20 percent protein, respectively, with about 70 percent usable by the body, twice our needs.[8]

If animal protein by itself is implicated in degenerative disease, then *too much* animal protein is adding fuel to the already roaring fire. Animal protein is implicated in osteoporosis, kidney disease, autoimmune diseases like rheumatoid arthritis and lupus, and cancers such as colon, pancreatic, bladder, and cervical.[9]

Although there is no life left in the chicken and fish we're consuming, there is still plenty of life left *on* them. One out of every 3 chickens contains salmonella.[10] Two out of every 3 contains campylobacter. Some gets cooked out—some doesn't. These pathogens kill 1,000 people and sicken between 6.5 million and 76 million people a year.[11]

Fish begins to breed bacteria the day it is caught. Roughly 65 percent of fish is beginning to spoil or has spoiled by the time it reaches the dinner table, often 2 weeks after being caught.[12] The result? Conservatively 325,000 cases of food poisoning every year.[13]

There is also more on the inside of chicken and fish than muscle, fat, and bone. Antibiotics, hormones, pesticides, and dyes in chicken; PCBs and mercury in fish.[14] These may be worse than the meat itself. And unlike the bacteria that might give us short-term food poisoning, some of these chemicals can contribute to long-term cancer.

Omega-3 fatty acids found abundantly in fish help reduce the risk of coronary artery disease as they thin the blood and reduce clotting. There is no doubt in that. However, it might help to read the terms, conditions, and limitations before filleting the sole.

The high quantity of Omega-3 fatty acids in fish oil can also increase the risk of cerebral hemorrhage.[15] And to get the Omega-3 fats in fish we have to take the good—with the bad and ugly—in the name of unwanted fats, proteins, contaminants, and bacteria. It pays to read the fine print.

Anyway, Omega-3s are not the sacred treasures of fish. They can also be obtained in various vegetables, legumes, nuts, and seeds.[16] Besides, fish get their Omega-3s from the plant kingdom too—the underwater plant kingdom—in the form of algae and plankton.

It seems to be the same old story. We eat animals high up on the food chain and thus receive excessive concentrations of nutrients, causing disease. In the case of cows and pigs, it's protein and iron, resulting in multiple risks. In the case of fish, it's Omega-3s, resulting in the risk of cerebral hemorrhage. At least we are consistent.

What we obtain from chicken and fish in adverse properties is only half the story. What we *don't* obtain from them might be just as bad. Chicken and fish have no fiber, complex carbohydrates, or phytochemicals, and they have few antioxidants, not to mention they are taking the place of foods, in the name of plants, that do have these qualities.[17] The average American eats 50 pounds of chicken and 12 pounds of fish every year.[18] That's 62 pounds of marine and land animals better left as they are.

Excessive fat, protein, and cholesterol. Salmonella, campylobacter, and other pathogens. Antibiotics, hormones, and pesticides. Mercury, dyes, and PCBs. No complex carbohydrates, fiber, and phytochemicals. These are the qualities in the foods we are replacing red meat with to improve our health.

Maybe the next time we are face-to-face with our critical doctor, healthy friends, and vegetarian acquaintances, it would be great if we could say, "I have stopped eating *all* meat. I only eat from the plant kingdom now."

22: Milk

WEIGHING THE PROS AND CONS

Milk has received a lot of bad press. Yes, the very milk that most of us grew up on and many of us still drink. Is milk necessary for the health and development of our children? Should milk be a staple for adults? Often we come to haphazard conclusions without objectively weighing the benefits and drawbacks, and reviewing the data in a detached and analytical manner.

Sometimes it helps to make a list of opposing points and compare them side-by-side, in black and white. To this end in order to help us answer the question—should humans drink milk?—a list of pros and cons have been compiled.

CONS:

- Children who drink too much cows' milk run the risk of iron-deficiency anemia.[1]

- Cows' milk can cause intestinal bleeding and blood loss in children.[2]

- Childhood otitis media (ear infection) affects 10 million children and is linked to cows' milk allergy.[3]

- One out of every 5 babies suffers from colic. Pediatricians have known for some time that cows' milk was often the reason.[4]

- Among children, canker sores, skin conditions, and post-nasal drip can be caused by dairy products.[5]

- The highest rates of leukemia are found in the children who consume the most dairy products. It is estimated that 20 percent of American dairy cattle are infected with the leukemia virus.[6]

- A specific cows' milk protein sparks an autoimmune reaction which is believed to be what destroys the insulin producing cells of the pancreas, causing insulin-dependent diabetes (Type I or childhood).[7]

- Infants who drink cows' milk often have colds, chronic diarrhea, rashes, and big tonsils.[8]

- Asthmatics can find a marked improvement in their condition by eliminating cows' milk from their diets.[9]

- Milk is deficient for human needs in iron, fiber, essential fatty acids, vitamin B_1, and vitamin C.[10]

- Cows' milk contributes to osteoporosis.[11]

- Osteoporosis is most prevalent in countries that consume the most dairy and milk products.[12]

- In one study, women who drank more cows' milk had a higher incidence of hip fractures.[13]

- Ovarian cancer has been linked to the sugar in cows' milk.[14]

- Cows injected with bovine growth hormone (BGH) can increase the risk for prostate and breast cancers.[15]

- Cows' milk contributes to the formation of kidney stones.[16]

- Cows' milk increases the risk of prostate cancer.[17]

- Cows' milk increases the risk of type II diabetes.[18]

- Cows' milk protein, cholesterol, and fat increase the risk of heart disease.[19]

- Antigen-antibody complexes in cows' milk are implicated in rheumatoid arthritis.[20]

- Cows' milk sugar, galactose, can lead to cataract development.[21]

- Ulcers are made worse by cows' milk.[22]

- Cholesterol in cows' milk leads to gallstones.[23]

- Cows' milk can lead to a calcium deficiency, because protein from milk washes calcium from the body.[24]

- Two percent cows' milk is 31 percent fat by calories; whole cows' milk is 49 percent fat.[25]

- Cows' milk contains roughly 80 antibiotics that result in increased bacteria resistance to them.[26]

- Cows' milk contains frequent contaminants, from pesticides to drugs.[27]

- If vitamin D, which is really a hormone, isn't properly mixed in cows' milk it can be toxic in 5 times greater the amount of standard fortification.[28]

- Given there are 4,000 species of mammals that all make unique milk, milk is probably species-specific.[29]

- Cows' milk is formulated to turn a 90-pound calf into a 450-pound cow in 1 year. [30]

PROS:

There we have it, a rundown on the pros and cons. We should now be better positioned to make an informed decision on the issue of milk consumption for us and our children.

Four thousand mammals produce milk to nourish their young. In 3,999 cases, mammals give *their* milk to *their* young during infancy until such a time they are capable of foraging for, and eating, solid food. In only one case, a mammal drinks another mammal's milk, and does so for a lifetime.

Nearly two-thirds of the human inhabitants of this planet—roughly 4 billion people—don't drink cows' milk, or any other mammal's milk.[31] There aren't any nutrients in milk that aren't readily available from a wide variety of plant-based foods, including whole grains, fruits, vegetables, legumes, nuts, and seeds.[32]

The difference between us and all other species is our higher level of intelligence. This intelligence gives us the ability to modify instinctive responses based on learned behavior, make rapid adjustments to new demands, and perform conscious thinking and planning to further evolve our species.

Given the 30 CONS and the zero PROS it might be time for us to take advantage of the differences.

23: Dairy Products

WE *CAN* DO WORSE

With a rap sheet a mile long we might think the worst thing we could do with milk is drink it. We can do worse. We can distill milk into a variety of more concentrated products, making milk spin-offs potentially more harmful than milk itself. The most beneficial component of the process, the water, we discard in favor of ingredients that will only augment milk's rap sheet of sickness and disease causing potential.

The average American consumes 586 pounds of milk and dairy products a year.[1] Given this substantial number it would stand to reason we would have intimate knowledge of these products. So just for fun let's see if that is the case.

Below are four descriptions, each a common dairy product. Guess the dairy product that best fits each description. The answers will be provided at the conclusion.

1. To make 1 pound of this dairy product we express 10 pounds of a cows' lactating secretion from her mammary glands. As it begins to coagulate we add lactic acid bacteria to sour it. Next we extract the gastric juice, rennin, from the fourth stomach of a slaughtered calf along with calcium chloride to curdle it. Then we add some potassium nitrate to inhibit contaminating bacteria and dyes for color. We spray it with mold-forming spores, wash it in alcohol, and then let it set for up to 2 to 3 years until it becomes firm, dry, crusty, and smelly.[2]

   This dairy product contains roughly 70 percent fat in calories.[3] Eighty percent of its protein is casein. Casein is also used as a glue to affix labels to beer bottles, and hold furniture together.[4] This protein is also a foreign substance to the body, thus it can create an antibody-antigen reaction that can cause a constant flow of mucus and phlegm, clogging the kidneys, spleen, pancreas, tracheal-bronchial tree, lungs, and thymus.[5]

For women, the suspended consumption of this product will reduce her risk of breast cancer up to 3 times.[6]

2. One story attributes the origination of this dairy product to King Charles I of England. The story goes that he introduced it at a formal banquet for family and friends. It was served after dinner for dessert and resembled fresh-fallen snow. The delicacy appeared to be a hit. However, in 1649 King Charles fell into disfavor with his people and he was beheaded.[7]

   Although no specifics were given for his demise one has to wonder if the people found out about the many health hazards of his concoction.

   It takes 3 gallons of milk to produce 1 quart of this product, which contains 49 percent fat.[8]

   More than 50 million Americans that have lactose intolerance find it hard to digest.[9] It's one of many foods that contribute to Irritable Bowel Syndrome.[10] The progesterone in this product is implicated as a factor in the development of acne.[11] The many proteins from it can lead to allergies, asthma, and ear infections.[12]

   It causes everyone to *SCREAM*, especially those having a coronary event.

3. This dairy product contains friendly bacteria called lactobacillus, although its beneficial effects have not been conclusively proven.[13] It contains 49 percent fat, and its low-fat version, 31 percent fat.[14] Being a product of milk it contains all the same inherent problems.

   Women who consume it have triple the risk of ovarian cancer as those who don't, thanks to the milk sugar galactose contained in this product.[15] Many have characterized this dairy product as a health food. It is often associated with the French, thus giving it sophistication. Of course, the French also eat snails.

4. This dairy product requires 21 pounds of milk to make 1 pound of it.[16] It contains a hefty 85 percent fat.[17] This dairy food dates back to 2000 B.C. However, it wasn't a food then. Then it was used as an ointment, medicine, or illuminating oil.[18]

Know the answers? If your answers match the ones below then you get 4 points. If you answered, how could any of these described items possibly be foods, then you get 8 points.

1. Cheese
2. Ice Cream
3. Yogurt
4. Butter

In addition to the already listed indictments, there is one other. The milk of any mammal was intended to go directly from the nipple into the mouth, never to touch the air or see the light of day. Because it doesn't, we have to keep the lid on a spectrum of organisms and bacteria such as mycobacterium tuberculosis, salmonella, staphylococcus, and listeria by applying heat (pasteurization), acids, salt, and preservatives to dairy products.[19] Most of the time this works but when it doesn't, add food poisoning, from mild to fatal, to the list of offending complications.

Many vegetarians continue to consume dairy products because:

- They think their protein needs won't be met.

- They think dairy doesn't contribute to the cruelty of animals.

- They view dairy as healthy and wholesome because of their calcium and vitamin D properties.

As it goes in baseball, it goes here too, three strikes and you're out, because:

- A good variety of plant-based foods will more than satisfy protein requirements.[20]

- The dairy cow is always pregnant and overstressed, her calves are taken from her at birth, and she is most likely made into hamburger after living only about 10 percent of her life.[21]

- According to studies, the calcium from milk is offset by the milk's protein, creating a negative calcium balance.[22] Vitamin D is more accurately classified as a hormone as it is made in sufficient quantities by the body from getting 15 minutes of sunshine, three times a week.[23]

When we think of dairy products, words that might come to mind are wholesome, healthy, parties, desserts, and snacks. Words that probably never come to mind are glue, illuminating oil, bacteria, mucus, and disease.

This huge disparity in perception might have us asking two questions: Who is doing the masterful PR job for these products? And could they have saved King Charles?

24: Eggs

PERFECT FOOD — FOR THE CHICKEN EMBRYO

The egg is often touted as Nature's perfect food. And it is—for the nourishment of the chicken embryo. In the same vein we could say that the human placenta is Nature's perfect food. And it is—for the nourishment of the human embryo.

Most likely after witnessing a human birth, and seeing the placenta expelled, our thoughts did not include the desire to cook up an omelet. But apparently we are able to disassociate the human birth experience with our ovum eating habits because the average American ingests the aggregate of 300 eggs a year.[1] Therefore, could there be any truth to the claim that the egg is Nature's perfect food? In a very narrowly defined and misleading way, there is.

The order and proportion of the amino acids makes the egg protein 94 percent usable by the body, more than any other "food" consumed.[2] Conversely, plant-based food proteins are between 40 and 70 percent usable by the body.[3] If we stopped here and didn't think about it too much, we might accept the "perfect food" claim. But it might be in our best interest to think about it.

A chicken embryo needs an all-in-one, highly efficient complete food very close at hand, as would any animal embryo, because its ability to forage for a variety of foods is exceptionally limited. However, *we* are not limited to one food. If we consume a variety of plant-based foods, then without too much trouble we can get the aggregate protein usability that is on a par with the egg—if that is even meaningful since usability refers to a single food that is not applicable to our diets. When we add a few other things we know about the egg to this information we can get a complete picture.

The nutrient ratio of our food should be roughly 80 percent carbohydrates, 10 percent protein, and 10 percent fat in calories. The egg is 3 percent carbohydrates, 32 percent protein, and 65 percent fat.[4] Three times the protein, 6 times the fat, and virtually no carbohydrates. The perfect food is beginning to appear a little less perfect.

A single egg contains 213 milligrams of cholesterol—213

milligrams more than the RDA of zero given the body produces 500 milligrams of its own cholesterol a day.[5] If we ate one egg per day, and had no other animal or animal byproducts in our diet, we would raise our blood cholesterol level by 12 percent and our risk of heart attack by 24 percent.[6] One could say, "an egg a day keeps the cardiologists' bank accounts A-OK." And it doesn't hurt the pediatricians' bank balance either because egg white is third on the list of pediatric food allergies.[7]

Most likely Mother Nature wouldn't have risked the demise of our species by creating one perfect food, placing it in a chicken egg, and hiding it under a hen where we might never find it. But some people must have thought she did—probably some very sick individuals. And if they weren't sick, they may well have become so after including unfertilized chicken eggs in their diets.

For those who like to cook and bake it would seem almost preposterous that eggs weren't meant to be a part of the human diet equation. They are used to bind, thicken, and lighten; they are used to add flavor, color, and texture. Eggs appear in so many recipes that to have to exclude them might cause many cooks to throw up their arms in frustration and go find new hobbies.

But where is it etched in stone that eggs were decreed as the food to perform these functions? Isn't the making of foods from Nature's raw ingredients a human contrivance, with no significance other than history, habit, and tradition? As it turns out there are many egg analogs derived from the plant kingdom that bind, thicken, lighten, flavor, color, and provide texture as good or better than eggs.[8] The only difference is that the egg analogs do it healthier.

Children yet to be indoctrinated by Madison Avenue, economic interests, and cultural conditioning, with their instincts still in tact, might have a different view of the egg.

A little boy, maybe 5 years old, sat down to breakfast one morning. In front of him was an egg prepared sunny-side up by his mother. The egg's consistency reminded him of the time he had a cold; the taste didn't improve his opinion of it. He refused to eat it.

As adults, many of us have come to believe that the egg is The Incredible Edible Egg. But if the 5-year-old boy had the language skills, he might have described it as: The Detestable Dispensable Egg.

25: Cholesterol and Fat

Unless we have been in a coma for the last decade, we probably know that cholesterol and fat are substances that can do great harm to our bodies. But do we have the whole picture? What better way to capture the whole picture than to paint it!

The painting will actually be five mini-paintings, all done on one canvas in oils, with lots of colors and contrasts. Each mini-painting will have its own theme and symbolic colors. This may seem like an odd way to present the information, but then again, a picture is worth a thousand words.

PAINTING No.1
TITLE: "I'll Make It Myself."
COLORS: Black and white

Humans and animals synthesize a waxy substance in their bodies called cholesterol to assist in hormone, bile acid, and vitamin D production.[1] Most of it is manufactured in the liver, but some in the cells. Humans make 500 milligrams a day and require no additional cholesterol from outside sources, say for instance, animals.[2] Plants have almost undetectable amounts of cholesterol, consequently when we eat from the plant kingdom we don't ingest it.

Humans do require fats in their diet, but only two—unsaturated linoleic and linolenic fatty acids—and they are only synthesized by plants.[3] It appears an optimal amount of fat intake is 10 to 15 percent of total calories, which just happens to coincide with the fat content in a representative sampling from the plant kingdom.[4]

It's as clear as black on white.

PAINTING No. 2
TITLE: "I'm Just Sick About It."
COLORS: Ashen and blue

Americans on average eat close to 40 percent of their calories in fat, and ingest another 500 milligrams of cholesterol a day more than what the body manufactures.[5] Our bodies aren't too happy about us eating the stored calories of another animal (fat), or a substance it already makes for cell maintenance (cholesterol). Consequently, our bodies rebel with the result being a wide variety of degenerative diseases, the most prominent, circulatory disease. For the white American a short poem might be in order:

> When we have good circulation,
> the skin is a pinkish hue.
> But when the circulation is not so good,
> the skin is ashen and blue.

PAINTING No. 3
TITLE: "Are the Cards Stacked?"
COLORS: Cloudy gray

Heart disease is virtually avoidable with a blood cholesterol level of 150 milligrams per deciliter (mg/dL) or better.[6] American vegans average 133 mg/dL.[7] Yet the "desirable level" we are told is 200 mg/dL. The average American has a blood cholesterol level of 205 mg/dL, and the average American dies of a heart attack every minute.[8] Some questions come to mind.

- Why is the level set at 200 mg/dL when the average American with a level slightly above that, is dying from heart disease every minute?

- Might this be a level that is set in the context of the American SICK diet?

- What do we tell the spouse of a heart attack victim, when he or she wonders how this could have happened given the deceased had attained a more than desirable level of 180 mg/dL?

- Many "official" organizations, groups, and individuals recommend we get no more than 30 percent of our calories from fat. The commercial diet center foods contain 20 to 30 percent of calories from fat, including animal fat.[9] Aren't these recommendations and foods slightly above the 10 to 15 percent ideal?

- Because they are calculated by weight, and not by percent of calories as they should be, many low-fat foods are not really low in fat. As an example, 2 percent fat milk when measured in calories becomes 31 percent fat milk.[10]

- Although chicken and fish have less saturated fat than pork and beef, they have twice the cholesterol when measured in calories. That is because cholesterol is found in the lean portion of meat.[11]

- The unprocessed, healthier, lower profit margin foods are usually found in the outer aisles of the supermarket, farthest from the door.[12]

Has our diet and health picture been clouded by economic interests?

PAINTING No. 4
TITLE: "A Perpetual Treadmill."
COLORS: Fool's gold

Despite the best efforts to get healthy, the average American's fat intake has not changed since the mid-eighties, and obesity has increased by 50 percent in the 1990s.[13]

All of the appetite suppressants, weight loss drugs, commercial weight loss centers, liposuction sessions, stomach stapling operations, trendy diet plans, cholesterol and blood pressure lowering drugs, exercise equipment, health clubs, angioplasty, self-induced vomiting, heart bypass surgeries, low-fat processed foods, and 1,800 diet books have not made a dent.[14]

Someone is hauling in the gold, and someone is being made the fool.

PAINTING No. 5
TITLE: "The Supermarket Outer Aisle."
COLORS: Deep greens, yellows, reds, and oranges

- With little effort, populations that subscribe to the WELL diet eating only vegetables, fruits, grains, and legumes—like those in rural China—maintain cholesterol levels between 90 and 150 milligrams per deciliter (mg/dL), and have little or no coronary artery disease.[15] Those monitored for 35 years in the Framington Heart Study with cholesterol levels below 150 mg/dL did not suffer one heart attack.[16]

- For every 1 percent reduction in blood cholesterol a 3 to 4 percent heart attack reduction is realized.[17]

- No matter how hard we try we can't produce atherosclerosis in a dog, a natural carnivore.[18]

- Arterial plaque can be reabsorbed and atherosclerosis reversed by changing to a plants-only diet.[19]

Most likely, Nature made our foods in deep, bright colors so we could easily find them, and color-coded them so we would obtain a variety of nutrients.

The painting is complete! Why don't we let it dry for now. Later we can find an appropriate place to hang it. Maybe over the kitchen table.

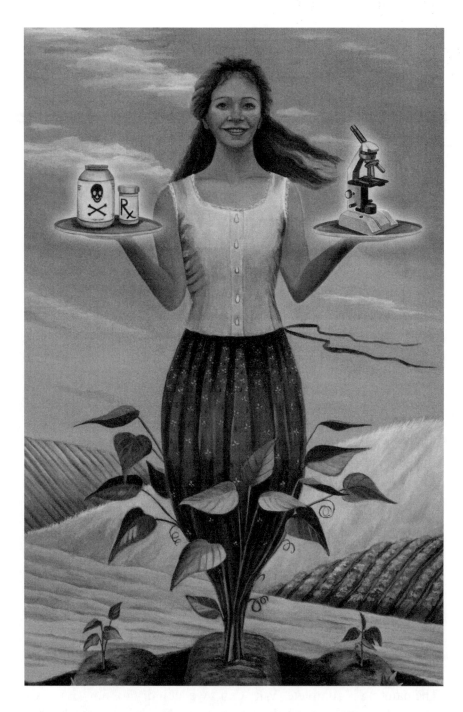

More Than "Meats" the Eye

∼ 4 ∼
Contaminants
MORE THAN FAT AND CHOLESTEROL

If we thought the inherent properties of animal-based foods—like fat and cholesterol—were all there was to worry about when sitting down to a meal of meat, fish, dairy, or eggs, we were mistaken.

Ahead in this chapter...

Why are the animals raised in factory farms consuming 8 times the ANTIBIOTICS that people do?[1] And why are there possibly 60,000 reasons that the meat-eater should care?[2]

No need to super-size that next hamburger value meal. It has already been taken care of down at the cattle and dairy farms with powerful growth HORMONES.

It's common to see long, exhaustive, warning labels on PESTICIDES. Where else might these warning labels be placed to benefit the consumer—the consumer of animal-based foods that is.

With no likable characters, little comic relief, far too many bathroom scenes, and a downer ending, it is no surprise that a movie about FOOD POISONING—*Sal Monella and the Seven Pathogens*—didn't fair too well at the box office.

A movie treatment was submitted to producers and rejected as being too far out and not believable. The title of the movie was, *MAD!—Mutually Assured Destruction*. Unbeknown to the producers, the movie was a non-fiction work about MAD COW DISEASE.

Take a 20 question true/false test to find out why MEAT INSPECTION may well be considered an oxymoron, and why fans of Robert Ripley ("Believe It Or Not"), and Dave Barry ("I'm not making this up."), will find this material right up their alley.

26: Antibiotics

TAKE WITH FOOD, NOT IN FOOD

Don't the instructions on the bottle of antibiotics say, take with food—not—take in food?

Apparently the factory farm producers of animal meat products have misread the label because they are dumping 24 million pounds of antibiotics a year into the feed of chickens, pigs, and cows.[1] Consequently, every time we sit down to a meal of chicken wings, pork chops, or New York strips we are also sitting down to a meal of tetracycline, penicillin, and vancomycin.

Why is farmer Fred feeding nearly 8 times the antibiotics to his animals that are used to treat human illness—and why should we care?[2]

In the close quarters of the factory farm environment antibiotics are necessary to prevent the spread of disease. The economic reality that diseased and dead animals do not bring as much money at market is probably a motivating factor. In addition to their use in disease prevention, antibiotics promote growth in the animals, increasing their weight by up to 12 percent.[3] Both these byproducts of antibiotic use translate into higher profits for the farmer and lower prices for the consumer. What could be wrong with that? For the farmer maybe nothing, but for the consumer maybe plenty.

Although consumers may be under budget in their food spending, there is every likelihood that they will go over budget in their healthcare spending. That's because the roughly 80 different antibiotics ingested daily as part of the Self-Induced Carnivorous Killer (SICK) diet creates antibiotic-resistant bacteria.[4] This can lead to effectively treating a bacterial infection as a tossup. However, that's not the only problem with antibiotic resistance.

The animals, like us, build up a resistance to antibiotics meaning they, too, are developing disease that becomes harder and harder to treat. Consequently, the "once animal, now meal" brings to the table along with its dead flesh, live bacteria like salmonella, E. coli, and campylobacter.

To better appreciate the adverse potential that bacteria-resistance has, let's place it in context. Where humans produce a new generation every 20 years, bacteria reproduce and evolve every 20 *minutes*.[5] Antibiotics kill most of their enemies, but those few bacteria that might survive the battle reproduce again in 20 minutes, and every 20 minutes thereafter. The second time around when Mr. Antibiotic comes looking for a fight these bacteria will be stronger, better prepared, and have a greater chance of winning the battle. For instance:

- 95 percent of staphylococcus aureus are now resistant to penicillin.[6]

- Between 1992 and 1997 infections in humans increased nearly 8 times because of antibiotic-resistant bacteria.[7]

- Drug resistance to campylobacter, the most common known cause of bacterial food-borne illness in the United States, increased from zero percent in 1991 to 20 percent in 1999.[8]

- In 1998, the Centers for Disease Control and Prevention found that salmonella was resistant to five different antibiotics primarily because they are used in livestock feed.[9]

- Hospital antibiotic use is 100 times greater than it was in the 1960s.[10]

- Each year up to 60,000 people die because their medications were ineffective in combating bacterial strains.[11]

The question that most likely comes to mind is this. If adding antibiotics to the feed of livestock is harmful to human health, and potentially catastrophic, why hasn't the practice been stopped?

Well it has. In Great Britain, the Netherlands, Sweden, Finland, Canada, Germany, Denmark, Japan, the European Economic Community, and the European Union.[12] However, the practice continues in the United States.

Are the agencies that are responsible for our health and welfare asleep at their posts? Or does the blame fall somewhere else?

- In 1977, the Food and Drug Administration (FDA) tried to ban antibiotics in the animal industries.[13]

- In 1997, the World Health Organization (WHO) called for a ban on feeding antibiotics to livestock.[14]

- In 1999, the Centers for Disease Control and Prevention (CDC) placed the blame for the dramatic rise in infections on the routine use of antibiotics in livestock production.[15]

- In 2001, the American Medical Association (AMA) recommended restricting antibiotic use in animals stating that the increase of antibiotic resistance is a threat to human health.[16]

- In 2001, legislation was introduced in Congress to curtail the use of essential antibiotics in livestock and preserve them for human use.[17] That legislation is pending.

Clearly, the agencies responsible for our well-being are doing all they can—at least for those who eat meat—to curb antibiotic use in animals. So why haven't they been successful after trying since 1977?

The agricultural and pharmaceutical industries have a lot to lose if antibiotic use is curbed in livestock. Apparently these industries and their lobbyists are a formidable force—organized, strong in numbers, and continually fighting off their opponents.

Oh sure, their membership doesn't reproduce every 20 minutes, nonetheless, a new antibiotic might be in order.

27: Hormones

WE DON'T NEED TO SUPER-SIZE IT

The next time we place our order at the fast-food drive-through window, and the friendly order taker asks if we would like our hamburger value meal super-sized, we can tell him, "That won't be necessary. It was already done back on the factory farm with the furnishing of growth hormones to cattle and dairy cows to increase their size and milk production."

We can bet he will never be without something to contribute to the conversation at family events again.

Hormones are chemicals that regulate body functions such as metabolism, reproduction, and growth. One can imagine that any substance that makes us grow has to be a very powerful and concentrated chemical. How powerful? We could taste a grain of sugar in a swimming pool if our taste buds were as sensitive to flavor as our target cells are to hormones.[1]

Growth hormones such as zeranol, trenbolone acetate, progesterone, testosterone, and estradiol are implanted in more than 90 percent of beef cattle in the United States to promote quick weight gain.[2] rBGH is a growth hormone given to 25 percent of dairy cows. It can more than double their milk production, from 20 to 45 pounds a day.[3]

Can these hormones that benefit us when produced in proper quantities by our own bodies do us harm when we ingest additional amounts from other bodies, that is, animals in the form of meat and dairy products? Can the same fire that gives us heat also burn our house down?

What could be more natural than injecting a growth hormone (rBGH) into a mammal, cows, to over stimulate their mammary glands to ensure a different mammal, humans, have enough of the other mammal's milk to drink. As natural as the results:

- rBGH has been shown to increase the risk of prostate cancer in men older than 60 by 8 times.[4]

- rBGH has been shown to increase breast cancer for pre-menopausal women by 7 times.[5]

- rBGH has been implicated in colorectal, thyroid, and bone cancer.[6]

There is some difference of opinion as to whether rBGH is killed by pasteurization, or broken down by enzymes before it ever has a chance to enter our bloodstreams. Scientists say it isn't; milk producers say it is. What could be more natural?[7]

rBGH is not the only problem-causing hormone found in cows' milk. There are at least four other hormones commonly found in processed milk that have been implicated in reproductive and lymphatic cancer.[8]

Then there is one last hormone in milk added *after* it has left the cow, presumably for our own good. It can be toxic in high doses. About 10 cases of toxicity are reported each year. It has been shown to produce abnormal ectopic tissue in rabbits fed 2 milligrams a day. Sufficient amounts are made in our bodies when we are exposed to 30 minutes of sunlight a week. The hormone is called calciferol. We know it better as vitamin D.[9]

Given the hormone participation in milk, maybe milk and cookies, should be referred to as, hormones and cookies.

Roast Beef au Hormone probably doesn't sound much better to the meat connoisseur. But given that beef, too, comes to the table well-stocked with a variety of hormones, this label might be better suited. The hormones implanted in beef are used to speed weight gain and growth in cattle, but they have a slightly different effect on humans:

- The hormone, 17 beta-oestradiol, is a complete carcinogen (has both tumor initiating and tumor promoting influence).[10]

- Lutalyse, given to female animals so they will ovulate all at the same time, can cause women to miscarry.[11]

- Estrogen can increase the risk of uterine and breast cancer.[12]

- Androgen may cause liver cancer.[13]

- Certain hormones can cause increased menstrual flow in women and reduced sperm count in men.[14]

However, there is some question as to whether these hormones end up in our meat in quantities significant enough to cause harm. Some research has found that it's difficult to determine at what level these hormones begin to start and advance cancer.[15] On the other hand DES (diethylstilbestrol), a synthetic hormone initially used to fatten animals, and later to prevent miscarriages in women, wasn't proven to be a cancer risk for 15 to 20 years after it was introduced.[16] It all sounds like hormone roulette—a game we may not want to play, just as the European Union decided *it* didn't want to play.

Since 1995, the European Union (EU) has banned giving growth hormones to cattle because of their potential to cause cancer and reproductive dysfunction in people. It also banned beef imports from the United States. When a ruling came down from the World Trade Organization requiring the EU to make payment of $150 million to the United States for lost profits, it indicated it would pay the price rather than have U.S. beef come into their countries.[17]

We can't see them, and we can't taste them, and when we talk about them there is every likelihood that it's within a sexual context. Hormones are probably the furthest things from our mind when we have a glass of milk or a roast beef sandwich. And if we are ever diagnosed with cancer, hormones again will probably be the furthest things from our mind.

However, next time fast-food is on our mind, and we roll up to the order window, we can tell the friendly order taker, "I'll have a garden salad and a large orange juice. Hormones and cookies, and Roast Beef au Hormone are not on *my* menu anymore."

We can bet he will have something new to add to the conversation at his next family event.

28: Pesticides

NO WARNING LABEL ON THAT SANDWICH?

At one time or another we probably visited the lawn and garden section of our local home improvement store to purchase a pesticide. We wanted to kill the aggravating bugs or insects in and around our home. After 30 minutes of reading the fine print on the labels explaining hazards, warnings, and dangers, we began to wonder whether the pesticide might not be worse than the pests themselves. So we left without a purchase.

On the way home we picked up a sub sandwich loaded with our favorite meats. Once home, we ate our sandwich and decided we could tolerate the pests. We were proud not to have brought dangerous pesticides onto our property.

So at least we thought. Too bad there wasn't a warning label on our sandwich.

Pesticides bring together all the right elements, for just the right disaster. We can't spell, pronounce, or describe them. We can't see, smell, or taste them. But they are potent, concentrated, and deadly. They make a lot of money for the manufacturers, they save a lot of money for the meat producers, but they can create a lot of sickness for the humans.

If there *was* a warning label on our meaty sub sandwich, the fine print might read something like this:

*****

WARNING! Please Read Before Consumption: This sandwich may contain multiple pesticides in unknown quantities. Pesticides are developed to kill living creatures. Some were originally developed to kill humans.[1] There are 21,000 commercial pesticides and a global consumption of 5.5 billion pounds, nearly 1 pound for every human being.[2] Pesticides are being produced 13,000 times faster than in 1950.[3] They can remain active for decades, even centuries, and they become increasingly more potent as they accumulate upward in the food chain.[4]

SPECIAL INFORMATION: The meat you are eating has accumulated pesticides in the following three ways:

FISHMEAL: Half of the world's fish catch is fed to livestock. Because of their long food chains fish accumulate toxic chemicals at a high rate. The EPA estimates that fish can absorb 9 million times the level of polychlorinated biphenyls (PCBs) from the waters in which they live. Additionally, more than 110 million pounds of DDT are in the oceans off North America.

LAND-GROWN FEEDS: These are heavily sprayed with pesticides.

DOUSING AND SPRAYING: Potent pesticides are used to kill parasites and fight flies in the factory farm environment. They are then absorbed, ingested, and retained in the fat of the animals.[5]

POSSIBLE RISKS:
- Women with high blood levels of PCBs have a higher prevalence of endometriosis.[6]
- Seven studies demonstrate that pesticides and other toxic chemicals often found in meat have been detected at elevated levels in violent criminals.[7]
- The concentration of pesticides in animal-based foods increases long-term cancer risk.[8]
- Of 150 known pesticides and drugs found in poultry and meat, 42 are known or are suspected to cause cancer.[9]
- Pesticide exposure can contribute to immune system diseases.[10]
- Dioxin, a potent pesticide, can cause tumors in lab animals in as low as 1 part per trillion.[11]

IF PREGNANT OR PLANNING A FAMILY:

- Pesticide exposure through meat and dairy foods may well contribute to other more subtle birth defects that present themselves as learning disabilities, ADHD, lower IQs, weakened immune systems, and emotional problems.[12]

- An omnivore mother exposes her unborn and new-born to the toxicity of pesticides by way of her placenta and breast milk, increasing his or her risk of cancer, and damage to the developing nervous systems.[13] (Note: In 1950 cancer was a rarity in children. Today, cancer is the second leading cause of death in children under 15.)[14]

- Of 150 known drugs and pesticides found in meat and poultry, 32 have been found or are suspected of causing the following: Birth defects (20), mutations (6), and adverse effects to fetus (6).[15]

- Percentage of mothers' milk in United States containing significant levels of DDT: Non-vegetarians 99 percent, vegetarians 8 percent.[16]

- Contamination of breast milk, due to chlorinated hydrocarbon pesticides in animal-based foods found in omnivore mothers, is 35 times higher than in herbivore mothers.[17]

- Of 17 pesticides tested from samples of breast milk, vegans had levels of 1 to 2 percent of the general population.[18]

- The principle reason for sterility and sperm count reduction of U.S. males is chlorinated hydrocarbon pesticides (dioxin, DDT, etc.). (Note: The average sperm count in the 1960s was 60 million per milliliter. In the 1990s it had dropped to 20 million per milliliter.)[19]

INSPECTION PROTOCOL: The USDA tests one out of every quarter-million slaughtered animals for toxic chemical residue, and then only 10 percent of the toxic chemicals known to be present in meat are tested for.[20]

HERBIVORE AND OMNIVORE COMPARISON: Chemical residues of pesticides in the diet: 95 percent comes from meat, fish, dairy, and eggs, and 5 percent from plant-based foods.[21] Meat contains accumulations of pesticides and other chemicals up to 14 times more concentrated than in plant-based foods. Dairy products contain accumulations of pesticides and other chemicals up to 5.5 times more concentrated than in plant-based foods.[22]

*****

If we bought a sandwich, and there was a label on it like this one, we would probably lose our appetite. Most likely we would throw the sandwich in the garbage. That's a good idea, but not the best solution.

The best solution would be to lay the sandwich down in the yard so the pests could feed on it.

29: Food Poisoning

SAL MONELLA AND THE SEVEN PATHOGENS

The Disney folks have created some magnificent animated features. An early classic was *Snow White and the Seven Dwarfs*. In the movie Disney capitalized on the concept of the poison apple as their chosen antagonist. However, as business enterprises often do, Disney went to the well once too often.

They produced a second movie attempting to cash in on the poison food concept. It bombed. Remember it? (You won't because it didn't happen, but work with me here.) *Sal Monella and the Seven Pathogens?* The stars were Sal Monella of course, and the seven pathogens were played by E. coli, Campylobacter, Trichinosis, Yersinia Enterocolitica, Clostridium Perfringens, Staphylococcus Aureus, and Listeria.

The movie appeared as though it was going to be a big hit as most people came out of the theater doubled over with laughter. But as it turned out they were doubled over for another reason. Each year the movie made 76 million people sick and killed 5,000.[1]

Disney came to the conclusion that the horror movie was not going to be its genre. Let's analyze the movie to see where it might have gone wrong.

*****

The movie begins on the factory farms where the eight characters were right at home. With 100,000 chickens living in close quarters, and cattle crowded into feedlots, they were assured a virtual bacterium playground.[2]

Sal and the Seven Pathogens' first threat was antibiotics. Although initially this nemesis had its way with the stars, in the long run it only made Sal and the gang stronger and more diversified.[3] After the animals were slaughtered Sal Monella and the Seven Pathogens went to work.

Sal's favorite food was chicken, with eggs a close second. Sal, like all the other pathogens, was able to reproduce himself by the millions every hour. This way he could spread himself all around, hitching a ride on 1 of every 3 chickens until he reached his final destination—the intestinal track of an unsuspecting human.[4]

Sal and his clones, too small to be seen by the naked eye, waved goodbye to the meat inspectors and were on their way to market. During the trip Sal bragged about the time in 1993 when he got into ice cream and sickened 224,000 people.[5] No time to rest on past laurels though, it was time to go to work.

When the unsuspecting human opened the cellophane wrapping, Sal Monella spilled onto the sink in the chicken juice. He hoped to spread himself around onto the sponge, utensils, and cutting board too, because he would often be killed during cooking.[6]

Sal was successful this time as he made two members of the family sick with abdominal pain, diarrhea, fever, nausea, and vomiting that lasted for 7 days.[7] He was a nasty fellow inflicting sickness on 2 to 4 million people every year. And when Sal was at his best he could kill 1,000 to 9,000 people annually.[8]

Around town the Seven Pathogens were also performing their ugly deeds. Most of the time—95 percent—they chose animals and their byproducts, usually high-protein foods as their targets. After all, they were predominately carnivores.[9]

E. coli was lurking in ground hamburger at a company picnic. He loved his burgers. He could be found in 50 percent of beef carcasses and in 89 percent of ground hamburger.[10] A prolific performer, E. coli made a minimum of 200 people sick every day by attacking their colons and making them bleed, inflicting severe stomach cramps and watery diarrhea.[11] His favorite targets were children because of their underdeveloped immune systems.[12]

E. coli was in luck today. The cook manning the grill had a few too many beers. The result was 12 undercooked burgers that caused four lengthy sicknesses and two serious hospital stays, one of which caused lung damage and kidney failure.[13]

Campylobacter has worked hard to become the number one cause of food poisoning.[14] Not getting top billing in this movie was quite a blow to him. "Campy" as his friends call him, was wreaking havoc at a wedding reception where chicken, his favorite food, was being served. Campy feasts on 2 out of every 3 chickens, sick-ens 5,000 people every day in the United States, and kills 750 a year.[15] He is also very sneaky because he doesn't normally cause symptoms until a week after he has been ingested, and in 20 percent of cases he will cause relapses.

Yersinia Enterocolitica and Trichinosis usually team up as a dynamic duo because of their love of pork.[16] Yersinia Enterocolitica can outdo anyone when it comes to diarrhea. (Many believe Yersinia would have gone further if she had adopted a shorter stage name.)

Trichinosis, called "Tricky" by close friends, was quite a worm in this movie. He lives by the motto, "Kill me now or you'll pay later." Tricky got into the intestine of one unsuspecting woman then headed for his favorite hangouts: the tongue, calf, and diaphragm. There he weakened his victim until she could barely move.[17]

Clostridium Perfringens is known as the "buffet bug," and although she has a minor role in this movie—since her repertoire is limited to mainly diarrhea—in other ways she is quite versatile. Her strengths include meat, poultry, sauces, gravies, casseroles, fish, and chili. In *Sal Monella*, she showed up at a residential highbrow social function. Unfortunately, the home had eight bathrooms foiling her attempt at any real fun.[18]

Staphylococcus Aureus's claim to fame is he can't be destroyed at normal cooking temperatures. He usually shows up in custards, sauces, potato salad, and pastries. In *Sal Monella* it was no different. A 7-year-old girl's birthday party was the setting. Twelve party dresses, twelve dry cleaning bills, a perfect score.[19]

The movie's blockbuster finish featured Listeria at an outdoor concert on a sweltering summer day in Southern California. Soft cheeses, hot dogs, deli meats, eggs, poultry, and rare meats were its playgrounds. Every year, 92 percent who become infected with Listeria require hospitalization and 20 percent die. Listeria had no problem living up to his reputation on this day. Some will never attend another concert.[20]

*****

It's no surprise the critics panned *Sal Monella and the Seven*

Pathogens. No likable characters, little comic relief, far too many bathroom scenes, and a downer ending.

Needless to say, Disney never featured Sal Monella and the Seven Pathogens again. This was undoubtedly a great relief to Donald, Mickey, and the rest of the beloved Disney characters. After all, Sal and his buddies can't do much damage to people without a solid cast of dead animal co-stars.

30: Mad Cow Disease

GOOD NEWS — BAD NEWS

Most writers secretly long to see their ideas and words brought to life on the big screen. One author recently pitched a movie treatment he knew couldn't miss to a few producers. But it did—by a mile. "Too far out," they laughed. "Not based in reality," they chided. "No one would believe it," they moaned.

Not willing to accept their criticism he is looking for a second opinion. He has asked us—because of our apparently high intelligence and perception—to provide it.

So let's sharpen our pencils and give him some feedback on his movie treatment titled: *MAD!—Mutually Assured Destruction.*

*****

The setting is the early to mid 1900s. A tribe of cannibals in New Guinea is dying off in large numbers after having each other for supper—and we do mean, having each other for supper. The corpses' brains are found to be perforated with holes.[1]

Fast forward to the 1980s. A growing number of cattle in England are staggering around as if they were drunk, becoming belligerent, and then falling over dead.[2] Their brains, too, are found to be perforated with holes. A few humans begin to exhibit the same symptoms, and they, too, perish. Their brains show the same spongiform (holes) in as the cattle and the New Guinea tribe. Apparently a germ is invading humans when they eat the carcasses of the infected animals (or other humans in the case of the tribe).[3]

Approximately 750,000 infected cattle have entered the human food chain, and no one knows who is stricken.[4] It turns out the germ is a protein, or prion, that is indestructible, always kills its victims, and can remain dormant for 10 to 30 years. And it strikes without warning.[5]

No scientists want to study it because of its deadly nature.[6] The only way to confirm for certain who has been stricken is to do a biopsy, rather autopsy, because it can't be done until the person is dead.[7] People who have been infected might exhibit these signs: dizziness, headaches, weight loss, slurred speech, loss of coordination, short-term memory loss, bladder and bowel incontinence, and dementia.[8]

Up to 18 million residents of Great Britain could be infected.[9] Cattle have been found in 12 other countries containing the microbe.[10] Who will be next?

*****

Not a bad concept. Nonetheless, if the critical reviews from the producers are any indication, this movie won't be coming to a theater near us, however we can't be so sure that it won't be coming to a meal in front of us.

The plot line, unfortunately, is all too true. It describes what has been termed, Mad Cow Disease, a form of Transmissible Spongiform Encephalopathies (TSE), a brain wasting disorder. In cattle it is called Bovine Spongiform Encephalopathy (BSE), and in humans it is called Creutzfeldt-Jakob disease (CJD). The disease has been most associated with the eating of beef that passes the disease to humans.[11] Maybe the "Mad" in Mad Cow Disease should stand for, Mutually Assured Destruction. We slaughter the animals, then they slaughter us.

However, as terrible as this all sounds there is always an upside to every bad situation, even this one: A silver lining in the cloud, or the glass is half full instead of half empty. In that spirit, listed here are 12 pieces of "good news" to go along with the bad news.

- The good news is, in 1997 our government banned the feeding of cows, to cows, to prevent Mad Cow Disease. The bad news is, they still permit the feeding of cows to pigs and chickens, and back to cows. The ban has as many holes in it as a brain riddled by the disease itself.[12]

• The good news is, for British people, 200,000 tons of beef were shipped out of Britain during the peak of Mad Cow Disease outbreak. The bad news for Americans is, 13,000 tons of it entered the United States.[13]

• The good news is, the United States has tested more than 12,000 cattle for BSE since 1990 and not one has tested positive. The bad news is, we only test 1 cow in 75,000. The Swiss test 1 in 60, and Ireland tests as many cows in one night as we test in 2 years.[14]

• The good news is, we have an agency responsible for ensuring our meat and dairy food safety, the United States Department of Agriculture (USDA). The bad news is, it also has the responsibility to promote meat and dairy food sales.[15]

• The good news is, medical personnel can find out if we have Mad Cow Disease by doing a brain biopsy. The bad news is, we have to be dead before they can do it.[16]

• The good news is, the British have burned and incinerated 2.5 million cows that had Mad Cow Disease. The bad news is, that will not kill the disease, and thus it can enter the earth and spread back into the food chain.[17]

• The good news is, the National Cattleman's Beef Association has said that what has been fed to cattle has been cooked at temperatures high enough to sterilize it. The bad news is, we can radiate it, soak it in formaldehyde for 10 years, boil it, freeze it, and cook it at 1,100 degrees—hot enough to melt lead—and we still can't kill the prions responsible for the disease.[18]

- The good news is, a Food and Drug Administration (FDA) spokesman has said there is no health problem with Mad Cow Disease in the United States today. The bad news is, it can take 10 to 30 years to show up in the body.[19]

- The good news is, we may have up to 30 years of life left after being infected. The bad news is, it is always fatal.[20]

- The good news is, an insurance company in France now offers discounts to vegetarians. The bad news is, 4,700 to 9,800 cattle in France have been infected with Mad Cow Disease.[21]

- The good news is, there have never been any cases of Mad Cow Disease confirmed in the United States. The bad news is, the disease is remarkably similar to Alzheimer's disease.[22]

How about we deliver the bad news first for a change, and wind up on a positive note.

- The bad news is, British politicians denied the problem of Mad Cow Disease for years to protect the cattle industry, consequently more than 1 million undetected BSE-infected British cattle have been eaten by animals and humans. According to one source, "every adult in Great Britain has already eaten 50 meals containing BSE-infected meat." The good news is, this could never happen in the United States.[23]

31: Meat Inspection

"BELIEVE IT OR NOT." "I'M NOT MAKING THIS UP."

If we eat meat, and have no interest in the inspection practices of our meat, then we can skip this section. If we eat meat, and we do have an interest in what is being done to inspect and ensure the safety of our meat, we should definitely skip this section.

Who then is this section for? Maybe those who enjoy Robert Ripley or Dave Barry, because this section falls under the heading of "Believe it or not," or "I'm not making this up."

The U.S. Centers for Disease Control and Prevention report that eating tainted food—of which 95 percent comes from animal-based foods—results in 76 million cases of gastrointestinal illness, 325,000 hospitalizations, and 5,000 deaths every year.[1] We're not suggesting we can attribute all these incidences to poor inspection practices. We're only suggesting we can't believe these numbers are so low.

How much do you think you know about meat safety and inspection? Take the following true/false quiz that includes 20 problems to find out. It's a *true* test of your knowledge, a tried and *true* test. Good luck.

TRUE OR FALSE?

1. Despite the fact that less than 1 percent of chickens are sampled for pathogens, *every* thigh, wing, and breast is stamped with the USDA seal of approval.[2]

2. In 55 studies it was found that, on average, 30 percent of chicken is contaminated with salmonella and 62 percent with campylobacter—two pathogens responsible for 80 percent of illnesses and 75 percent of deaths associated with meat consumption. Note: When in 1993 the head of the USDA was asked about warning labels to alert the public

that poultry products might contain pathogens, he responded, "We wouldn't do anything that might hurt sales."[3]

3. As of 1996, there were 1,370 inspector positions that remained unfilled.[4]

4. There are no requirements or regulations for factory farms to be tested for E. coli, campylobacter, salmonella or any other diseases that can make people sick or kill them. The U.S. meat industry has opposed legislation and it still prevails.[5]

5. The meat, dairy, and egg producers suggest that the problems resulting from the pathogens is not their fault. It is the fault of the consumers for not cooking and handling the foods properly.[6]

6. An E. coli breakout in 1993 that poisoned many children, killing some, prompted the USDA to begin testing for E. coli. The American Meat Institute sued the USDA on the basis that the testing would make consumers assume meat was safe, causing them to be less vigilant in proper cooking and handling practices.[7]

7. The meat industry fought long and hard to keep cooking and handling instructions off meat because they believed the warnings would alarm consumers.[8]

8. The Secretary of Agriculture does *not* have the authority to make a recall on meat.[9]

9. Food and Drug regulation officials inspect seafood companies only once a year, essentially to inspect paperwork and review voluntary procedures.[10]

10. The inspection system is only slightly better now than when it was instituted in 1910.[11]

11. A new system of inspection, HACCP (Hazard Analysis of Critical Control Points), implemented in 1996 required workers to be responsible for food inspection and for the inspectors to monitor the workers. The system prohibited the inspectors from removing vomit, feces, and metal shards from meat.[12]

12. In 2000, the USDA imposed new inspection rules that reclassified the following problems in meat as safe for human consumption: cancers, pneumonia, tumors, lymphomas, infectious arthritis, open sores, and diseases caused by intestinal worms.[13]

13. The large recalls of meat we hear about might make us think someone is on top of meat safety. However, most meat recalled is never recovered. One recall included 170,000 pounds of meat, but only 3,000 pounds were recovered. Another three recalls added up to 3.1 million pounds recalled of which only 1.3 million pounds were recovered. We can assume the rest of the meat was eaten.[14]

14. In the cases of recalled meat it is not unusual for the beef companies to avoid fines and make their usual profits for all tainted beef that was eaten before it could be recalled.[15]

15. A newspaper investigation found some meatpacking plants were allowed to continue operating even after being cited more than 1,000 times for safety violations.[16]

16. Carcasses on the inspection line can move past inspectors at 140 to 160 per minute.[17]

17. According to the Government Accountability Project (GAP), a chicken slaughterhouse may contain the following filth on walls, floors, equipment, transport tubs, conveyor belt, and in coolers: oil, grease, animal excrement, glass, plastic, wood chips, rust, paint, cement, dust, rodent feces, maggots, and larvae.[18]

18. Slaughterhouses that are supposed to be inspected once per shift can often go 2 weeks without inspection.[19]

19. The president of the National Joint Council of Meat Inspection Local (2000) ate very little to no meat, just sardines and other fish. He was trying to get his wife to stop eating meat.[20]

20. For 20 years the USDA used violet dye #1 to stamp on meat that it was safe for human consumption. In 1973, the USDA had to stop using it. It was determined the dye caused cancer.[21]

How did you do? The answers? Let's put it this way:

If you answered 20 as true, you got the clue.
If you answered any as not, we're sorry a lot.

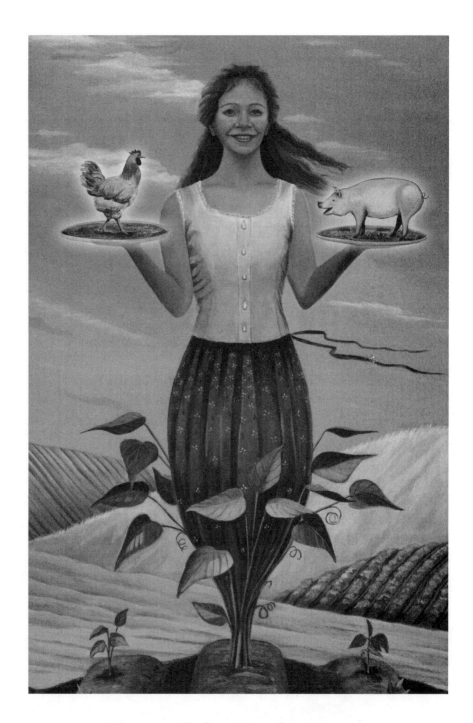

Beyond the Euphemisms

～ 5 ～
Animals
JUST WHO ARE WE EATING?

It's understandable we don't want to look beyond the euphemisms, slick advertising, and supermarket meat cases for fear of seeing sensitive and intelligent animals—or maybe worse, seeing cruel and heartless humans—but we must.

Ahead in this chapter…

Live through the eyes of a cow named Lucky, and see if meat, milk, and leather are still the only things that come to mind when we think of THE COW.

We associate THE PIG with so many negative attributes, that most people are highly offended to be called one. Find out why people should instead be highly flattered.

THE CHICKEN undoubtedly crossed the road to flee the factory farm. We should cross the road, too. Because on the other side we will find the truth about this species—a truth that is far different than our perception.

Dumb, a four-letter word we often apply to animals, might best be suited for us if we don't tune into nature and recognize that ANIMAL INTELLIGENCE is anything but an oxymoron.

We think of being VEGAN as the last and most perfected attainment of vegetarianism, but maybe this is where we should start given its very simple precept: respect for all life.

FACTORY FARMS do produce inexpensive meat, but they also generate expensive costs not considered in the equation. And if "what goes around comes around" holds true then we might someday have to pay the greatest price of all.

If we require truth in advertising shouldn't the menu read this? "VEAL AND FOIE GRAS—Previously Living Organs and Tissue from Sentient Creatures That Have Been Monstrously Altered by Torturous Means."

There are two sides to every story and even HUNTING is no exception.

32: The Cow

YOU CAN CALL ME LUCKY FOR NOW

"Oh, hello. My name is Elsie, but my friends call me Lucky, because so far I have been able to avoid the hamburger patch. That's the place we all go when our milk production slows. It's not really a patch, we just call it that because many of your children have been led to believe that's where hamburgers come from. We know better.

"I understand we have a life expectancy of nearly 25 years, but no one around here has seen anything close to that.[1] After continually being pregnant, and producing milk at 10 times the rate Nature intended, we wear out at 3 or 4 years of age.[2] I guess it might not be so bad if they didn't take my babies away from me right after birth. You would think with all the extra milk I'm producing they would allow me to give just a little to my baby, but I guess it cuts into profits.

"It was really upsetting when I had a boy. When he was 4 months old, they took him away to make something called veal. Since he can't produce milk they punished him by chaining him at the neck, and depriving him of solid food. I only hope he gets to make this *veal* out in a sunny green meadow with plenty of space and room to romp, but somehow I doubt it.

"My quarters aren't so luxurious either. I've spent most of my life on a concrete slab, chained in a stall so small that I can barely move. I've been fed hormones and high-energy feed to bolster my milk production.[3] Maybe I shouldn't complain because my friend, Buck the steer, lives in a 12-foot by 15-foot pen along with a dozen of his friends.[4] He has been castrated to increase his fat content, dehorned to minimize damage to other cattle in the overcrowded feedlots, and fed sawdust, shredded newspaper, and processed sewage to fatten him up the cheapest way possible.[5]

"Maybe some day we can live the long life we were meant to live, to be the social creatures that Nature intended, to nurture our young, to enjoy the sunshine, to lie down with the herd in a green meadow and nibble the grass after a spring rain. But it doesn't appear that day will be anytime soon. As I understand it, 90,000 of us in the United States are killed every day for food and clothing. Many are dairy cows like myself who can no longer give you enough of our milk.[6]

"It seems a shame you believe it necessary to use our muscle and fat as a food source, when it has no more to offer you than food made from plants, and can make you sick in so many ways.[7] It seems unnatural that you would want our babies' milk for your children and adults—milk designed for calves' growth, not human nutrition. It saddens me that after we are gone you turn our skin into clothing when you have so many alternatives.

"I know you see us as only milk-and-meat machines, but like you, we are living creatures with the same breathing life force and will to live. We differ from you less than you might think. Our central nervous and endocrine systems are virtually the same as yours. The biochemistry of our physiological and emotional states differ little from yours.[8]

"The philosopher Descartes said, because we were animals, and could not speak, we had no feelings.[9] Well, I'm here to tell you that we feel love and affection, pleasure and pain, fear and contentment just as you do. We don't want to be an Oscar Mayer wiener, or do our best for Jerseymaid, we just want the freedom to live our lives.

"I know you see us as just dumb, clumsy animals. Maybe it's our big lazy brown eyes and slow movements that make us appear that way. Did it ever occur to you that these traits might be characteristic of patience, gentleness, and a desire to tune into the rhythms of the earth? Just because we don't speak your language doesn't mean we are unintelligent either. As I understand it, Darwin, Edison, Newton, Picasso, and Einstein were all considered dumb and stupid at one time because they were different.[10]

"I know you think our species can also be mean. You only have to attend a rodeo to see us kick and fight to believe that. But you might behave that way too if someone placed a tight strap around your genital area, and an electric prod on your bottom.[11] We are really very docile creatures who wouldn't hurt a flea. We are vegetarian you know.

"I've often wondered how things got to be this way. Surely God didn't intend dominion over us to mean that we are to be exploited for food, clothing, and entertainment while suffering immense pain and cruelty at your hands.

"Mahatma Gandhi once said the greatness of a nation, and its moral progress, will be judged by the way its animals are treated.[12] I don't know who this man is, I only wish he were beside me now because it appears my time has come.

"It's time to stop calling me Lucky. Guess I'll see you at dinner."

33: The Pig

IF YOU CALLED ME A PIG, THEN THANK YOU

Porky Pig, Babe, Miss Piggy, Arnold, and Piglet. All beloved television, movie, and cartoon pigs. They make us laugh, they make us cry, and in the case of Porky and Miss Piggy get on our nerves at times. But that's OK. In fact, we love 'em all the more because of it.

Then there are some pigs we've probably never heard of before. Mr. Snort, Binki, Tootie, and Penelope are their names. They are just a few of the many pigs across the country evoking some of the same emotions as their celebrity friends. But they do it for only small groups of people. They are household pets.

In stark contrast to what pigs do for their masters is what 90 million pigs a year do for the majority of Americans—satisfy their hunger pangs.[1] Often three times a day as smoked bacon for breakfast, ham sandwiches for lunch, and pork chops for dinner. Bacon? Ham? Pork? Sorry, it's a pig no matter how we slice it. And it's best we didn't.

Pigs have become celebrities, puppets, cartoon characters, and pets for a very good reason. They are as friendly, sociable, and loyal as dogs.[2] They are as clean as cats. They are as intelligent as chimpanzees.[3] And with profound irony they have saved human lives.[4] They are sensitive creatures that feel pain, pleasure, fear, and happiness just like humans do.

This portrayal might not be quite in line with our perception of the pig. We often view the pig as an animal that is dirty, fat, and mean. Why such a huge disparity between the perception and the portrayal? Maybe here is why.

Pigs were kept dirty because at one time people in Europe believed that dirty pigs tasted better.[5] Pigs are fat because they are overfed to bring a higher market price. Pigs are mean because of the living conditions they are forced to endure while being raised for food.

We might get a little bent out of shape too if we had to endure the life that the pig does down on the factory farm. What would we have to endure? The best way to know is through empathy.

*****

So take off your clothes, go to your coat closet, and step inside. You'll find it has been modified a bit. The floor has been remodeled to only 7 square feet with metal slats on all sides, including top and bottom. Get comfortable. This will be your home, 24 hours a day, for the rest of your life.

You will have company as there will be more closets around you; above, below, and on all sides. You will be in the dark most of the time. Your food will come from automatic feeding machines, and it will be the same food every day. It will include recycled waste, arsenic, hormones, and antibiotics.

Do you have to go to the bathroom? Go ahead. You just go where you stand, as will your roommates directly above you. That's the reason for the metal slats, to funnel off the waste. The stench of ammonia-saturated air will permeate your lungs. After a time your body will start to cripple and you will begin to go insane. What a surprise. This will cause you to start biting at your neighbor's bottom (tails in the case of pigs), as other people will do the same to you. This damages the goods. To curb this behavior your bottom (tails in the case of pigs), will be cut off and your teeth chipped off. Sorry, no anesthetic will be provided.

It probably goes without saying, but you will be in pain most of the time. You will have an 80 percent chance of contracting pneumonia, and a 20 percent chance of dying before The Big Day.

If you survive those conditions, once you have gained enough weight, you get to leave your coat closet of misery and be given a nice shower. Could things be looking up? Unfortunately, no.

You will be escorted to a large facility where you will be hung upside down. There you will die by having your throat slit. Later you will be cut up and served as food on the plate of some higher civilized being.[6]

*****

James Cromwell, the actor who played Farmer Hoggins in *Babe*, learned about meat production at the same time he was experiencing firsthand the sense of fun, intelligence, and personalities of the pig and other animals on the set. It's not surprising that he changed his food habits and became a vegan.[7]

Before we sit down to breakfast tomorrow and dig into a slab of bacon, let's do two things: Watch the movie *Babe*, and spend some time in the coat closet. When we're done, we'll go to the store and buy a box of cereal.

34: The Chicken

LET'S CROSS THE ROAD, TOO

Why did the chicken cross the road? Undoubtedly to flee the horror of the factory farm.

The chicken living in the pastoral setting with a red barn and a weather vane, scratching serenely in the dirt, happily making eggs for our consumption or passing the time until it can provide us a nutritious meal, might only be found in a child's picture book.[1]

No doubt this is our perception of how a chicken lives. But it couldn't be further from the truth.

There are a number of misperceptions we have when it comes to the chicken. Perception often substitutes for truth because we lack information, or we prefer not to know the truth. But as it pertains to the chicken, the information is readily available. And since it is always in our best interest to know the truth, let's cross the road ourselves and see if we can find it—the truth that is—on the other side.

THE ATTRIBUTE: Courage.
THE PERCEPTION: Chickens are *chicken*.
THE TRUTH: Chickens are anything but.

- A mother hen will fight to the death to protect her chicks from harm; the rooster is proud and assertive.[2]

- Chickens startle easily but this is because of their highly successful evolutionary survival strategy.[3]

- In China, the rooster is regarded as a symbol of good fortune and is also the protector of the family.[4] In France, the rooster is the national bird.[5]

THE ATTRIBUTE: Intelligence.
THE PERCEPTION: All they do is bob, peck, and scratch the dirt.
THE TRUTH: They can do things humans can't.

- Because of their excellent vision and alertness, chickens were used by some armies during World Wars I and II to detect and announce approaching airplanes.[6]

- Chickens, 100,000 strong, were used by China to fend off a locust infestation. They were trained to hunt and eat locusts at the sound of a whistle.[7]

- Many people believe chickens can predict when it's going to rain.[8]

THE ATTRIBUTE: Maternalism.
THE PERCEPTION: Sitting on eggs is but a simple instinct.
THE TRUTH: As devoted to motherhood as any species.

- Mother hens perform an elaborate sequence of behaviors while searching for a nest site, building the nest, and laying eggs.[9]

- Mother hens communicate with their chicks through soft chirping and clucking while they are still in the egg.[10]

- Mother hens will scratch and peck more at the ground when they see that their chicks are eating food they believe to be of poor quality.[11]

- Mother hens have been known to hatch the eggs of other species and proceed to meet that species' needs with the proper food and training.[12]

- The expression, "taken under someone's wing" comes from a hen's nurturing and caring qualities.[13]

THE ATTRIBUTE: Social Behavior.
THE PERCEPTION: Chickens don't even acknowledge each other.
THE TRUTH: Might be more sophisticated than some humans.

- Chickens are highly social animals. Adult chickens can recognize and remember about 100 other chickens, based primarily on features of the head and neck.[14]

- Chickens keep themselves very clean by taking baths in the dust.[15]

- Chickens love to watch television and listen to music. Their music of choice? Vivaldi's *The Four Seasons*.[16]

- When a hen and rooster are courting, they dance around each other in a ritual called "waltzing."[17]

THE ATTRIBUTE: Living Conditions.
THE PERCEPTION: Red barn in pastoral setting.
THE TRUTH: Indoors and inside cages.

- One factory farm can house 80,000 chickens.[18] Broilers (the ones we eat) will live their lives crammed four to five in a 16-by-18-inch cage.[19] Imagine living our total life in an elevator with 20 other people.

- Often layers (the ones that produce the eggs) are driven insane from living in close quarters, evoking the cannibalistic pecking of other birds. To reduce the damage, chickens' beaks are partially removed.[20] Imagine having our fingernails torn off.

- Beak removal hurts their ability to eat and drink and can result in starvation. If they don't starve this way, often their toes grow around the wire cages, keeping them from food and water; their toes must be cut to free them.[21]

- Artificial lighting, forced molting, and laboratory food are introduced to quicken egg production and weight gain.[22]

This often leads to birds getting too large for their skeletons and becoming crippled.[23]

- Chickens have a life expectancy of 13 to 14 years. A broiler lives for 2 months. A layer for 2 years.[24]

- The deaths of the 14,000 chickens slaughtered for food every minute in the United States—7 billion a year—parallel their grim existence as they are shackled upside down, and their lives ended with the slice of an automatic blade.[25]

What we learned about chickens when we crossed the road to find the truth was quite different from our perceptions. Chickens are smart, nurturing, proud, brave, and sociable.

Wouldn't we be lucky to know *people* with those qualities.

35: Animal Intelligence

WHO MIGHT BE THE DUMB ANIMAL?

Animals are just a bunch of reflexes and instincts. Sure they feel pain, but it doesn't mean the same to them as it does to humans because, after all, animals don't have souls. Animals don't have the compassion, love, and reverence for life that humans have. They are dumb creatures placed on this earth for human food, multiple products, and entertainment. Since we are superior to animals it's not wrong to exploit them.

We may never articulate that, or even give it much thought, but if we didn't believe it somewhere down deep, we probably wouldn't be able to do the things we do to animals, not the least of which is to turn their lives into our food.

Is this a fair appraisal of the animal kingdom, including the animals we eat? Do animals not have a reverence for life, capability to love, and compassion toward others? Are they dumb, and are we superior?

Our daily "To Do" list usually doesn't include: tune into nature. Therefore, provided here are some stories exemplifying animal behaviors that we might have observed if we *had* included this item on our list. Maybe in the future we will.

REVERING LIFE: Would the act of saving a human life qualify animals as revering life?

- Carletta, a cow, rescued an elderly Italian farmer, Bruno Cipriani, from being gored to death by a wild boar. She mooed loudly and attacked the animal, saving the farmer's life.[1]

- LuLu, a pig, saved the life of Jo Ann Altsman's in Presque Isle, Pennsylvania. When Jo Ann was suffering a heart attack, LuLu managed her way through the doggy door and went into the street, where she laid down and played dead until a passing motorist stopped. She gained the attention of the motorist, then LuLu got up and led the motorist to the house, to find Jo Ann on the floor in pain.[2]

LOVING ANOTHER ANIMAL: Do animals show love for each other on a par with humans?

- A man in England sold a cow and her calf to two separate farms. During the night the mother cow broke away from her new home, going through a hedge to a road. The next morning, the cow was found 7 miles away at the farm where her calf had been taken—a place she had never been—happily suckling her hungry calf.[3]

- Gordon Haber, who had studied wolves for decades, documented a case where a wolf had been seriously wounded by a caribou and went into a vacant cabin to die alone as animals sometimes do. But every night another wolf came to the cabin to feed his friend with pieces of meat until the wolf recovered.[4]

COMPASSION FOR HUMANS: Even if animals had the capacity to be caring toward humans, would they exhibit this trait given how we often treat them?

- When Reverend O. F. Robertson of Tennessee started to lose his eyesight, his cow Mary, began nudging him around with her nose to make sure he didn't bump into things. As his eyesight worsened, Mary's diligence increased until she would accompany the reverend wherever he went. After he became almost completely blind, the reverend depended on Mary as his only help. Until his death, the two were inseparable.[5]

- Crisco is a chicken that helps sick and elderly patients recover more quickly at a St. Louis, Missouri, healthcare center. He is the favorite among all the animals, which include rabbits and dogs.[6]

- In 1975, a shipwreck victim was aided by a giant sea turtle. The sea turtle went without food and stayed on the surface of the water for 2 days carrying the woman until she could be rescued.[7]

EXHIBITING INTELLIGENCE: Can animals be intelligent if they don't speak our language?

- In Bensalem, Pennsylvania, a police officer driving down the road tried to veer away from a duck that kept walking around in circles to block the vehicle. When the curious officer got out of his car, the duck led him to a drain where her baby ducks were trapped.[8]

- Emily, a cow, aware of the fate awaiting her made a successful escape from the slaughterhouse. She foraged in the woods with a herd of deer. Her actions impressed the slaughterhouse owner and she was released to The Peace Abbey in Sherborn, Massachusetts, where her gentle disposition was put to use working with special-needs children.[9]

- When ostriches sit on their eggs their long necks make them vulnerable targets to their enemies. In order to protect themselves, they lay their long necks across the sand. From a distance they appear as a small hill of sand.[10] (And here we assumed the dull-witted ostriches were sticking their heads in the sand.)

EXCEEDING HUMAN CAPABILITY: Are we superior to animals, or is it the other way around? Maybe superior is the wrong word to use. Maybe each species has a strength, enabling everyone to make a unique contribution to the planet.

- Ants can lift 50 times their own body weight. Many animals have 40 times the smelling sense, and 10 times the hearing sense that humans have.[11]

- A cat traveled from New York to California to find its owner and was successful.[12]

- A couple moved from Des Moines, Iowa, to Denver, Colorado; their German shepherd preferred Des Moines and found its way back across 750 snow-covered miles.[13]

- Many animals including beavers, wolves, penguins, and geese mate for life, with an unequalled commitment. (Beats the 50 percent human divorce rate by a bit.)[14]

- Spiders and birds engineer complex nests and webs. Ants work around the clock with a teamwork precision we would have a tough time emulating.

Our reaction to these 15 to 20 examples, if we want to hold on to our "dumb animal" perception, is that they are isolated or exaggerated incidences. If we don't, then let's imagine that because we pay such little attention to nature, we miss seeing demonstrations like these, which turn out to be common and consistent.

The only connection many of us have with the animal world is to our companion pets, most often dogs and cats. Think about the personalities, sensitivities, and intelligence they have, the loyalty and the enrichment they bring us. Why couldn't any animal have this potential—including the ones we designate as food?

Humans have the capacity for logical, rational, and analytic thought, good judgment and sound sense. Let's use these gifts we have been given to reconsider our perception of animals so we won't qualify as dumb animals.

36: Vegan

VEGAN BECAME BEGAN

> He began to type vegan,
> but vegan became began.
> The spell checker didn't know the word,
> that's the current state of Man.

Some computer word processor spell checkers don't recognize the word *vegan* and so automatically change the word to *began*. This single word exclusion from the database tells us volumes about ourselves.

Vegetarians don't eat meat, and pure vegetarians don't consume meat, dairy, and eggs. Vegans take this one step further, and because of their reverence for all life, don't use animals for any purpose.

Given humankind's insensitivity to, and exploitation of animals, we can excuse the spell checker's negligence, but not ours. We also must fault the spell checker for not being consistent when it includes the word humane. After all, the word is derived from human, and until we gain a reverence for all life how can we, as humans, be considered humane?

The following two sections attempt to capture what humans do to animals, and what animals go through when humans do them.

THE HUMAN EXPERIENCE:

- Eat their tissues and dine on their organs (food)
- Feast on their eggs and drink their milk (food)
- Wear their skins (clothing and shoes)
- Take their food (honey)
- Rub them on our faces (cosmetics)
- Confine them in cages (zoos)
- Make them run (horse and dog racing)
- Make them perform (circuses)

- Ride on their backs and tie them up (rodeos)
- Hold them captive (marine parks)
- Snatch them from the water (fishing)
- Shoot at them (hunting)
- Burn their eyes (product testing)
- Slice their flesh (dissection)
- Mutilate them (lab experiments)
- Splice their genes (genetic manipulation)
- Torture them (factory farms)
- Kill them (slaughterhouses)

THE ANIMAL EXPERIENCE:

- Pain
- Terror
- Suffering
- Isolation
- Panic
- Fear
- Depression
- Rage
- Anguish
- Exhaustion
- Fright
- Agitation
- Claustrophobia
- Frenzy
- And finally, and thankfully, nothing

It might be hard to imagine what our lives would be like without all the seemingly necessary commodities provided by animals. We have come to take their use for granted as if it was ordained. But were animals placed on this earth for our unbridled use, pleasure, and nourishment, or were they placed here as part of the complex web of nature, here as we are for their own purpose?

Let's explore this question by way of logic, and see if we can make headway into the mystery by playing the, If/Then game.

- *If* Nature had wanted us to exploit animals, *then* why were they equipped with senses that cause pain and suffering?

- *If* animals were to be nourishment for humans, *then* how does one account for the woeful byproducts: chronic disease, environmental destruction, mass starvation, and economic consequences that result from their consumption?

- *If* the zoo takes animals away from their natural habitats and families, deprives them of personal space and comfort, prevents them from playing and exploring, and suppresses most of their basic physical, social, and behavioral needs, *then* what can we really learn about them in this environment?

- *If* the animals always lose or at best break even, *then* how can fishing and hunting be considered sports?

- *If* there are multiple alternatives to dissection such as video, films, models, computer simulations, slides, and transparencies, *then* why not utilize these life-affirming aids, rather than promoting scientific discovery through suffering?[1]

- *If* the law does not mandate that products first be tested on animals before they can be used by humans, and there are reliable alternatives to determining toxicity, *then* why is it necessary to put animals through the suffering that ensues?[2]

- *If* entertainment means having animals poked, prodded, whipped, humiliated, abused, and trained to perform unnatural acts, *then* what does it say about our character and moral fiber?

- *If* we have more effective and beneficial alternatives to the use of animals for food, clothing, sport, entertainment, and testing, *then* why don't we utilize those options?

- *If* we eventually could see the wrong and abolish the once-acceptable behaviors of slavery, child labor, segregation, and women's oppression, *then* why can't we make the same progress when it comes to animals?

- *If* we are the strongest and the smartest species, *then* does that give us the right to take advantage of all other species?

- *If* we once assumed that our earth was at the center of the solar system and were wrong, *then* is it possible we could also be in error about our superiority on this planet?

- *If* we are going to survive as a species, *then* don't we need to evolve?

37: Factory Farms

HUMANS WILL BE IN STORES NEXT WEEK

It sounds like a plot from a bad science fiction movie...

> A few selected species of sensitive and innocent crea-
> tures that love to romp, forage, and play are confined
> mostly indoors, with no sunshine or fresh air, by a
> superior group of beings.
>
> They are shackled so they can't move; their every
> instinct, urge, and need squashed. They are filled with
> pesticides, hormones, antibiotics, and laboratory food.[1]
> They are mutilated by beak searing, tail docking, ear
> cutting, and castration.[2] They are driven insane.
>
> They are hoisted up, their throats are slit, they are
> cut into pieces, and then distributed to grocery stores.
> Other parts are made into goods and distributed to
> malls.
>
> The superior beings take the animal parts home.
> They eat the tissues and unfertilized eggs, drink the lac-
> tating secretion, and wear the skin.

Of course this could only happen in a movie. No one would ever
believe this could happen in real life.

The days of green pastures, red barns, grazing cattle, chickens scratching in the dirt, and pigs wallowing in the mud are mostly gone.[3] Today animals—or more accurately production units—are
raised in the smallest possible space, at the lowest possible cost, to
maximize productivity and profits for the producers.[4]

Welcome to, appropriately coined, the Factory Farm. The
factory farm is a place that is like...it's like...how can it best be
described. Well, let's try this:

- Have you ever been stuck in an elevator or felt claustro-
  phobic?

- Have you ever been handcuffed or incarcerated?
- Have you ever felt isolated or unloved?
- Have you ever been physically abused?
- Have you ever been mentally ill?
- Have you ever been obese, crippled, or chronically ill?
- Have you ever been the victim of racism or sexism?
- Have you ever had your child taken from you?
- Have you ever lost a loved one prematurely?
- Have you ever had a body part severed or watched someone die?
- Have you ever heard first-hand what it was like to be confined in a concentration camp or affected by slavery?

If we had all these experiences, day in and day out, then we would have near perfect empathy for the factory farm animal.

No human, with any compassion, wouldn't feel some sympathy for these creatures. However, most people who subscribe to the Self-Induced Carnivorous Killer (SICK) diet realize the reality: If they want to purchase their meat, dairy, and eggs at the lowest cost possible, then the factory farm approach is the price that must be paid.

But is the cost really that low, and is the price that has to be paid, the only price? Let's explore the Greater Price / Added Cost economics.

GREATER PRICE: The crowded feedlots and high-speed processing of the factory farm has led to increased contamination of food with such pathogens as E. coli, salmonella, campylobacter, and Mad Cow Disease.[5] The meat from a single E. coli-infected cow can contaminate 16 tons of ground beef.[6] There were 26 active meat recalls, affecting 1.2 million pounds of beef, due to bacterial contamination in 1999.[7] Every year, 76 million people get sick, and 5,000 people die from food poisoning.[8]

ADDED COST: Medical expenses and potential funeral expenses.

GREATER PRICE: Factory farms produce 5 tons of animal waste for every person in the United States.[9] Animal wastes are transformed from what could serve as valuable soil nutrients into hazardous waste that pollute waterways and contaminate drinking water.[10] Pfiesteria in the North Carolina coastal plain and Chesapeake Bay, and the Dead Zone in the Gulf of Mexico are but two examples.[11] Only 2 percent of poultry operators who are required to purchase discharge permits under the Clean Water Act have done so. This might help explain why agriculture is the leading source of water pollution in the United States.[12]

ADDED COST: Diminished water quality for recreation and consumption. Increased water bills. Increased taxes for cleanup.

GREATER PRICE: Pesticides are required in hopes of repelling the flies and other insects that naturally flock to the crowded and filthy conditions found in factory farms. Antibiotics are used to combat disease that is multiplied many times by the animals' close living quarters.[13]

ADDED COST: Increased cancer risk. Greater resistance to disease. Medical expenses.

GREATER PRICE: Factory farm animals have as much as 30 times more fat than pasture-raised animals due to lack of exercise, and the producers' goal of fattening the animals quickly and inexpensively.[14]

ADDED COST: Degenerative diseases. Medical expenses.

GREATER PRICE: Factory farm animals, which are conscious, living, breathing, and feeling creatures suffer at the hands of humans.

ADDED COST: Abandonment of our compassion, moral compass, and humanity.

Factory farming is the logical progression—really perversion—of an animal-based diet. Often the clue to how wise or smart it is to pursue an action or process can be found in its byproducts. The aforementioned consequences of this distorted approach to food production should give us a clear indication about the intelligence—or lack of intelligence—demonstrated by the Factory Farm approach.

There is a logic to the universe. A balance and order. It can be observed at all levels. From the movement of the stars and planets, to the movement of protons and neutrons, and everything in between. For every action there is an equal and opposite reaction. Garbage in, garbage out. Debits equal credits. Karma. What goes around comes around. Etcetera, etcetera.

Given the nature of the universe then, it might not be surprising to see the following headline someday from the *Cosmic Galaxy Register* (formally, *The New York Times*):

FOOD SOURCE DISCOVERED

Today, a new planet was discovered in the Milky Way. The current inhabitants, humans, call it Earth.

Food Procurement from G Sector has determined that the humans, who at first count number 6,214,779,243, can provide our population proper nutrition. Currently the food source is being collected, categorized, and processed at facilities being erected every 3 minutes.

The first available humans will be in our stores early next week.

38: Veal and Foie Gras

We're in the hospital about to give birth to our first child. We don't care whether we have a boy or a girl. After a few hours of hard labor we have a healthy boy. We have never had such an over-whelming feeling of love. We can't take our eyes off our precious child as we suckle and stroke him, oblivious to the world around us.

The next day a nurse comes to our bedside and takes our new baby away without explanation. She takes him down the hall and shackles him in a crib. There he will spend the next 4 months unable to move, kept in total darkness except for feeding time, and then fed only iron-deficient formula. Our breast milk is expressed every day, and we often wonder whether any of it finds its way to the child we have not seen in such a long time.

Maybe it's better we are focused on the milk, instead of our child, because at 4 months of age he was slaughtered and prepared as the main course for a casual business dinner of another species.[1]

OK, so this will never happen to us and our babies, but it does happen to more than 1 million male calves and their dairy cow mothers every year.[2] And although they are a different species, they are still mothers and babies that share the same love and insepara-ble bond as humans.

Their offspring, the male calves, are useless to the dairy industry, but useful to the veal industry because many Americans consider their pale, tender flesh a delicacy that the restaurateur can charge a hefty price for. Consumers pay the steep price with their wallets; calves pay it with their lives.

Prior to World War II, the expendable male calf was slaugh-tered at his birth weight of 150 pounds, before he exercised his muscles and ate anything but mother's milk, in order that his flesh remained pale. After the war, a method was devised to get his weight to 350 pounds while still maintaining the pristine muscle tissue.[3]

To meet this goal, the calf is taken from its mother within 24 hours. It is chained in a 22-inch stall so it cannot move or lie down. It is fed no solid food, only skim milk, and so becomes anemic. It is kept in the dark except for feeding time. It lives—or more accurately exists—in this state for 4 months until it reaches the desired weight, at which time it is slaughtered.[4] Some of the products of this cruelty are Veal Oscar, Veal Scaloppini, and Veal Piccata, fancy names for nothing more than the anemic, underdeveloped, atrophied muscle tissue from a four-month-old cow. Some delicacy.

It's hard to imagine a worse atrocity that an animal could endure in the name of human eating pleasure than veal, but there might be.

*****

There probably isn't a man, woman, or child who can't help but watch as a mother duck leads her ducklings into a pond. The way she guides them into the water with military precision by her purposeful quacks. The efficient manner in which they move their webbed feet, barely disturbing the water. The way she teaches them to dip into the water for a bite to eat, their colorful feathers repelling the water as they bob up and down.

There also probably isn't a man, woman, or child who can't help but *not* watch as a duck is raised for the delicacy, foie gras. We can bet a food that doesn't sound remotely like a food should raise our suspicions about its origins.

Foie gras is really liver pâté. Which is really liver. Which is really *the* liver, an internal organ that secretes bile and removes toxins. Which is really the duck's liver that is enlarged up to 10 times its normal weight—while the duck is still using it.[5] And how is this accomplished?

The male duck is caged so it cannot move, and then force-fed 6 to 7 pounds of grain three times a day with an air-driven feeder tube down its throat. This process lasts for 28 days until the liver has swollen to the desired size, or the stomach bursts (10 percent of the time), whichever comes first.

The 25 million ducks and geese raised for this delicacy each year are then slaughtered. Given that the feeding process causes tears in the esophagus, severe breathing difficulties, internal bleeding, and multiple bone fractures, most likely they are thankful to be killed.[6]

The result of this barbaric process is a diseased liver that many consider a delicacy. It is rich in poisons and cholesterol, and contains 85 percent fat in calories.[7] Although the process is outlawed in the United States, the treat can be found at many of our finer restaurants for about $50 for a serving of four. Also at upper-class social functions.

We might wonder if the demand would go down if instead of finding these items on a restaurant menu: Veal Oscar, Veal Scaloppini, Veal Piccata, Foie Gras, and Liver Pâté, we found this on the menu: Previously Living Organs and Tissue from Sentient Creatures that have been Monstrously Altered by Torturous Means.

Maybe restaurants shouldn't have a choice. After all, there is such a thing as truth in advertising.

39: Hunting

THERE ARE TWO SIDES TO EVERY STORY

Hunters are some of the most ingenious and resourceful individuals ever to inhabit our planet. The cerebral capacity required to rationalize the cruelty perpetrated on innocent animals as sport, has to be immense. Of all the behaviors that make it hard to look at ourselves in the mirror, hunting would have to be near the top.

Most likely hunters have no problem standing tall and proud while looking at their reflections. In their view, hunting develops the noble qualities of self-reliance, ruggedness, discipline, and courage.

As they say, there are two sides to every story. And although hunting appears to be an endeavor bringing into question the civility of the human race, to be fair we should try and see the hunters' side.

With that in mind, let's compare the perspective of the untrained eye of the individual who does not hunt, with the point of view of the hunter.

UNTRAINED EYE OF NON-HUNTER: Men and women dress up in camouflage clothing, hide in trees and behind bushes, deceptively lure animals with mating sounds, mating smells, and bait, and then ambush the animals by shooting them in the back with high-powered riffles as they run, or fly, for their lives.

HUNTER: Men and women carry out an innate, time-honored tradition of challenging and conquering the elements of nature and the savvy of animals for food and clothing while developing courage, also resulting in the thinning of herds to minimize starvation, and protecting the public from traffic mishaps and property damage.[1]

UNTRAINED EYE OF NON-HUNTER: Human sacrifice, slavery, and child labor were also once time-honored traditions.

Humankind stopped hunting for food 10,000 years ago when agriculture became exceedingly more efficient.[2]

Since only 6 percent of the population hunts it doesn't appear to be in our nature.[3]

Nature naturally controls animal populations by weeding out the sick and weak; hunters often kill the largest and strongest.[4]

Herds are artificially increased by forest clearing and gender manipulation designed to increase targets for hunters.[5]

Innovative reflectors and inexpensive repellents can humanely control deer that damage our property—the property that once belonged to the deer on which we have encroached.[6]

However it must take a certain amount of courage to hunt because every year roughly 150 people are killed and nearly 2,000 are injured in hunting accidents.[7] The animals, though, are rarely a threat.

HUNTER: Hunters pay good money for licenses and thus have the right to get a return on their investment.

UNTRAINED EYE OF NON-HUNTER: On federal land alone, more than 200 million animals are killed by hunters every year. Since 94 percent of U.S. citizens don't hunt, should hunters be allowed to kill animals that belong equally to everyone and on land, the majority of which is, maintained by non-hunters?[8]

Given the agencies are called, Department of Wildlife Conservation and Department of Natural Resources, maybe most of the license money should go toward wildlife *conservation* and preservation of *natural resources*, rather than preserving the recreational sport and economic-boosting industry of hunting.[9]

HUNTER: Animals may feel pain on a physical level, but it isn't the same type of pain humans feel, because animals don't attach emotion to it.

UNTRAINED EYE OF NON-HUNTER: Just because the animals don't have the same facial expressions as we do, and can't describe the pain, agony, and stress they feel, doesn't mean they don't experience what we would feel if we were terrorized—ahhh, hunted.

Animals have a brain, nervous system, and the same five senses we do. And because their senses are more finely tuned, their level of pain may well exceed ours.[10] Rough estimates are that 30 percent, or 60 million animals in addition to the 200 million killed, are merely wounded and left to suffer, starve, and die every year.[11]

HUNTER: God has given humans dominion over animals to be used for whatever purposes we see fit.[12]

UNTRAINED EYE OF NON-HUNTER: It would be hard to imagine that *any* God intended dominion to mean for us to use our power to abuse, mistreat, and kill animals, often leaving their babies orphaned and the adults widowed. Is it possible that dominion means responsibility and shepherding to further all living beings best interests?

HUNTER: Hunting provides parents the opportunity to bond with their children, instill values, and commune with nature.

UNTRAINED EYE OF NON-HUNTER: The values that hunting would appear to instill are that concern for the suffering and death of animals is a sign of weakness, and that killing is enjoyable.[13]

Given that animal cruelty is linked to violence, it might be more constructive for parents and children to bond and commune with nature by camping, bird watching, hiking, and shooting the animals—with a camera.

As we can see there *are* two sides to every story. But when we bring the two stories together side by side, one story appears to be the kind that children tell when they are trying to avoid getting into trouble. It's called a lie.

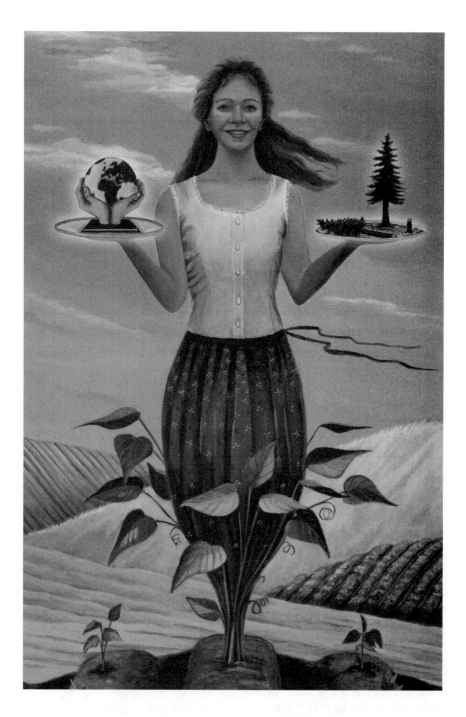

It's Dependent On What We Eat

∽ 6 ∽
The Environment
WHAT DOES IT HAVE TO DO WITH DIET?

When we think of doing our part to help the environment we think of protecting the oceans, the wilderness, and the forests, conserving energy and water, halting water pollution and soil erosion, and saving endangered species. The last thing we would think about doing is giving up our carnivorous habits—but it should be the first thing. Because our environment's health, like our health, is greatly dependent on what we choose to eat.

Ahead in this chapter...

We limit our shower time to help with WATER DEPLETION, but doing without one fast-food hamburger saves the equivalent of 40 showers.[1]

We carpool to conserve oil resources to help with ENERGY DEPLETION, but animal agriculture consumes the same amount of energy as our automobiles.[2]

We worry about urban sprawl's impact on SOIL DEPLETION and THE LAND, but because of livestock agriculture, deserts are expanding globally by 27,000 square miles annually.[3]

We are concerned about oil spills in THE OCEANS, but changing to a plant-based diet would do more to clean up our nation's water than any other single action.[4]

We recycle paper to save a tree, but a vegetarian saves 1 acre of THE FORESTS every year.[5]

We worry about sewage spills polluting our waters, but ANIMAL WASTE contributes 10 times the water pollution as the human population.[6]

We focus on a select group of endangered species, but don't realize that animal agriculture is accelerating SPECIES EXTINCTION to the point that we may soon have to add ourselves to the select group.

40: Water Depletion

A HAMBURGER OR FORTY SHOWERS

It was once a seemingly abundant resource. It is now seen as a real threat to the stability of the world. Numerous countries are in dispute over its supply. The seeds of future wars are beginning to germinate.[1] Stress in the Middle East revolves around this nonrenewable resource. It is an ominous obstacle to peace as Israel's economy relies heavily on its use.[2] Civilizations have collapsed due to its scarcity. And as we begin to see our country's reserves depleted, we must change our course, or face potentially grave consequences for our nation's security and our own survival.[3]

It might be hard to believe the preceding paragraph does not refer to oil. But it doesn't, it refers to water. Water is the resource that should scare us most. After all, with oil there are energy alternatives; with water there are no substitutes.

Maybe we have never looked at water in this way. Maybe now we will be more vigilant in conserving it. What steps could we take?

- Pledge to finish our shower before the hot water runs out.

- Promise to wash our car only when it's covered with enough dirt to write, "Please wash me."

- Badger our absent-minded neighbor to turn off his automatic sprinklers when it's raining.

- Go without water when brushing our teeth.

If we all pitched in and applied this attitude toward water conservation is it possible we could eliminate our water shortage problem? While our enthusiasm is admirable, the impact is negligible, because our personal water consumption is just 5 to 8 percent of our total water usage.[4] Our water is going elsewhere, but where?

- Instead of taking shorter showers, we could forego one fast-food hamburger, since it takes the equivalent of 40 showers worth of water to produce the meat in one burger.[5]

- Instead of waiting to wash the car until we could write in the grime, we could forego meat and dairy products for one day, and conserve 3,700 gallons of water.[6]

- Instead of brushing our teeth without water, we could forego steak dinners for the family once a month for 1 year, since it takes the equivalent amount of water to service all the needs of a family of four for 1 year.[7]

- Instead of jumping on our absent-minded neighbor for his flagrant waste of sprinkler watering—oh go ahead, he deserves it.

As it turns out, 70 percent of our total water consumption goes to support agriculture, and 80 percent of that water goes to support animal agriculture. This includes irrigation water for grassland and feed growing, water for drinking, and water for sanitation.[8] This means that more than 50 percent of our total water usage goes toward meat, dairy, and egg production to support our Self-Induced Carnivorous Killer (SICK) diet habit. In essence, one-half of it goes to satisfy our craving for baloney and cheese sandwiches.[9]

"So what." some might mutter. "There seems to be plenty of water on this planet. And besides isn't water a recyclable resource?"

Of all the water on this planet, we have access to only one ten-thousandth, of 1 percent.[10] The rest is inaccessible in oceans, ice caps, or deep underground.[11] The evaporated water from irrigation does come back to earth as rain, but most of it falls in the ocean or somewhere else where it is no longer accessible. Thus, it is only partially recyclable.[12]

Maybe the following examples will bring the point home.

- Most of the water used for irrigation in the United States is in the underground Ogallala Aquifer, the largest body of fresh water on the earth. At the current pumping rate of 13 trillion gallons a year, estimates are it will be gone by the year 2030 simply because groundwater drawdown is 25 percent higher than its replenishment rate.[13]

- Texas has used up 25 percent of its underground water since 1975. Consequently, it has lost 14 percent of its irrigated land in that time.[14]

The next logical question might be: Could the continuing depletion of water be reversed if Americans made the switch from a meat-based diet to a Wholly Eating Leaves to Live (WELL) diet?

- Where it takes 2,500 gallons of water to produce 1 pound of beef, it takes:[15]

  - 25 gallons to produce 1 pound of wheat.
  - 24 gallons to produce 1 pound of potatoes.
  - 33 gallons to produce 1 pound of carrots.

- The following amount of water is required to produce a one-day food supply for the average American:[16]

  - The SICK diet: 4,000 gallons.
  - The WELL diet: 300 gallons.

It boils down to this: If all Americans adopted a vegetarian diet, irrigated agriculture would be unnecessary and our water losses would be reversed.[17] We could go back to long showers, clean cars, and wet toothbrushes, and not feel guilty. We could even get back on good terms with our neighbor.

When we do the math we find that vegetarians save more than a million gallons of water a year. But do they really *save* it? Maybe it's more accurate to say they have used water per Nature's plan—a plan that included an ample supply of natural resources sufficient to support all life…on our planet…always.

41: Energy Depletion

Fill up *Our* Tanks with Greens and Beans

It might be difficult at first blush to see the connection between the eating of meat and the depletion of our energy resources in the name of fossil fuels. We can't imagine that the energy required to cook hamburgers on an outdoor grill would be a big hitter in the energy use department. And although there are a lot of turkeys logging long hours in our ovens at Thanksgiving, it's only once a year. Slow-cooking stews, ribs, and chicken require some long-term heat, but if our energy problems revolve around our desire for tenderized meat, then we must be running out of fuel faster than we thought.

The use of energy as it relates to meat obviously doesn't occur in its cooking. The demand for energy as it relates to meat is required for its production.

Food production in the United States uses nearly one-fifth (20 percent) of our energy in the name of fossil fuels. Animal agriculture uses 75 percent of the 20 percent. Therefore, a full 15 percent of our energy resources are used to support the SICK diet.[1]

Now, 15 percent may not sound like a large share until we bump it up against another energy user: automobiles. They, too, use 15 percent of U.S. fossil fuels.[2] Theoretically then, switching from a meat-based diet to a plant-based diet would have the same impact on energy conservation as switching from a gas combustion automobile to a 15-speed bicycle.[3] In essence, putting greens and beans instead of ham and lamb in *our* tanks has the same impact on our fossil fuel use as going without automobile transportation.

How, then, is energy used in animal agriculture, and why do we need so much?

Pigs and cattle don't get to the sizes they do, as fast as they do, from nibbling on pasture grass. They require feed and lots of it. Electricity, coal, gasoline, and other petroleum products are used to produce feed that includes the following activities:

- Nitrogen fertilizers for growing
- Pumping water for irrigation
- Tractors for clearing the land
- Planes for spraying
- Combines for harvesting

Given that 80 percent of the agricultural land is used to grow feed for the animals, and it provides just a 10 percent return, most of this food and the energy to produce it would not be required if we all transitioned to the WELL diet.[4]

Other demands for energy include:[5]

- Transporting feed and antibiotics to animals
- Temperature and lighting control in hog and chicken confinement buildings
- Movement of animal waste
- Transporting animals to the slaughterhouse
- Assembly line machines for slaughtering and packaging
- Refrigeration
- Transportation of goods to market

When we multiply the fuel requirements against 10 billion land animals slaughtered for food every year in the United States, then we can begin to understand how animal agriculture can be the energy giant in utilization that it is.[6]

Conversely, the fuels required for the production of plant-based foods is an energy midget. Let's quantify the comparison based on three measurements: CALORIES, PROTEIN, and INPUT-OUTPUT.

CALORIES: One calorie of fossil fuel will produce the following food calories:

- Corn: 1.80
- Wheat: 1.71
- Soybeans: 1.45
- Chicken: 0.07
- Feedlot beef: 0.03
- Milk: 0.14

The practical meaning of these figures is that for the same amount of fuel, corn produces 13 times the calories as milk, wheat 24 times the calories as chicken, and soybeans 48 times the calories as feedlot beef.[7]

PROTEIN: To obtain one gram of protein requires the following calories of fossil fuel:

- Corn: 3.5
- Wheat: 3.5
- Soybeans: 2.0
- Milk: 36.0
- Chicken: 22.0
- Feedlot beef: 54.0

The practical meaning of these figures is that milk requires 10 times the fuel as corn, chicken 6 times the fuel as wheat, and feedlot beef 27 times the fuel as soybeans.[8]

INPUT-OUTPUT: The energy requirements for our food production can best be summed up in the input-output equation. The production of all plant-based foods gives us MORE energy output than energy input. The production of all animal-based foods gives us LESS energy output than energy input. Any business that ran itself this way would eventually go bankrupt.

We, too, are conducting a business of sorts on this planet—the business of survival.

If this country phased out the production of animal-based foods, 30 percent of all raw materials currently consumed in this country and their accompanying energy requirements could be saved.[9] A 20 to 50 percent savings in hydroelectric and wood energy resources would result.[10] And it would mean little or no reliance on either oil imports or nuclear power.[11]

Although the figures are impressive we might be skeptical, because after all, our cars still start, our showers always deliver hot water, and our televisions never fail to come on. Why should we be worried about our energy state?

Here are but a few reasons for concern:

- Increased risk of war
- Protecting our freedoms
- Nuclear plant mishaps
- Increased taxes
- Higher energy bills
- Quality of life
- Economic recession
- Our country's security
- Our children's future

The input-output equation of food production might also apply to the productivity of our machine, the human body. Meaning that the input of plant-based foods as fuel will always exact a positive output, and conversely, the input of animal-based foods will always exact a negative output.

Let's enjoy a bean salad tonight, ride our bicycles to work tomorrow, and think of all the possibilities.

42: Soil Depletion

THE SAHARA WASN'T ALWAYS A DESERT

If it looks like a tomato, smells like a tomato, and tastes like a tomato, then it probably is a tomato. Well, maybe not.

The tomato of the past, grown in rich organic soil contained an average of 71 milligrams of calcium, 109 milligrams of magnesium, and 29.8 milligrams of iron, plus trace elements rich in zinc, copper, and selenium. The tomato grown today with predominately chemical fertilizers contains 13 milligrams of calcium, 14 milligrams of magnesium, and 0.5 milligrams of iron, plus a comparable depletion of trace elements.[1]

As far as the mineral content goes, the tomato has lost close to *90 percent* of its nutritional value. Maybe it would be more accurate to call today's version of this fruit a "shamato."

Most people don't give much thought to soil. Some see it as the covering for our big ball of dirt—the earth. Others see it as a material to hold plants up so they don't fall over. But what it should be seen as is a brew specially formulated by Nature. A blend of rock and mineral particles, organic decaying plant and animal debris, and water and gases.[2] A well thought out concoction of topsoil intended to support the lives of animal and man. A recipe that yields 1 inch every 300 years.[3]

There were 21 inches of topsoil 200 years ago. Today, on average, there are 6 inches.[4] Did Nature miscalculate our needs or miscalculate our deeds?

The deed is raising animals for human food. The earth contains 1 billion cattle, with a combined weight that doubles the human population of this planet. When we add the rest of the livestock (pigs, chickens, etc.) raised for food to the cattle they take up 50 percent of the earth's mass as pastureland.[5]

The equation breaks down—or better said—the soil breaks down as follows: Cattle trampling the land + Cattle eating the vegetation + Clearing forests for grazing + Growing corn and soybeans for animal feed + Rain and wind = Soil erosion that is occurring at 7 to 13 times Nature's sustainable rate.[6]

The result is, we lose 4 million acres of cropland to erosion in the United States each year, or 3 to 6 billion tons of topsoil.[7] The topsoil ends up in our lakes, streams, and rivers making it difficult to use for growing plants.[8] Although we still get something out of it: A $44 billion annual bill in taxes and higher food prices to pay the cost of water purification.[9]

Sixty percent of rangeland is overgrazed and one-third of the topsoil is gone in major farming states.[10] For every inch of topsoil that we lose, 6 percent fewer crops can be grown.[11] Sort of.

Chemical fertilizers are ostensibly picking up the slack for the continuing loss of topsoil. The fertilizers normally contain a combination of nitrogen, phosphorus, and potassium.[12] They help plants grow fast and tall, however, to the detriment of our health the minerals that were once delivered to us by way of plants have been significantly depleted by the loss of topsoil.

The chemical fertilizers further degrade the soil by leaching the nutrients and necessary bacteria.[13] And if all this damage wasn't enough, in order to manufacture the fertilizers we are becoming increasingly more dependent on foreign sources for ammonia, potash, and phosphates.[14]

Things would be much easier for human beings if we could just bury our legs up to our knees in the dirt for an hour or two a day and absorb all the nutrients we need from the soil. But we can't. Nature left it up to plants to perform that job for us, and there is hope they might again be able to perform it, because there is some light at the end of the topsoil-rich formed tunnel.

An alien just arriving to our planet might get the impression that organic farming and foods are a new craze, a blossoming overnight industry, when in fact it's just natural farming that didn't before need a name. A switch to a vegetarian-based economy would eliminate 90 percent of the erosion caused by our current meat-based economy, do away with the need for artificial growth stimulants in chemical fertilizers, and allow us to refer to organically grown fruits and vegetables as—fruits and vegetables.[15]

Topsoil, now just on average 6 inches deep, is a complete and delicately balanced ecosystem. It was intended to support our lives, probably not support the weight of innumerable cattle and other livestock raised for food. If we continue to follow the path we're on—the eroding topsoil path—Nature's special brew will likely become history. Yes, history, a good choice of words.

Just 10,000 years ago there was a 3 million square mile mass of fertile land filled with vegetation in Africa. Most scientists believe that overgrazing by livestock, rather than climate, was the chief cause of the land's demise. The land no longer supports life.

Back then the land had but one name: Sahara.[16] Today it is referred to by two names—Desert follows Sahara.

43: The Land

THE RELATIVE SIZE OF THE EARTH

The earth is a big planet, approximately 110 billion acres of land and ocean. Certainly it's large enough to support a meat-based diet for all its inhabitants.

Of course 71 percent of the earth is ocean. But that still leaves 29 percent, or 32 billion acres of land.[1] With a population of 6 billion people that's 5 plus acres of land per person.

Of course 2 acres of land per person would be required to grow feed, mostly for livestock.[2] No problem, that still leaves 3 acres of land per person, more than enough for a house, lawn, and garden.

Of course 4.4 acres of land per person would be required for livestock grazing.[3] No problem...wait a second! We're out of land!

Given there is currently less than 15 billion acres of cropland and pastureland, and the requirement for land on a meat-based diet for everyone is 38 billion acres, a quick calculation indicates a lot of people are going to go hungry if all 6 billion humans on the planet are eating meat regularly.[4]

Fortunately, that is not the case. Only one-third of the world consumes a meat-based diet. Given that's the case, should we still be concerned that we don't have enough land to feed everyone? Well at least 1 billion people are concerned; that's the number of people underfed and malnourished.[5] Maybe the earth isn't so big after all.

What has the United States and other countries done with the land to support the carnivorous habits of the one-third?

- In the United States 90 percent of agricultural land and more than half the total land area is devoted to livestock agriculture.[6]

- Half of the forests in the United States have been leveled, much of it for livestock grazing.[7]

- Much of the public land has been turned over to ranchers, with 50 percent of the land in the Western United States designated wilderness grazed by livestock.[8]

- Two-thirds of the land in Central America that is agriculturally productive is used for livestock production at the expense of the poor.[9] (The meat is eaten by the rich or exported.)

- Nearly 70 percent of the Amazon Rain Forest has been burned for cattle pastures.[10]

- Half of the world's forests have been cleared for livestock grazing and continue to be cleared at a rate of 13 million acres a year.[11] (For every 1 acre of land cleared for urbanization 7 acres are cleared for grazing.)[12]

The impact of the SICK diet on our food supply is not the only consequence of choosing to use the land as we have. The impact on the land itself may prevent us someday from producing *any* kind of food, animal or vegetable.

- Because of livestock agriculture, deserts are expanding globally by 27,000 square miles every year.[13] As a result, approximately one-third of the earth's land has been desertified to some extent.[14]

- Roughly 40 percent of the world's agricultural land is degraded and 5 million acres of cropland is being lost each year.[15]

- In the United States, during the past 150 years, the soil resources have been reduced by 50 percent.[16]

In essence, our life-support system, the earth, is shrinking daily. Is it possible to pump some air into our planet and reverse the trend?

PEOPLE FED: On 2.5 acres of land the number of people that could be fed a particular food.[17]

- 1 person beef
- 2 people chicken
- 15 people whole grains
- 20 people a variety of vegetables
- 22 people potatoes

OATS VERSUS BEEF: On 1 acre of land oats can provide this number of times the nutrients as beef.[18]

- 8 times the protein
- 16 times the iron
- 25 times the calories
- 6 times the niacin
- 12 times the riboflavin
- 84 times the thiamine

BROCCOLI VERSUS BEEF: On 1 acre of land broccoli can provide this number of times the nutrients as beef.[19]

- 10 times the protein
- 24 times the iron
- 11 times the calories
- 11 times the niacin
- 79 times the riboflavin
- 85 times the thiamine
- 650 times the calcium

POTENTIAL TO FEED: Currently we are short food for 1 billion people. If the remaining third of the planet became vegetarian tomorrow, estimates are that the following number of people could be fed.[20]

- 10 billion people
- 3 times the current 6 billion population
- 14 times more than a meat-based diet

It appears the planet has plenty of room to expand.

Is there any way of knowing where our planet is headed if we continue with animal agriculture? Historians always tell us that history repeats itself. But no earths have gone before us, at least to our knowledge, to learn from. However, past cultures and populations, serving as microcosms, might provide some insight.

- Early Roman, Greek, Arab, and African civilizations all put great emphasis on livestock agriculture with considerable social and economic consequences.[21]

- The meat eating Indus Valley civilization went belly-up; extensive deforestation existed in the area.[22]

- Many communities in the Mediterranean region suffered decline or collapse from overgrazing and deforestation.[23]

- During the Middle Ages, Spain and Italy relied heavily on sheep herding with destructive consequences.[24]

- Ethiopia experienced catastrophic drought and famine because of the clearing of 90 percent of its forests and subsequent overgrazing and soil erosion.[25]

Americans account for only 4 percent of the earth's population but consume 23 percent of the world's beef.[26] There seems to be plenty of room to expand the relative size of our country's land and its resources to grow and prosper by embracing the WELL diet.

Or might our country someday be referred to as the American Desert, nothing more than a footnote in the history book of another country—one that subsisted on a plant-based diet.

44: The Oceans

IF IT DOESN'T FLUSH, IT'S NOT A TOILET

When we think of ocean pollution, most likely we think of things like oil spills, sewer mishaps, and industrial runoff. It is probably most unlikely that a meat-based diet is the first thing that pops into our heads, if it comes to mind at all. But maybe it should be our first and foremost thought. Because the spills, mishaps, and runoffs pale in comparison to the ecological impact a flesh-eating diet has on our oceans.[1]

Our choice to include livestock and fish in our diets translates into three assaults on our oceans: The pollution generated by livestock agriculture, the pollution generated by aquaculture (the ocean version of livestock factory farming), and the pollution generated by conventional fishing. Together these three activities are turning our oceans into a global toilet.

So what is so coveted about large bodies of salty water, some might ask. How do we know they're polluted, and how do we know it's our flesh-eating diets that are responsible? What do the oceans do for us now, and what might they do for us in the future? Let's get wet and find out what's below the surface.

The oceans dominate our planet. Because water makes up 71 percent of the earth's surface, it might better be said that humans and animals live on floating islands on a watery globe. The world's oceans contain 328 million cubic miles of seawater.[2] The United States alone has more than 95,000 miles of coastline and more than 3.4 million square miles of ocean.[3]

Living in the oceans are 58 species of sea grasses, 1,000 species of sea anemones, 1,500 species of brown algae, 7,000 species of echinoderms, 13,000 species of fishes, 50,000 species of mollusks, and a vast amount of life yet to be discovered and classified.[4] The oceans are a planet within a planet.

It's hard to imagine that pollutants, no matter what their volume or where they came from, could have a significant impact on the massive oceans. But apparently they do, because:

- The loss of shellfish due to pollution in the Chesapeake Bay is indicated by how long it now takes to filter the pollutants. Back when the Europeans were exploring the bay it took 8 hours. Today it takes the few remaining shellfish a full year to do the job.[5]

- Swimmers across the United States were chased from the oceans by the 11,270 closings and advisories issued in the year 2000.[6]

- The catch of U.S. fishermen is reduced because a 7,000 square-mile area of gulf waters off Louisiana can no longer support most aquatic life.[7]

- Oceanographers have calculated that 40 percent of estuarine and coastal waters are polluted, and 65 percent of coastal rivers and bays are contaminated.[8]

A spit in the ocean it's not. What are the contaminants and where are they coming from?

LIVESTOCK AGRICULTURE: Of all the ocean contaminates, 75 percent are from land-based sources.[9] Phosphorous, nitrogen, and bacteria runoff from livestock farming, which comes from waste, fertilizer, and pesticides, produces algae that takes oxygen away from plants and fish.[10] Topsoil runoff smothers eggs, blocks sunlight, and kills plants.[11]

FISH AQUACULTURE: Fish farming, the ocean's version of factory farming is the practice of raising fish in mass, in cages. This method of fishing now accounts for one-third of fish consumed.[12]

To carry out this activity the highly rich inland mangrove forests and coastal wetlands are exploited, cleared, and drained.[13] Fish farming then creates further chaos by removing the lower food chain fish from the oceans for feed.[14] The ecosystems are further compromised when non-native fish escape into local waters disrupting the balance of nature.[15]

The intensive farming practice, not unlike its land counterpart, generates pollution from feces, uneaten feed, massive antibiotic dosing, and pesticide washing.[16]

COMMERCIAL FISHING: There are 13 million fishers in the world that can typically get 80 to 90 percent of a fish population out of the oceans in any one year.[17] This has caused the extinction of many species, threatened the extinction of many others, and disrupted the predator-prey relationships.[18] Parts of ocean floors have been turned into marine deserts leaving nowhere for fish to spawn.[19]

The prevailing attitude about our use of the oceans might go something like this: Fewer fish in the water, more fish in cages, and some unclean water. Seems like a fair trade-off to put meat and fish on our plates. Besides, we don't live in the ocean, we don't drink from it, so why should we get excited about its ecosystem balance?

Let's change that attitude by highlighting 10 contributions of the oceans we might have overlooked.

- The ocean provides recreation in the name of boating, surfing, diving, and swimming.

- The ocean gives 180 million people who visit America's coastlines each year vacations they will treasure forever.

- The ocean gives us beauty and aesthetic qualities that have inspired some of the world's finest paintings, poetry, stories, and music.[20]

- The ocean provides leading edge anti-inflammatory drugs and potentially life-saving cancer treatments from fish and marine organisms.[21]

- The ocean gives us food besides fish. Experts predict that the sea can yield about 25 percent more organic food than it does now.[22]

- The ocean is continually sharing its secrets in the name of new ecosystems that might be the basis of future drugs and medical treatments.[23]

- The ocean provides natural services such as carbon storage, atmospheric gas regulation, and nutrient cycling.[24]

- The ocean furnishes coral reefs, mangroves, and kelp forests to protect coastal areas from storms.[25]

- The ocean yields marine algae that contributes nearly 40 percent of global photosynthesis.[26]

- The oceans regulate the world's climate. We need healthy oceans for the planet to survive.[27]

The fact that the oceans cover two-thirds of the earth indicates they have important roles to play in the success of our planet. They are already playing those roles. And no doubt the roles will expand as time passes. Unique plant-based foods? Critical medicines? Fresh drinking water? Human living quarters? It's hard to know what the future holds. But we do know some things about the present.

We know the indirect and direct byproducts of our land animal and sea animal diets are damaging the oceans. We know that the damage will only get worse if we continue our flesh-eating habits. And we know that the oceans weren't designated to be the global toilet, because if they were, we could flush and fill them up with clean water.

45: The Forests

THE EARTH'S VITAL ORGANS

Rain or tropical, pines or oaks, scenery or landscape, Gump or Sherwood.

The word "forest" brings to mind a variety of words and images. However, there are some words and images we probably never associate with forest, such as: livestock agriculture, cut down and clear, ecological disaster, vital organs, or survival. Maybe it's time that we did.

Because of our desire for fast-food burgers, T-bone steaks, and prime rib roasts, we have had to alter the earth's landscape. We have had to cut down and clear away more than half of the world's forests and rain forests, including 300 million acres in the United States, in order to accommodate livestock grazing and feed production.[1]

And the practice is not static, as forests are cleared at a rate of approximately 13 million acres a year. At the current rate of deforestation the earth's forests will eventually become the earth's deserts.[2]

The forests, themselves, are not static either. Half of all species, and 80 percent of the earth's vegetation, lives and grows in the rainforests.[3] Each time we consume one fast-food burger we also consume and dispose of 55 square feet of rainforest, 100 insect species, 25 plant species, and a dozen bird, mammal, and reptile species.[4] And here we thought our fast-food hamburgers came cheap.

The life we kill off in the forests may not be the only life impacted by our meat-based diet habit.

The forests perform a number of critical roles for the earth, not unlike various organs do for the body. If we begin to remove organs from the body, eventually it will cease to function properly. If we begin to remove the forests from our earth eventually *it* will cease to function properly. Whether it's our bodies or the earth, the result is the same for us: We will cease to exist.

Let's look at how the forest provides life-support for the earth, and see if we can make some analogies with our body's life support system.

- LUNGS: The forests process carbon dioxide and oxygen.

- KIDNEYS: The forests recycle and purify water.

- HYPOTHALAMUS: The forests regulate the earth's temperature. (If we continue as we are, by the middle of the century we will have raised the earth's temperature 5 to 7 degrees, which will create a number of ecological disasters.)[5]

- BLADDER: The forests hold watershed.

- CELLS: The forests contain much of the life on our planet.

And if we can stretch the analogy a bit, then...

- SKIN: The forests supply wood to build our homes that enclose and protect us, as our skin does.

- PROTEIN: The forests assist in the growth and repair of the soil, as protein does for our tissues.

- LYMPH SYSTEM: The forests directly support our body's defenses by supplying 25 percent of the raw materials for our medicines, and the potential for more as we have only tested 1 percent of the forest's treasures.[6]

- METABOLISM: The forests supply the cooking fuel for much of humanity, which in turn provides our fuel, food.

- BEAUTY: The forests draw 240 million people to our national parks each year for their beauty, solace, and inspiration, as the physical beauty of our bodies attract people to us.[7]

The forests are an integral player in the health of our earth—and thus our health. Each acre of forest that is cut and cleared is the loss of one more cell or tissue that diminishes our planet's efficiency.

It takes 10 times the land to produce food for the SICK diet as it does for the WELL diet. We can choose to produce 165 pounds of beef from 1 acre of land or we can choose to produce 20,000 pounds of potatoes from the same acre. We often hear the expression, "Recycle and save a tree." But how often do we hear the expression, "Become a vegetarian and save an *acre* of trees." Because an acre of forest can be saved every year by embracing a plant-based diet.[8]

If we have children, our daily list of chores probably includes items that we need to do for them such as: Give kids a bath. Buy kids new shoes. Help kids with homework. Think about kids' future with regard to forest destruction.

Well, the last item probably isn't included, but maybe it should be. Because if we don't look beyond the day-to-day details to see the larger picture, the routine things we do for our children today aren't going to matter much.

One could say that as adults, if we can't see the forest for the trees, then our children won't see the forest *or* the trees.

46: Animal Waste

NOT AN END RESULT — A BEGINNING PROBLEM

Have we ever asked ourselves what happens to the excrement generated by the animals raised for food? Given that we probably don't give much thought to even the animals, it's most likely we haven't explored the question.

Animals raised for food produce 2 billion tons of excrement a year—5 tons for every man, woman, and child in the United States, and 130 times more waste than Americans produce.[1] To place this number in perspective, it breaks down to 7.6 million pounds every minute.

The word "waste" implies an end result. And being an end product should mean that we are finished with it. So what is there to discuss?

Given the impact that animal waste has on our waters—rivers and streams, oceans and lakes, and maybe most of all drinking—it's not an end result, but a beginning catastrophe. Instead of calling it animal waste, maybe it should be called animal *worst*.

Because animals are housed in feedlots and confinement buildings there is no economically feasible way to return the manure to the soil.[2] Therefore, much of it is kept in large lagoons, with some portion of it sprayed back onto the fields.[3] This may sound pretty benign in terms of the damage it can cause. Then again...

- It's not uncommon for these pools to leak into the groundwater.[4]

- The waste sprayed back onto the field is generally too much for the plants to uptake, so the excess often runs off into surface water of streams and rivers.[5]

- Ammonia gas emitted from the open lagoons returns to earth in subsequent rainfalls polluting surface waters.[6]

- Not all of the waste is systematically stored or sprayed. Some is deliberately dumped into waterways.[7] But how common can this be given our strict clean water and waste laws? Then again...

When the Clean Water Act went into effect in 1972 agriculture was exempted.[8] Although we have strict laws governing human waste, the laws governing animal waste are lax or non-existent even though the pathogens, in at least hog waste, are 10 to 100 times greater than human waste.[9]

Bacteria, wormy parasites, virus, cholera, chlamydia, E. coli, heavy metals, nitrogen, phosphorous, mercury, nitrates, ammonia, fecal streptococci, and fecal coliform are among the contaminants found in animal waste.[10] It goes without saying that these are not the type of elements we want in our waters; it *doesn't* go without saying what their impact is on them.

- According to the U.S. Senate Agricultural Committee, 60 percent of rivers and streams are impaired by agricultural runoff, the largest contributor to waterway pollution.[11]

- The Environmental Protection Agency (EPA) says most of the nation's 127 estuaries show nutrient pollution.[12]

- Resources for the Future, an environmental research center, indicates that 40 percent of nitrogen and 35 percent of phosphorous that pollute U.S. waterways are due to agriculture.[13]

Given that animal waste is responsible for 10 times as much water pollution in America as the human population, these statistics shouldn't surprise us.[14] But the specific damage it can do as demonstrated by the following examples just might.

- A hog lagoon spill in North Carolina waterways and chicken waste pollution on land near the Chesapeake Bay have activated an organism called Pfiesteria. It has killed millions of fish and been the most likely cause of fishermen, coastal residents, and tourists becoming ill.[15]

- A "dead zone" of 7,000 square miles in the Gulf of Mexico off Louisiana can no longer support most aquatic life because of severe oxygen depletion from animal manure pollution.[16] It's probably no coincidence that 80 percent of U.S. farms are on or near waters that drain into the Mississippi River, which ultimately feeds the Gulf.[17]

- In Milwaukee, a pathogen from dairy manure infected drinking water that killed 100 people and sickened 400,000.[18]

- In Indiana, the LaGrange County Health Department identified six miscarriages among women living near hog farms; their drinking water wells had been contaminated with unsafe levels of nitrates.[19]

- In Missouri, swine factory farms have been the biggest culprit in polluting 150 miles of Missouri's streams, killing more than a half million fish and increasing respiratory illness among its residents.[20]

- In Milford, Utah, where a hog plant does business, residents have 20 times the state average rate of diarrheal illness.[21]

- According to EPA tests, 17 states have groundwater that is impaired by feedlot manure containing fecal streptococci and fecal coliform bacteria. The result is that 39 million people in rural America are drinking water that may be unsafe.[22]

Are these examples of isolated cases exaggerated by environmental extremists, or do they represent the tip of the iceberg brought to our attention by altruistic patriots? If we can use as a barometer the amount of money spent annually by Americans for bottled water and tap water treatments, then we might have our answer. That figure is $2 billion.[23]

Producing 1 pound of meat generates 17 times more water pollution than producing 1 pound of pasta.[24] So it is no surprise that a plant-based diet would do more to clean up the nation's water than any other single action.[25]

Fresh water is not a renewable resource, nor is it completely recyclable. Eventually we will have to make the choice between a piece of meat or a glass of clean drinking water. One we must have, the other we don't need.

Let's not waste the opportunity to make our choice now. Time is wasting.

47: Species Extinction

THE SPOTTED OWL OR HUMAN BEINGS?

It's fun to remember back to the carefree and fun-filled days of our youth, until our brain stumbles across something like pop quizzes. They were pesky annoyances then. What about now?

Let's take out a No. 2 pencil, put our books away, and find out.

1. Living organisms are becoming extinct 100 to 5,000 times faster than they used to, at a rate of 1 every 10 minutes, or roughly 50,000 every year.[1] What is the predominate cause?

   a) flooding
   b) drought
   c) pestilence
   d) none of the above

2. According to some scientists, the extinction of which species should we be most worried about?

   a) Spotted Owl
   b) Blue Whale
   c) Mountain Gorilla
   d) none of the above

3. Some scientists predict that the end of our civilization will occur sometime before the end of this century.[2] The most likely cause will be:

   a) nuclear holocaust
   b) climate change
   c) meteor collision
   d) none of the above

If we hadn't studied our lessons in school, but we had a little savvy, we might choose "none of the above" more often than not figuring it greatly expanded our answer pool. If that was your logic here, then congratulations, you made a perfect score. If you knew the actual answers to be,

>   (1) livestock agriculture,
>   (2) human beings and,
>   (3) species extinction,

then you need to stop fooling around with pop quizzes and No. 2 pencils and spend your idle hours working for the future of our planet and civilization.

Let's discuss the answers to learn why they might not be as surprising as they first appear.

LIVESTOCK AGRICULTURE: Since the advent of Homo sapiens the normal extinction rate that should run 10 to 25 species a year has accelerated dramatically.[3] Animals, plants, trees, plankton, bacteria, fungi, and insects are included in the speed up.

Man's choice to raise animals for food has resulted in 20 billion livestock (cattle, pigs, chickens, etc.) grazing on one-half the planet.[4] Of all man's engagements with the planet, this pursuit has been the most devastating to living organisms and the earth's ecological web. One-half of endangered species, according to the Endangered Species Act, is due to cattle ranching.[5]

It is estimated that producing 1 pound of beef is 20 times more damaging to wildlife habitats than producing 1 pound of pasta.[6] A total of 11,046 species of plants and animals are currently threatened, facing a high risk of extinction in the near future.[7] Fortunately, the ant is not one of them.

The ant?

Ants turn and aerate much of the earth's soil, break up 90 percent of small, dead creatures as part of the soil-nutrient cycle, pollinate plants, and prey on insects. Their extinction would cause the demise of multiple species and the decimation of some ecosystems.[8] Imagine the effect on the destiny of the ant having 20 billion livestock stomping around the planet.

HUMAN BEINGS: Putting our collective energies toward saving a few of the more highly evolved animals and mammals shows we have our hearts in the right place, but not our heads.

Our focus should be on our own survival, with our attentions on the destructive effects of the SICK diet habit on other living organisms and their delicate ecological webs. If we soon don't realize our species is dependent on the survival of other species, then we won't be around to help save any species.

We rely on the estimated 1.75 million species on earth to maintain hydrological cycles, regulate climate, contribute to the process of soil formation and maturation, store and cycle essential nutrients, absorb and break down pollutants, and more.[9] Losing a species is like losing a tooth on a gear of the human machine.

Already enough teeth have been lost to have an effect. Ebola and AIDS, along with respiratory and epidemic disease, skin cancer, malnutrition, and natural disasters have their roots in ecological destruction.[10] When enough teeth on enough gears are gone, our machine will cease to run.

SPECIES EXTINCTION: It is theorized that five mass extinctions have occurred during the last 500 million years on this planet, the last one being 65 million years ago with the extinction of the dinosaurs.[11]

According to biologists surveyed by the American Museum of Natural History, we are now in the midst of our sixth extinction, the fastest in Earth's history.[12] Some believe that our civilization, due to the elimination of species and subsequent ecological breakdown, will complete the sixth extinction by the end of the century.[13]

Humans alone have been responsible for nearly every loss of species in the past few thousand years.[14] At the rate we are going some scenarios predict we will lose nearly 50 percent of all living species by the year 2050.[15] If this prediction holds true, could the scales tip and bring to a close the human chapter in this planet's history?

It's anybody's guess, but everybody's choice.

It should humble us to realize that we are dependent on other species for our existence, and no species is dependent on us. If ants become extinct the planet is in dire straits. However, if humans become extinct the planet would prosper; the atmosphere would stabilize, endangered species would blossom, forests would return, and so on.[16]

Few Americans would argue with the principle that life is sacred. Shouldn't this fundamental precept apply to *all* life? If we are willing to say that it does we could be well on our way—well on our way to putting off indefinitely the sixth mass extinction.

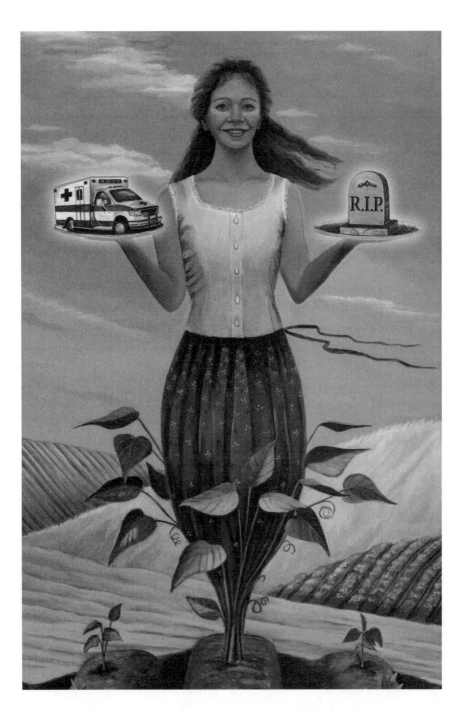

Just One Name Would Suffice

∼ 7 ∼
Disease: Killers
ONE CAUSE — ONE DISEASE

The diseases go by many different names. But given their singular cause maybe they should go by one: the SICK disease.

Ahead in this chapter...

It's no secret that HEART DISEASE is our number one killer, but it *is* a secret that it's virtually avoidable, even reversible.[1]

ATHEROSCLEROSIS does to our vital organs what a crippled Interstate Highway System would do to our cities.

It's not likely that 50 million Americans have HYPERTENSION because Mother Nature didn't have the engineering background to design our circulatory system.[2]

Because PROSTATE CANCER shortens a man's life by 9 years it deserves more respect than to be the butt of jokes.[3]

Studies suggest 95 percent of COLON CANCER cases have a nutritional connection, yet only 2 percent of Americans believe eating less meat can reduce the risk.[4]

It's time to put down the pink ribbons, pick up the green vegetables, and take a different look at BREAST CANCER.

Wouldn't Mother Nature have made the ovaries impenetrable to outside threats—like OVARIAN CANCER—to ensure the survival of our species? Maybe she did.

CANCERS are not a mysterious, random occurrence; something has to initiate them and something has to promote their growth.

DIABETES might bring to mind sugar and thirst, when it should bring to mind predator and killer.

Our kidneys were built virtually indestructible, yet 20 million Americans have urinary and KIDNEY DISEASE.[5]

The acceleration of AGING is greatly determined by whether we feed weapons to the good guys or the bad guys.

Is ALZHEIMER'S DISEASE a whole other ballgame, or the grand finale of degenerative diseases?

48: Heart Disease

DADDY DOESN'T FEEL WELL

It was a balmy October Saturday night as the TV show *Leave It to Beaver* was winding down. A mother called to her 8-year-old son that it was bedtime. The child proceeded down the hall to bed, holding his mother's hand, and carrying his Yogi Bear stuffed animal.

Before he turned into his room he caught a glimpse of his parents' room where he saw his dad sitting still and quiet on the side of the bed. He asked his mother if Daddy was going to tuck him in. His mother replied, no, Daddy doesn't feel well.

During the night as the little boy went in and out of sleep he heard sirens in the distance, and later commotion in the hallway outside his closed door.

When the boy awoke Sunday morning the first thing he saw was the minister from his church sitting by his bedside. The first thing he heard was his mother crying from another room. He knew he would never see his Daddy again. He soon learned his father had died of a heart attack.

*****

Coronary artery disease takes the lives of more than a half million Americans 35 and older each year. That's roughly a life every minute. Another 12.4 million Americans are waiting in the wings to have their coronary event.[1]

Let's forget for a moment we are talking about heart disease. What if we said there was an unknown disease killing an American every single minute, and there were more than 12 million of us that might be next. Would this not be the lead story on the evening news? Would this not be the number one topic of discussion all over America? Would Americans not be concerned and scared? Would Americans not be mobilizing in an attempt to conquer the menace?

Instead our response to heart disease is: hardly any response at all. The prevailing attitude is that it's part and parcel of America's riches and lifestyle. A function of stress that goes along with our progressive, technological society. The feeling is that our diets have some influence, but so does our family history, and who knows what else. It's the bad that we have to take with the good. It's an inevitable part of aging.

Given what we actually know about heart disease the prevailing attitude might be more frightening than the disease itself.

Let's review a few, but compelling, tidbits of evidence that exist about heart disease. Maybe they would make a good lead story for the evening news.

THE FIRST 3 MILLION SUBJECTS: To prevent food shortages during World War I the Danish government began to feed its grain to the populace, rather than to the livestock. The reduction in meat consumption translated into a 34 percent reduction in mortality rate due to disease, including circulatory diseases.[2]

A BLESSING OF WAR? During World War II Norway was occupied by Germany. Their supply of meat was virtually cut off. The correlation between the reduction of fat consumption and circulatory disease in Norway from 1938 to 1948 was almost identical.[3]

LOOK WHAT'S INSIDE: During the Korean War when soldiers who were killed were autopsied, more than 77 percent of the young American soldiers had blood vessels narrowed by atherosclerotic deposits, while the opposing forces subsisting on a predominately vegetarian diet showed no such damage.[4]

BEYOND OUR SHORES: In 1964, Dr. Dudley White, who treated President Dwight Eisenhower's heart attack, tested and studied a culture of people in Kashmir, the Hunzas, after learning that they subsisted on a pure vegetarian diet. He found they had no trace of coronary artery disease. The study included 25 men who were older than 90.[5]

Another population that subsists on grains, legumes, vegetables, and fruits is the rural Chinese. Coronary artery disease is virtually unknown among them. Their normal adult cholesterol levels are between 90 and 150 milligrams per deciliter (mg/dL).[6]

IT'S NOT OUR FAMILY'S FAULT: Further studies done during the Korean War placed South Korean soldiers, who normally subsisted on a virtually vegetarian diet, on the U.S. Army diet and found they developed atherosclerosis.[7]

When the Japanese, known for their predominately vegetarian diet, moved to other parts of the world and changed their eating habits a direct correlation developed between their diet and heart disease.[8]

The famous heart surgeon, Dr. Michael DeBakey, suggests that heredity accounts for about 5 percent of heart disease.[9]

PUT TWO AND TWO TOGETHER: The Framington Heart Study showed that when people kept their cholesterol levels below 150 mg/dL they were virtually assured of never suffering a heart attack. This was tracked for more than 35 years and not one person suffered a heart attack during that period.[10] The average cholesterol level for U.S. vegans is 133 mg/dL.[11]

REMOVE THE THORN; THE WOUND HEALS: Dr. Dean Ornish's program, based on a low-fat whole-foods vegetarian diet, has shown to reverse atherosclerosis in 75 percent of people, with 80 percent being able to avoid surgery after 1 year on the program.[12]

Dr. Caldwell Esselstyn's program, using a low-fat near-vegan diet, is just as impressive. Those that came to him had suffered 48 serious cardiac events before they entered the program, and after 12 years on the program had zero events.[13]

Lifestyle, stress, heredity, aging, or an unknown entity. In light of the data, in the overwhelming cases of heart disease it would be hard to blame any combination of these factors in its cause and promotion. It appears we have to look no further than diet. A Wholly Eating Leaves to Live (WELL) diet keeps heart disease from starting and reverses it when it is started by the Self-Induced Carnivorous Killer (SICK) diet. Could it be any simpler? Is there any controversy in this assessment?

The American Medical Association doesn't argue with it. It stated in its journal that a vegetarian diet could prevent 97 percent of coronary occlusions.[14] The year it was printed? 1961. Just in time for a particular father to hear about it.

Maybe he did, maybe he didn't. Maybe the media didn't report it; maybe the father chose not to heed it. But try to explain this to an 8-year-old boy who lost his father.

When the 8-year-old boy became an adult, married, and had children, he vowed he would do everything in his power so his children would not have to grow up without a father like he did. Thus on the day of the birth of his first child, he became a vegetarian.

And 14 years later, as this book is being written, the children still have their father.

49: Atherosclerosis

MAINTAINING *OUR* STREETS AND HIGHWAYS

Each of us houses a blood vessel system that if placed end-to-end would stretch 100,000 miles, twice the length of the U.S. Interstate Highway System, or 4 times around the earth.[1]

In some form, everything we breathe, drink, and eat winds its way through our body's highway system of veins, capillaries, and arteries. The arteries, an integral part of the system, are responsible for moving oxygenated blood to all of our vital—and presumably not-so-vital—organs. If the arteries are damaged and the blood is impeded, then each and every organ has the potential to be harmed.

It seems unlikely, given our body's highly evolved restorative and defense capabilities that a disease like atherosclerosis could ever happen—a disease that can destroy the principal components of our circulatory system. Then again, the body probably had no idea what it was going to have to contend with.

As it turns out the body *does* have an efficient way to deal with unwelcome visitors to the arteries. When an injury occurs in an artery wall the body goes into action to repair it, dispatching platelets and white blood cells to the site as it would for a sore on the skin. If the problem is short-term, scar tissue forms healing the area making it even stronger than before. But if the offending invader keeps hammering away at the location, the body can't keep up with the repairs. That's when problems begin.

Fat and cholesterol are foes of our arteries. If we subscribe to a meat-based diet, then we are dumping a daily and steady flow of these substances into our bloodstream opening up sores on the artery wall. The body goes to work healing the damage, but it can't keep up and close the sores fast enough. Thus, the sores remain open, and fat and cholesterol continually enter the arterial wall mixed with scar tissue, platelets, and white blood cells. This recipe makes a plaque. The plaque are fibrous and hard, and they continue to multiply until either we shut off the troublemakers—fat and cholesterol—or they shut off our blood flow.

Given that a meat-based diet is the diet of choice in this country, the latter occurs far more often contributing to 1 million U.S. deaths a year, 1 every 30 seconds.

Because fat and cholesterol can go anywhere in the body by circulating through its 100,000 mile highway system, every artery is a potential target of atherosclerosis. It can restrict or shut off blood flow in the arteries that feed the heart, brain, or kidneys, resulting in heart attack, stroke, or kidney failure.[2] Or it can do the same to less vital arteries creating other health problems such as eye disease, hearing loss, senility, leg cramps, gangrene, and impotence.[3] No artery is safe. No organ is exempt.

Many view atherosclerosis as a disease of aging because the symptoms and damage usually don't show up for decades. But that doesn't mean it doesn't begin with the first bite of animal flesh, the first drink of cows' milk, or the first swallow of chicken eggs.

- Children show fatty streaks in their arteries at 9 months, signs of the disease at 3 years, and scar tissue formation in the teen years.[4]

- In one study of 2-to-15-year-olds that died of trauma, 50 percent had fatty streaks and 8 percent had fibrous plaque in their coronary arteries.[5]

- Of 21-to-39-year-olds, 85 percent had fatty streaks and 69 percent had fibrous plaque in their coronary arteries.[6]

- Of American soldiers in their 20s who were autopsied during the Korean War, 35 percent had fibrous plaque in their coronary arteries.[7]

- X-ray angiography done on high-risk men younger than 40 showed that one-half had at least 1 out of 3 coronary arteries narrowed by 50 percent.[8]

Do we find atherosclerosis in animals we know to be carnivorous? Russian physiologists, way back in 1908, wondered that very thing.

So they fed egg yolks to herbivore rabbits, and carnivore dogs and cats. The rabbits produced atherosclerotic plaque similar to those occurring in humans. They couldn't produce a single atherosclerotic plaque in the dogs and cats.[9]

If atherosclerosis is in fact a disease of a fat and cholesterol-laden diet, then we would expect that changing our diet would allow the body to catch up on repairs, thus curing the disease. We also would expect no other remedies to work.

- Garlic pills, fish oil, vitamins, angioplasty, surgery, aspirin, cholesterol-lowering drugs, exercise, and stress reduction can all help, but none of them will cure the disease, and all come with minor to major side effects.[10]

- One study showed that a low-fat vegetarian diet reduced cholesterol 24 percent (roughly 60 points) in 12 months, and caused 82 percent of the arterial plaque to shrink.[11]

- Other studies have shown that on a low-fat vegetarian diet, patients after 3 weeks suffering from angina have a 91 percent reduction in chest pain. After 5 days leg cramps have improved. And after 4 months hearing loss improved.[12]

- People who thrive on rice, potatoes, corn, beans, and wheat-based diets are almost immune from atherosclerosis.[13]

- Stress, lack of exercise, and heredity have little to do with the disease.[14]

If the SICK diet was on trial for perpetrating the crime of atherosclerosis the prosecution would rest now, fully confident it had proven its case beyond a reasonable doubt. We would expect the jury to return expeditiously with a guilty verdict.

In the penalty phase we would seek the punishment of death on the basis that an eye for an eye would be most appropriate.

It's time to remove the menace of the SICK diet from society. It is time for everyone to breathe a little easier. It is time to make our streets and highways safe again.

50: Hypertension

HE ANSWER IS RIGHT UNDER OUR NOSES

Maybe the worst part of this disease is its name, hypertension. Since hypertension has little to do with being hyper or tense, its name is misleading. It leads us away from the serious nature of the disease.

Hypertension increases our risk of stroke by a factor of 7, congestive heart failure by a factor of 4, and dying from a heart attack by a factor of 3.[1] Fifty million Americans have hypertension and less than half of Americans have optimal blood pressure.[2]

A name change might do more to help curb the incidence of this killer than any other measure. Maybe giving it a name like, Disaster Warning, would give the disease the respect it deserves.

What also seems to be misleading about the disease is our perception of its cause and treatment.

- We are led to believe it is a disease of the elderly, yet 1 in 8 American children have blood pressure that is too high.[3]

- We are led to believe, based on the fact that prescriptions are written 9 out of 10 times for the disease, that drugs will solve the problem, yet only 1 in 100 with mild hypertension will derive some benefit from medication.[4]

- We are led to believe that diet plays little role in hypertension, given we largely ignore it in favor of pharmaceutical therapy, yet we have had proof for more than 100 years, since the early 1900s, that diet plays a role.[5]

- We are led to believe that the disease is incurable, yet 58 percent in one study came off their medication after changing to a vegetarian diet.[6]

- We are led to believe it is primarily a disease of too much salt, yet even without reducing our salt intake we can lower our blood pressure by as much as 10 percent by changing to a vegetarian diet.[7]

If we learn that we have high blood pressure readings, an emergency alarm should blare in our heads. In life when an alarm sounds we quickly react to it hoping to avert a potential disaster. The last thing we would think of doing would be to disable the alarm and completely ignore what caused it to sound.

But that's what 9 out of 10 Americans do with high blood pressure. We go to the doctor for a prescription of beta-blockers, diuretics, or dilators to throw at the alarm to stop the noise.

For those with mild hypertension (diastolic of under 105), from which the majority of the 50 million suffer, there is little evidence that drugs will improve survival rates and reduce the risk of stroke and heart attack.[8] But what they *can* do is cause side effects such as failing memory, fatigue, increased cholesterol levels, impotence, increased heart attack rate, depression, headache, dizziness, low blood pressure, upset stomach, muscle cramps, joint pains, and heart arrhythmias.[9]

We never go looking for the problem, but it's easy to find. It's right under our noses. In our mouths.

There is nothing mysterious about the cause of hypertension for the overwhelming majority. The fat and cholesterol from our meat and dairy cuisine narrow the arterial walls with sludge and plaque, and iron and sodium make a secondary contribution.

- One study with 155 subjects showed vegetarians having a lower systolic reading of 9 percent, and lower diastolic reading of 18 percent, than meat-eaters.[10]

- A study of Seventh-Day Adventists, half of which are vegetarians, showed lower readings of 9 and 8 points respectively, compared against Mormons who ate meat.[11]

- Very high blood pressure is 13 times more likely in meat-eaters.[12]

- Blood pressure has shown to be lowered in just 2 weeks with 8 to 10 servings of fruits and vegetables a day.[13]

- High blood pressure is uncommon or absent for those cultures, both in the East and West, eating a diet low in sodium, fat, and animal-based foods, and a diet high in fiber and potassium.[14]

- Of the senior citizens in the United States, 50 percent have high blood pressure; senior citizens in countries subsisting on plant-based diets have virtually no high blood pressure.[15]

- In African societies where hypertension is unknown their descendants in the United States experience hypertension that is epidemic.[16]

- In Third World societies where strokes and heart attacks are unheard of, those in their 80s have the same blood pressure as teenagers.[17]

A blood pressure value associated with long life, with little chance of heart and blood vessel diseases, should be about 110 over 70, or less.[18] If our blood pressure reading exceeds that number regularly, then we should hear the alarm sound loud and clear.

When it goes off we will know exactly what we have: Disaster Warning. And we will know exactly what to do: Take a stroll down the produce aisle and take the pressure off.

51: Prostate Cancer

Nine More Exams Wouldn't Be So Bad

The prostate is a walnut-size gland located just below the bladder in men. It produces about 30 percent of the fluid portion of semen. Men usually don't give the prostate a second thought until they are in a doctor's office having a routine yearly physical examination. Then they probably wished the gland was located behind the left ear.

When the doctor gloves-up, prostate cancer is probably not the man's main concern. But maybe it should be. Prostate cancer is the number one diagnosed cancer in men with 198,000 cases a year in the United States.[1] It is the third most fatal cancer in men causing 31,000 deaths a year. Maybe focusing a little more effort on its cause, and a little less effort on prostate-inspired butt jokes, would be a more productive pursuit for American men.

Like breast cancer, prostate cancer is hormone-dependent. Higher levels of androsterone and testosterone circulating in the bloodstream will produce a higher incidence of the cancer.[2] Animal fat is known to promote higher levels of these hormones in the bloodstream, either by way of the over-production of hormones or lack of fiber in the diet. It also could be a combination of the two.[3]

A meat-based diet is low in fiber, and fiber is instrumental as the catalyst of waste disposal in the body, which includes the excretion of sex hormones.[4] But whether it's over-production or inefficient excretion it doesn't matter. Either way the finger still points—we'll forgo the humor here—to just one source: the SICK diet.

- A study involving 6,500 men indicated that the risk of developing prostate cancer was increased by 3.6 times in men who ate eggs, cheese, and meat.[5]

- The risk of prostate cancer for Seventh-day Adventist vegetarian men is one-third that of the general population.[6]

- American men who consume a higher amount of dairy products increase their risk of prostate cancer by 70 percent, while those that fill up with tomatoes (lycopene), carrots (beta-carotene), and cruciferous vegetables such as broccoli and cabbage, decrease their risk by 41 percent.[7] While the plant kingdom is full of fiber, meat contains *none*.

Let's increase the study population to include other countries and cultures. A different kind of evidence but the same kind of result.

- In an analysis of 30 countries plotted on a graph, the United States ranked 3rd in daily animal fat consumption and 3rd in death rates due to prostate cancer.[8]

- In an analysis of 28 countries plotted on a graph, a 67 percent correlation existed between daily animal fat consumption and the incidence of prostate cancer.[9] Put another way: An animal-based diet directly influences the start of prostate cancer in 2 of every 3 cases.

- For every 10 men who die of prostate cancer in Western Europe only 1 man dies in Asia. Western Europeans consume 4 times more animal fat than Asians.[10]

- A man from Sweden will be 8 times more likely to die from prostate cancer than a man from Hong Kong. A Swedish man's fat intake is twice that of a Hong Kong man's.[11]

The evidence is persuasive that animal fat, as part and parcel to a meat-based diet, is prostate cancer's best friend. But if we ask the average American about the friendship most don't know that it exists. In a Cancer Awareness Survey just 2 percent of men were aware there was any link between diet and prostate cancer.[12]

It's hard to believe such a huge gap between perception and reality exists. Maybe men don't want to admit the link because they have something to gain. Certainly they don't want to give up their flesh-eating habits, but there might be something more. Androsterone and testosterone in the bloodstream increase the sexual drive and need for sexual release.[13] Given a man's motivational priorities, this might be part of the logical explanation for the surprising survey results.

It's ironic that the increased pleasure meat may bring within the context of sexual potency, also may bring increased pain— that of prostate cancer. However, the irony is not over. If a man contracts prostate cancer that requires surgery and radiation, the treatment can commonly cause impotence. A circumstance that no amount of steaks or ribs will ever undo.[14]

One in 6 men will develop prostate cancer in their lifetime.[15] The average man will lose 9 years of a normal lifespan who contracts the disease.[16] Although a routine yearly physical is not the high point of any man's day, any man would gladly accept the chance to complain about nine more prostate exams.

52: Colon Cancer

If lung cancer is the disease of cigarette smoking then colon cancer might be the disease of meat consumption. Both cancers are simple to understand. Smoke regularly sits in the lungs. The smoke contains contaminants and carcinogens foreign to the body. The lungs get sick. Meat regularly sits in the colon. The meat contains contaminants and carcinogens foreign to the body. The colon gets sick.

The cultural statistics and international studies sustain the logic. In a tabulation of 37 countries, an 82 percent correlation exists between the amount of daily animal fat consumed and the death rate from colon cancer.[1] International studies suggest that fully 95 percent of colon cancer cases have a nutritional connection. A non-confrontational, scientific way of saying that if we consume meat, dairy, and eggs, and we contract colon cancer, we shouldn't be surprised.[2]

Is this to say we *will* get colon cancer if we regularly consume these foods? Who knows. Will a car coming the other way eventually hit us if we regularly run stop signs? It's anybody's guess. But what we can say is this: Every 4 minutes an American will be diagnosed with colon cancer and every 10 minutes an American will die from it. This translates to 135,000 new cases a year and 56,000 deaths.[3] Apparently a lot of people get hit by cars.

The human intestinal structure and colon are quite different from those of natural carnivores. Our colons are very long, winding, and deep-pocketed. Carnivores' intestines are very short, smooth, and relatively straight. It wouldn't be a big stretch to conclude that these fundamentally opposite systems might have been designed to process fundamentally opposite foods.

Colon cancer is cancer of the lower intestine, the last 5 feet of conduit where water is absorbed, and solid waste material collects until it's excreted. Let's take a bite of meat and see what goes on in our digestive track.

WITCHES' BREW: Because of its density, the fat from the meat requires the body to produce an excess of bile acids to break it down. This acid combines with the bacteria in our intestines to produce powerful carcinogens. The protein in the meat increases the production of fecal ammonia, which is implicated in tumor promotion also.[4] A witches' brew has now taken up residence in the colon.

SOUP CAN UNDER THE SINK: The piece of meat contains no fiber. Fiber has two functions to perform. One of the jobs of fiber is to act as a sponge and absorb the carcinogens. The other is to act as a transporter to move the waste out of our bodies. Given that fat is solid at body temperature, the mass sitting in our colons might look like the contents of the soup can meat-eaters often keep under their kitchen sink to collect fat from the skillet.[5]

SNAIL IN MOLASSES: The human intestinal system is 25 feet long, with a structure of deep pockets and hairpin turns. This creates further obstacles to waste elimination. Where it typically takes plant-based foods 35 hours to reach daylight, the waste matter from meat can take as long as 83 hours.[6] A portion of that time the carcinogenic mass snuggles up to the colon walls.

It's easy to understand why natural carnivores have shorter, smoother, and straighter digestive tracks to quickly expel waste matter.[7]

CLUES, RIGHT UNDER OUR NOSES: Although we aren't aware of the process going on inside our digestive tracts that could potentially lead to colon cancer, there are some outward signs that might be trying to tell us something.

Feeling sluggish, bloated, and constipated, straining to eliminate, popping out hemorrhoid and varicose veins, and jarring the olfactory lobe with unpleasant odor, is not the way it is supposed to be. A plant-based diet produces none of these byproducts of elimination. Yes, even the odor. Leave a dead animal on the kitchen floor. Do the same with a dead plant. Then compare the odors after 3 to 4 days. What occurs in the body is not much different.

Even if we contract colon cancer it is not necessarily deadly. Surgery can often be performed to remove the cancerous colon and a substitute is available to take its place—a sporty colostomy bag that can easily be nestled between one's beeper and cell phone.

Despite the evidence, and logical basis of the disease, only 2 percent of Americans believe that eating less meat can reduce the risk of colon cancer.[8] Among them might have been John Morgan, president of Riverside Meat Packers. He was quoted as saying, "Beef is the backbone of the American diet. To think that meat causes cancer is ridiculous."

We can't debate it with him though. He died. Of colon cancer.[9]

53: Breast Cancer

PINK RIBBONS OR GREEN VEGETABLES?

In 1971 America began the War on Cancer. Then a woman had a 1 in 20 chance of contracting breast cancer. Thirty years and billions of dollars later, a woman has a 1 in 8 chance of contracting breast cancer.[1] With casualties increasing there is no doubt we are losing the war.

Often wars are lost because the wrong weapons were used, or the enemy was not well understood. Could both these reasons apply to the war on breast cancer? Let's retreat, lick our wounds, find out where we've gone wrong, and consider redrawing the battle plan.

Breast cancer is diagnosed in 184,000 American women each year, with 44,000 deaths attributed to the disease.[2] It seems terribly unjust, and ironic, that the most prevalent cancer in females would turn the symbols of womanhood—personifying beauty and nurturing—against her as a weapon in her own demise.

No one could argue that the medical profession and women haven't done everything in their power to try and combat this disease. First by detection, such as sophisticated mammography, regular self-exams, awareness walks, and pink ribbons. And second by treatment, such as powerful chemotherapy drugs, precise surgery, and pinpoint radiation.

So why, then, are we not winning the war?

A breast cancer cell doubles every 100 days. A mammogram can't detect a tumor until it reaches one-half centimeter in size.[3] It takes one-half billion cells to reach one-half centimeter. It takes more than 8 years to reach one-half billion cells. In most, if not all, cases by the time cancer is detectable by a mammogram the cancer has already entered the bloodstream and spread to other parts of the body, where half the time it will metastasize, growing a new tumor.[4] Rarely does a woman die as a direct result of a tumor growing in her breast.[5]

The mammogram, instead of being a device to detect cancer before it has spread so a cure might be possible, appears to be a device to detect cancer that has been growing for 8 years and has already spread. What does the National Cancer Institute have to say about the mammogram?

"Adding an annual mammogram to a careful physical examination of the breasts does not improve breast cancer survival rates compared to getting the examination alone."[6]

Although the cancer has spread beyond the breast, we fortunately have chemotherapy to destroy the cancer no matter where it lurks in the body. What does the British medical journal, *Lancet*, have to report about chemotherapy?

"Chemotherapy has only a limited effectiveness against any tumor that is large or has spread; its successes are generally with small, early tumors." Several studies indicate that chemotherapy has no survival value in breast cancer. Survival may even have been shortened in some breast cancer patients given chemotherapy.[7]

It's not a wonder we are losing the war. We can't catch it early, and we can't kill it after it's begun. What else can we do? We have given detection and treatment our best effort. What about *prevention*?

The National Cancer Institute stated in 1995 that, "Breast cancer is simply not a preventable disease." The American Cancer Society announced in 1997, "There are no practical ways to prevent breast cancer, only early detection."[8] The company that has sponsored Breast Cancer Awareness Month since 1984, Zeneca Pharmaceuticals, motto is "Early Detection is your Best Protection."

Apparently prevention is not an option. At least not an option within the context of the diet most Americans subscribe to.

Breast cancer is a hormone-dependent cancer: The more estrogen in the breast, the more likely cancer will develop and influence the rate of growth.[9] How then does diet play a part in promoting higher estrogen levels, and what are the rates of breast cancer for those eating the WELL diet versus the SICK diet?

- After estrogen circulates through the body it leaves through the intestines. However, dietary fat inhibits absorption leaving more estrogen in the body.[10] It should be no surprise then that estrogen levels are 50 percent higher in omnivore women, and herbivore women excrete 2 to 3 times more estrogen in the feces than their diet counterparts.[11]

- Menstruation starts 4 years earlier and menopause begins 4 years later for women eating diets that are higher in fat. That's 8 years of higher levels of estrogen circulating in their bodies. The cumulative effect translates to double the risk in their lifetime of getting breast cancer.[12]

- Body fat promotes estrogen stimulation, which would mean obese women should have higher incidences of breast cancer. And they do. Their risk is twice that of women who are not obese.[13]

- When daily animal fat consumption was plotted against breast cancer incident rates for 37 countries, a 76 percent correlation was indicated. Put another way: An Animal-based diet is implicated in 3 of every 4 incidences of breast cancer.[14]

- Affluent women in Japan who eat meat have an 8.5 times greater risk of contracting breast cancer than do poorer Japanese women who can't afford meat.[15]

- A study of premenopausal women older than 40 found that the risk of postmenopausal cancer decreased by 54 percent with a vegetarian diet.[16]

Given the strong evidence implicating meat and animal fat in the promotion of breast cancer, one has to wonder why diet has not been given much, if any, recognition. One has to wonder why all the focus is on mammograms, pink ribbons, chemotherapy, and the like, and not on prevention by way of the foods we eat. One has to wonder why after 30 years of regress instead of progress, the fundamental approaches to conquering breast cancer haven't changed.

One has to wonder how long it will be before we realize that one green—money—is undermining the need for a different green—the green in the produce aisle.

54: Ovarian Cancer

SHE DID HER BEST TO PROTECT OUR EGGS

The ovaries produce eggs, the reproductive cells responsible for the propagation of our species. We would think Mother Nature would have made the ovaries impenetrable to outside threats ensuring the viability of our species. Maybe she tried.

Of the big three cancers that are hormone-dependent—prostate, breast, and ovarian—ovarian cancer has but 12 percent of the incidences of the other two, with 23,400 diagnosis a year.[1] Mother Nature also made *two* ovaries, possibly to increase our odds of success. We might say she was smart enough not to have placed all her eggs in one basket. It appears then she *has* tried.

Somehow though, humans have still found a way to gum up the works. No doubt Mother Nature accounted for this too by making this cancer one of the most lethal. Maybe this was her way to get our attention so we might be motivated to figure out what we were doing wrong. Because even though American women have only a 1 in 55 chance of developing ovarian cancer in their lifetime, if they do contract it, 3 of 4 women will see less than 5 more years of life. The disease claims 13,900 lives a year.[2]

Let's heed her warning and go figure it out.

Unlike prostate and breast cancer, ovarian cancer seems more prone to be initiated by dairy and eggs, than by meat. Eggs? A profound irony or merely a coincidence. The seven risk factors, foods implicated in the increased risk of contracting ovarian cancer are: eggs, milk, cottage cheese, yogurt, animal source calcium, animal fat, and cholesterol.[3] The ovaries are strongly influenced by sex hormones particularly estrogen, and omnivore women have 50 percent higher estrogen levels circulating in their bloodstreams.[4]

What do a sampling of studies reveal about the causes of ovarian cancer?

- A case control study in Canada found that ovarian cancer was associated with saturated fat intake, particularly egg consumption. Women who ate eggs three or more times a week, were 3 times more likely to get ovarian cancer than vegetarian women.[5]

- A study of 16,000 women in Norway showed that those who drank two or more glasses of milk a day had a substantially higher risk of ovarian cancer than women who drank less.[6]

- The process of breaking down the lactose (milk sugar) into galactose evidently damages the ovaries.[7]

- In 1989, Harvard University researchers noted that women with ovarian cancer had low blood levels of transferase, an enzyme involved in the metabolism of dairy foods.[8]

- The risk for ovarian cancer increases up to 3 times with the consumption of yogurt and cottage cheese.[9]

- A study of dietary factors and epithelial ovarian cancer from *The British Journal of Cancer* reported a significant dose-response relationship between the intake of fat from animal sources and the risk of developing ovarian cancer.[10]

- A comparison of 30 countries showed that ovarian cancer death was associated with higher per capita consumption of total fat, in particular, animal fat.[11]

- A study in *The Journal of the National Cancer* Institute found that the higher the women's cholesterol level, the greater their risk of ovarian cancer.[12]

These studies add up to a compelling argument, one that would be difficult to ignore. Yet even vegetarian women, fearful they are not receiving enough calcium or protein, often compensate with an increased consumption of dairy products and eggs. This would appear to be a grave error, with grave the operative word.

In contrast to foods from the animal kingdom, foods from the plant kingdom significantly lower the circulating levels of estrogen in women.[13] Fiber, antioxidants, and phytochemicals present in plants have shown to have a protective effect against ovarian cancer. A study done in California of Seventh-day Adventists found they had a lower risk of ovarian cancer than the general population.[14]

When we hear about the risk factors of ovarian cancer, diet is often not mentioned, or if it is, it's given secondary status. Other risk factors such as, earlier menstruation, later menopause, Caucasian race, Jewish culture, family history, and never having children, are more prominently declared, deflecting the focus from diet.[15]

Can this apparent contradiction be explained? Let's take a shot.

MENSTRUATION AND MENOPAUSE: Women on higher-fat diets start menstruation earlier and begin menopause later increasing the span of time that they have higher levels of estrogen in their bodies.[16]

CAUCASIAN RACE: The white race generally inhabits western countries, the United States and Europe, which have a much higher intake of fat than do Eastern cultures.[17]

JEWISH CULTURE: The Holiday meals for the Jewish culture include foods such as shank bone of a lamb, brisket, kugel, latkes, roasted egg, and the traditional fried foods of Hanukkah. Is the day-to-day Jewish diet also an animal fat, meat-based diet?

FAMILY HISTORY: Environment may have more to do with family history than genetics. Children generally eat the same foods as their parents for 18 years and then carry those learned habits on into adulthood.

NO CHILDREN: There is a strong correlation between animal fat and infertility.[18] In how many cases did couples not have children because they *couldn't*? The same diet that can cause infertility can also cause ovarian cancer. So rather than being a causal relationship, it's a parallel circumstance.

The annual death toll of 12,000 due to ovarian cancer will not threaten the extinction of the human species. Therefore, despite our behavior in the name of diet, Mother Nature has succeeded in her design and our survival. However, for 12,000 women every year there is not success and survival has a different meaning.

Mother Nature got our attention and we figured out where we went wrong. It seems safe to say now, when it comes to choosing our diet, we can put all our eggs into one basket.

55: Cancers

MAYBE NOT SO RANDOM AND MYSTERIOUS

There are many diseases that we can contract, but no disease scares us more than cancer.

We have come to think of cancer as a mysterious, random occurrence, striking anyone, at any age, at any time. A shadowy dark phantom floating through the air attaching itself to 1.3 million Americans every year, killing more than a half million.[1]

With other diseases we feel we have at least a modicum of understanding and control over their cause and treatment, so they aren't so unsettling as cancer. Our stereotypical perception of other diseases runs along these lines:

- A virus, even though it might strike at random, usually runs its course then goes away.

- An infection is usually contained in one place and can be controlled with drugs.

- A lifestyle disease, like a sexually transmitted disease or liver cirrhosis, although sometimes deadly is often a function of choices made.

- A circulatory disease, although twice as deadly as cancer in total numbers, at least progresses slowly, often provides warning signs before it does major damage, and can be improved with adjustments to lifestyle.

But cancer seems to be the exception to reason and logic. It can attack any body part, spread at will, and end a life in a matter of months. One would expect a random act to be low in incidences, but 1.3 million a year? A person diagnosed every 25 seconds?

Do we really have a runaway demon on our hands or have we grossly misjudged the disease?

According to the National Cancer Institute, 80 percent of cancers are due to factors that have been identified and are within our control.[2] According to Dr. Robert Hatherill, 90 percent (60 food and 30 smoking) of cancers are due to factors that have been identified and are within our control.[3]

What these two sources are saying in essence is: 8.5 out of 10 people who contract cancer did so due to factors within their control, most often through food or smoking. The other 1.5 people contracted cancer due to viruses, genetics or environment.

Hardly a mysterious and random occurrence—clearly a comprehensible and logical consequence—most definitely an erroneous and gross misjudgment on our parts.

Let's look at a few excerpts from studies and see what effect foods and their components have on the risk of the following cancers: lung, pancreatic, bladder, brain, lymphoma, Hodgkin's, melanoma, various skin, cervical, esophageal, childhood cancers, childhood leukemia, testicular, mouth and throat, and all cancers.

- LUNG: (Even if one smokes.) The risk is reduced with the consumption of fruits and vegetables. The risk is increased with high levels of cholesterol.[4]

- PANCREATIC: The risk is reduced by eating citrus fruits, lentils, beans, and soy. The risk is increased by fat, animal protein, and cooked meat and fish.[5]

- BLADDER: The risk is reduced by eating fruits and vegetables. The risk is doubled by consuming meat and excess animal protein.[6]

- BRAIN: The risk is increased by meat, fish, and poultry, and by cured meats such as ham.[7]

- LYMPHOMA: The risk is reduced for women by the higher intake of fruits and cruciferous vegetables. The risk is increased by dairy protein and red meat.[8]

- HODGKIN'S: The risk is increased by beef and dairy proteins.[9]

- MELANOMA: The risk is reduced by calcium, vitamin D_3, carotenoids, and vitamin E.[10]

- SKIN: The risk is reduced by vitamin E, vitamin C, and carotenoids.[11]

- SKIN BASAL CELL CARCINOMA: The risk is reduced with a well-rounded intake of all vitamins.[12]

- SKIN BASAL CELL AND SQUAMOUS CELL: Skin cancer patients put on a low-fat diet for 2 years reportedly showed a significant decrease in the number of new skin cancers compared with patients who maintained a high-fat diet.[13]

- CERVICAL: The risk is reduced by antioxidant nutrients from vegetables and fruits. (Antioxidant nutrient levels were deficient in women with cervical dysplasia.) The risk is increased by fat and protein.[14]

- ESOPHAGEAL: The risk is reduced with pasta, rice, raw vegetables, and citrus fruits.[15]

- CHILDHOOD CANCERS: The risk is doubled with the consumption of hamburgers, or hot dogs at least once a week.[16]

- CHILDHOOD LEUKEMIA: The risk is increased 10 times with a high consumption of hot dogs.[17]

- TESTICULAR: The risk is reduced by lycopene, the principal carotenoid in tomatoes that has powerful antioxidant activity.[18]

- MOUTH AND THROAT: The risk is reduced for people who eat relatively high amounts of whole grains.[19]

- ALL CANCERS: The risk is reduced with high fruit and vegetable consumption as a result of carotenoids, folic acid, vitamin C, flavonoids, phytoestrogens, and isothiocyanates.[20]

How did we come to view cancer as a frightening, mysterious entity that was beyond our control, rather than as a disease so deeply rooted in diet? Did we conclude that something so complicated couldn't possibly have a simple solution? Why not? How many times in life have we solved challenging problems with simple solutions—the more difficult the problem, the simpler the answer?

We can't blame the medical or scientific communities for lagging behind. Diet and cancer were first linked more than a hundred years ago, cited in an article from *Scientific American* in 1892.[21] In the 1920s, Dr. Max Gerson, believed the root of cancer was the Western diet, so he treated his cancer patients with a vegetable and fruit diet with excellent results.[22] In the 1970s, Dr. William Donald Kelly, produced long-term remission in his patients with diet and nutrition.[23]

Our body is too fine a machine to go reeling out of control, killing an American once every minute, without a logical and sound reason. It just wouldn't make any sense. Nor would it make any sense to fear something that we have 80 percent or more control over.

Most likely, overcoming our fear of cancer will occur at the same time we overcome another fear—our fear of change.

56: Diabetes

FAT MEN GUARDING THE DOORS

Dreams seem to be nothing more than random neural firings. But one night a man had the following dream that may have had symbolic meaning. He described it like this:

"There were 20 or 30 of us men, all dressed in white, at our first day on the job. We were going down a long, red hallway. We didn't know where to go, but fortunately some nice young ladies appeared. They said they were escorts, and they all had on nametags that said, Lynn. They were assigned to take us men to our workstations. They told us how sweet we were, and then they took us by the arm.

"As we walked down the hallway there were doors every 10 feet or so. Some doors were blocked by big fat men, others weren't. We sensed the workstations were through the doors, but there weren't enough unguarded doors to let everybody through. The hallway began to fill up with more men and escorts. After a while some men were without escorts, apparently the company had run out of them. The scene became chaotic. Anybody that couldn't get through a door was fired and sent down a yellow hallway that led outside the building…"

It was then that the man woke up.

The dream was later interpreted as a dream about adult-onset type II diabetes.

Diabetes is officially the 7th leading cause of death in the United States taking 193,000 lives annually, however some place it third due to its capacity to instigate and complicate heart disease, kidney disease, stroke, and other diseases.[1] There are 15.7 million diabetics in the United States, with 798,000 new cases reported each year.[2]

What's going on in the diabetic's body, and what does the dream have to do with it? Let's analyze the dream's symbolism and see.

> The sugar (sweet white-attired men) in the bloodstream (red hallway) is headed to cell membranes (workstations) escorted by insulin (escort girls named Lynn) by way of insulin receptor sites (doors) to perform fundamental metabolic processes (the job).
>
> Because fats (big fat men) in the body are hiding the insulin receptor sites, the efficiency of the metabolic processes is greatly reduced. Thus, sugar and insulin begin to build up in the bloodstream, where they are eventually excreted (fired) in the urine (yellow hallway). The result of this scenario is diabetes.
>
> After a time the problem worsens because the body's thermostat makes the pancreas produce more insulin to make up for the inefficiencies. Eventually it wears out and produces less insulin (men without escorts) making the diabetes even more serious.[3]

The point of the dream is to demonstrate that adult-onset diabetes, generally perceived as a disease of too little insulin, is more precisely a disease of too much fat.

We know that the SICK diet contains close to 40 percent of its calories in fat, when the WELL diet contains close to 10 percent of its calories in fat. We know from viewing photomicrographs that fat is hiding insulin receptor sites.[4] When we replace the 30 percent of excessive fat calories, with complex carbohydrates and accompanying fiber calories, insulin can do its job again.

- One study that placed subjects on a low-fat vegan diet saw their blood sugar levels drop 28 percent.[5] Fiber has shown to slow absorption of sugars into the bloodstream, better synchronizing with insulin.[6]

- One study placed 10 patients on a 70 percent carbohydrate, high-fiber diet. Sixteen days later, 9 of the patients were able to stop insulin.[7]

- One study placed 80 patients on a low-fat diet, and 60 percent were off insulin in 6 weeks. Two more studies had 75 percent success rates.[8]

- Diabetes is rare among Africans, Asians, and Polynesians; these cultures subsist on plant-based diets.[9]

Type I childhood diabetes is a different *animal*. The cow maybe—with its milk as the problem?

   This diabetes *is* the result of the pancreas failing to produce insulin. Strong evidence indicates that the protein in cows' milk stimulates antibodies that destroy the insulin-producing pancreatic beta cells. Cows' milk protein can be obtained directly by drinking milk, or through breast milk if the mother drinks cows' milk. One study found antibodies to cows' milk protein present in all 142 diabetic children at the time the disease was diagnosed.[10] Animal proteins are implicated as the cause of many autoimmune diseases. Childhood diabetes may be just a different book from the same author.

   Diabetes, of either type, is often viewed as a disease that causes thirst, excessive urination, and the need for a candy bar now and then. This perception masks the true nature of the disease—that of a predator and a killer.

- Diabetics have a 2 to 4 times greater risk of heart disease and stroke.[11]

- Diabetics, at a 60 to 70 percent rate, have high blood pressure and nervous system damage.[12]

- Diabetics account for 12,000 to 24,000 new cases of blindness each year.[13]

- Diabetics have an 18 times greater risk of kidney disease, and 100,000 undergo dialysis or kidney transplantation each year.[14]

- Diabetics, as a consequence of the disease, incur dental problems, complications from pregnancy, amputations, and coma.[15]

To underestimate this disease is to underestimate a freight train bearing down on us.

We can change our eating habits now. We don't have to wait until we have a dream that includes guys in white clothes, men who are fat, and girls named Lynn, before we wake up.

57: Kidney Disease

NOT QUITE MAINTENANCE FREE

We would never consider ignoring a clogged toilet, or not paying our waste disposal bills. We generally don't neglect changing our car's oil filter, or our home's furnace filter. But how often do we give *our* waste disposal and filtering system—the kidneys—any attention?

The majority answer might be: "We don't have to think about them, they don't require maintenance, filter changes, or unclogging."

If our furnace or car breaks down, or the toilet or trashcans overflow, we have options, and we can live with it. If our kidneys do the same, we have few options, and we can't live. Period.

Fortunately for us, Mother Nature, possibly anticipating our apathy, and recognizing the crucial role of the kidneys, designed these organs to be virtually indestructible. And just to be on the safe side she gave us two of them.

They are able to filter 50 gallons of blood per day, 1.4 million gallons in a lifetime.[1] This volume is a testament to the design and durability of the kidneys. Even if 75 percent of the kidneys' tissues are destroyed and turned to non-functioning scar tissue, they will continue to operate showing little systemic evidence of disease.[2]

Consequently we should see few, if any, problems with these marvelous machines.

- Americans who are at risk of developing chronic kidney and urinary tract disease—58 million.[3]

- Americans who will form kidney stones—33 million.[4]

- Americans who have kidney and urinary diseases—20 million.[5]

- Americans who have to take dialysis treatments to stay alive—245,000.[6]

- Americans who will die of kidney and urinary illnesses each year—66,000.[7]

- Americans who are currently awaiting life-saving kidney transplants—50,000.[8]

Maybe Mother Nature didn't anticipate everything. Such as a diet of animal-based foods. Let's run some of the components of this diet through the kidneys and see how they do.

PROTEIN: The American SICK diet includes 2 to 3 times the protein the body requires.[9] Excess protein in our diet makes the kidneys work harder by excreting more water, raising the fluid pressure that causes tissue damage and loss of kidney function.[10] And because proteins are not stored in the body they must be eliminated quickly, which increases the filtration rate.[11]

PROTEIN AND KIDNEY STONES: Twelve percent of the population will form kidney stones, a process not unlike an oyster forming a pearl, but not as coveted.[12] Kidney stones are 99 percent diet related and are virtually unknown in countries where people consume few animal-based foods.[13]

Too much protein, which is acidic, raises the pH in the blood. This requires the alkaline calcium from our bones to neutralize it. All this extra calcium has to exit the body. And it does by way of our kidneys often forming stones before it bids farewell.[14]

Apparently giving birth to a kidney stone is on a pain scale with giving *birth*. But the kidney's product doesn't make the pain seem as worthwhile.

DAIRY PROTEIN: Animal protein from dairy products, especially milk, cross-react with our body's protein-generating antibodies. These antigen-antibody complexes are trapped in the tiny blood vessels of the kidneys causing inflammation and damage.[15]

FAT AND CHOLESTEROL: Fats are toxic to the kidneys. High-cholesterol levels can contribute to kidney disease.[16]

PHOSPHATES: Phosphates from meat and dairy are thought to damage kidneys.[17]

OTHER DISEASE: Diabetes and hypertension, both byproducts of a meat-based diet habit, can destroy kidney function.[18]

The connection between diet and kidney disease is not a new revelation. Since the 1940s this information has been documented in medical journals and reported to physicians.

- A study from 1946 found that of the 100 patients placed on a low-protein diet, 65 showed objective improvement in kidney function.[19]

- A study from 1984 found that when 228 kidney patients were placed on a diet that only moderately restricted protein intake, their kidney disease slowed 3 to 5 times more than patients that were not placed on the diet.[20]

- A study from 1991 found that for one type of renal disease, nephritis, a vegan diet improved kidney function.[21]

As rugged and invulnerable as our kidneys are, when greater than 95 percent of their functionality is gone, then it is time to go looking—looking for a kidney transplant, dialysis machine, or gravesite.

The first is tough to get, and the last one we would rather not think about. The second option, dialysis, is the most likely. This process requires a commitment of 3 to 4 hours at a time, three days a week, if we want to stay alive.

We spent a lifetime ignoring our kidneys, claiming that they didn't require maintenance, filter changes, or unclogging. Well, the dialysis machine we are hooked up to now *does*. Let's hope the dialysis operator isn't as negligent as we once were.

58: Aging

FEEDING WEAPONS TO THE GOOD GUYS

There is a constant struggle going on between good and evil—good guys versus the bad guys. In this case though it's not the world we live in, it's the world that lives in *us*. A world comprised of 100 trillion cells, each cell having a life of its own. A life that entails eating, working, reproducing, and dying.[1] Just like us.

How our bodies age and how long our bodies live is greatly dependent on whether we feed weapons to the good guys or the bad guys. And "feed" is the operative word. Because on average humans eat 5 pounds of food per day, 140,000 pounds of food in a lifetime.[2] Is there a quantifiable way to measure how well we are doing in the struggle?

According to program and damage theorists, humans have a genetically programmed maximum life expectancy of 120 years.[3] That means the average American, in theory, is falling 40 years short of a full life. And given that 1 out of every 3 Americans has a degenerative disease, the quality of the last 10 to 20 years of the 80 years makes that life even less full.[4]

Apparently we must be feeding weapons to the bad guys. Who are the bad guys, who are the good guys, and what are the weapons?

The bad guys are free radicals. The good guys are antioxidants and phytochemicals. Let's explore what these substances are, where they come from, and what effect they have on aging and disease.

FREE RADICALS: Free radicals are natural byproducts of our metabolism, and some are products of outside sources such as food. In both cases they are unstable oxygen molecules looking for trouble. They attack and do structural damage to our healthy cells causing destruction throughout the body. The result is the development of disease and the acceleration of aging.

Some of the foods that add to the free radical load are fats, oils, milk, and iron.[5] Iron might be the worst offender. It is the catalyst for the formation of free radicals. When it combines with oxygen it affects the body the way rust affects metal. Meat provides an overabundance of the more absorbable iron that the body accumulates and can't get rid of.[6]

ANTIOXIDANTS AND PHYTOCHEMICALS: Antioxidants are protective chemicals that neutralize the free radicals and the tissue oxidation that they cause. Some examples are vitamin C, E, beta-carotene, and folic acid.[7] Virtually all come from the plant kingdom.

Phytochemicals include at least 1,000 active compounds such as tocotrienols, limonoids, and glucarates found only in plants. They inhibit carcinogens, fight disease, and strengthen the immune system.[8]

Eating from the plant kingdom not only provides us weapons to neutralize free radicals and combat disease and aging, but these foods also replace animal-based foods that increase the body's production of free radicals.

When we haven't armed our allies sufficiently to keep the enemy in check, there are some real-life consequences of the minute chemistry going on inside of us. For example:

SKIN: The aging of our skin is due to the sun. Plants spend much of their time in the sun, but have we ever seen a wrinkled leaf? Beta-carotene is the reason why. It can protect our skin from free radical damage as it does the plants.[9] Carrots and sweet potatoes contain ample amounts.

EYES: Cataracts form in the eyes due to constant light exposure and possibly milk lactose.[10] Vitamins A, C, and beta-carotene neutralize the free radicals. One study found that 3.5 servings of fruit and vegetables a day could reduce the risk of cataracts by 6 times.[11]

ALZHEIMER'S DISEASE: When free radicals attack the brain cells, message transmission is impeded resulting in memory, concentration, and motor skill degeneration, increasing the risk of Alzheimer's.[12] Blueberries, which have strong antioxidant properties, have shown to significantly improve motor and memory skills in rats as they age.[13]

AUTOIMMUNE DISEASES: When free radicals attack immune cells the immune system weakens. This diminishes the ability of the immune cells to distinguish between friend and foe. When they attack friends—healthy tissue—autoimmune diseases like lupus, multiple sclerosis, and rheumatoid arthritis can result.[14]

CANCER: Free radicals can bully their way into the DNA of a cell and kill it, or worse, cause it to replicate abnormally giving rise to cancer. If the immune system cells have also been compromised by free radicals then their ability to recognize cancer as a foe is diminished, allowing the cancer cell to multiply at will.[15]

OTHER DEGENERATIVE DISEASES: Cumulative free radical damage can also take its toll on our arterial cells furthering atherosclerosis, the hardening and clogging of the arteries.[16]

Kidney disease, liver disease, Parkinson's disease, stroke, and hypertension are all more likely because of the unchecked activity of free radicals.[17]

Can we show the cumulative effect of the battle—translating cell success or failure into human success or failure—based on which weapons are employed?

The Hunzas of Kashmir, who subsist on a 99 percent vegetarian diet, work and play at age 80 and beyond, have no cavities, father children, and have no heart disease into their 90s. They are active at age 100 and maintain 20/20 vision. Their broken bones heal in 3 weeks and they usually die of natural causes.[18]

Conversely, Eskimos who live primarily on meat and fish rarely exceed 30 years of age. The Kirgese of Eastern Russia, who at one time lived chiefly on meat, rarely survived past the age of 40.[19]

Armed with all this knowledge, it wouldn't be too surprising for us to have the following experience someday.

*****

One day while strolling down the produce aisle at our local grocery store, stockpiling ammunition against the ongoing fight against free radicals, we bump into the store manager. It's the fifth store manager we've known since shopping there. The other four have passed on. He asks how we are doing and we tell him not so well. Not so well because the store has run out of birthday candles. Why is that a problem? Because now we won't have enough to celebrate our birthday on Saturday: our 116th.

59: Alzheimer's Disease

GRAND FINALE OF DEGENERATIVE DISEASES?

Alzheimer's disease might well be the fifth dimension, a place that falls between life and death. Or it could be a nightmare we never wake up from. We don't know. We can only speculate because those who are afflicted can't tell us. And because they can't tell us, we are left to characterize the disease as best we can.

Is it directly related to the aging process? Perhaps a new strain of pathogen yet unclassified? Maybe a disease somehow tied to the technology age? No matter how it's portrayed, most would agree it's a unique and puzzling disorder like no other disease seen before.

Or maybe not.

Could Alzheimer's disease be yet another variation on the theme. That of a degenerative disease, perhaps the grand finale, brought on by a lifelong diet of flesh eating?

Why couldn't it be?

Let's see if there's evidence to support the possibility.

- A study revealed that Alzheimer's patients have low blood levels of the vitamin folic acid and high levels of the protein building block homocysteine.[1] Homocysteine is converted from methionine, a protein 2 to 3 times more prevalent in meat.[2] Folic acid found in green leafy vegetables and whole grains prevents methionine from being converted to homocysteine.[3]

- A study revealed that the homocysteine levels dropped 13 to 20 percent in just 1 week after the subjects switched to a vegan diet.[4]

- A study revealed that people who remained free from any form of dementia had consumed higher amounts of beta-carotene, vitamin C, vitamin E, and vegetables, than the people in the study who developed Alzheimer's disease.[5]

- A study revealed that subjects who ate meat, including poultry and fish, were nearly 3 times as likely to suffer from some form of dementia as their herbivore counterparts.[6]

- A study revealed that cox-2, an enzyme linked to the autoimmune driven arthritis, is also active in the brains of people who have Alzheimer's.[7] Autoimmune diseases may well have their roots in animal protein.

- A study revealed that people who suffered mini-strokes were at greater risk of contracting Alzheimer's.[8]

- A study revealed that reduced blood cholesterol levels (in this study cholesterol was lowered by drugs), lowered the risk of developing Alzheimer's disease and other forms of dementia by 73 percent.[9]

- A study revealed that high blood pressure increases the risk of Alzheimer's.[10]

- A 10-year study revealed a link between the incidence of diabetes and Alzheimer's.[11] Diabetes may well have its roots in animal fat.

- A study revealed that free radicals interacting with iron, ever so present in the damage to other parts of the body, also play a part in the development of Alzheimer's.[12]

At least within the context of these studies, Alzheimer's disease doesn't appear to be much more than the final chapter in the book of degenerative diseases.

Is it possible that Alzheimer's disease only *appears* to be a new and evolving menace? That in reality it's a function of catching up to the disease through knowledge and advanced diagnostics bringing it onto our radar screen?

Alzheimer's disease has been diagnosed in 4 million Americans. Roughly 10 percent of those older than 65, and 50 percent of those older than 85 have the disease.[13] Many doctors are seeing an increase in Alzheimer's patients in their 40s and 50s.[14] By the year 2040, 14 million Americans are expected to be stricken with the disease.[15]

The last chapter of our lives, like the first chapter of our lives, requires knowledge of the three R's. But the second time around the R's are different. They are: Remember, Reminisce, and Recognize. To remember our accomplishments, to reminisce about the good times, and to recognize our surroundings and children. Alzheimer's disease does not subscribe to the circular theory of life. It doesn't care.

When we think of degenerative disease we think of deterioration of the *body*. We don't think of deterioration of the mind. But the brain is no more, or no less, vulnerable to the ravages of our diet. The components of what we eat don't just circulate below the neck.

Because of this perception, and because the degeneration of the mind seems more profound and tragic than the degeneration of the body, we see Alzheimer's disease as a whole different ballgame.

But there is only *one* ballgame, and if we want to continue to play it, we may want to change our thinking—while we still can.

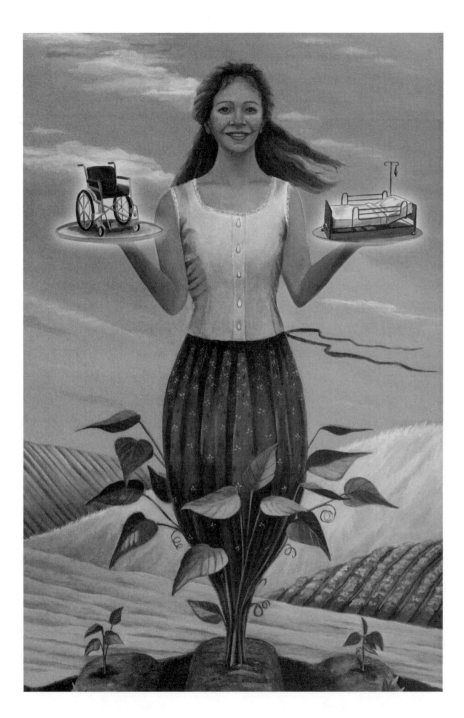

Food Does Not Discriminate

∾ 8 ∾
Disease: Hardships
100 TRILLION CELLS — NONE ARE SAFE

Because the wrong foods don't discriminate, no cell is safe.

Ahead in this chapter…

Does Britt Tilbones have OSTEOPOROSIS because of too little calcium intake, or too much protein intake? Get "just the facts" from an unlikely source.

Find out what Dr. Endd and Dr. Dometri might learn from others about the cause and cure of ENDOMETRIOSIS.

Is HEARING LOSS the result of aging, or is it only the personification of aging?

Can the green food chase away the white cane? The causes of VISION LOSS appear to be as clear as 20/20.

For a certain segment of the population IMPOTENCE, INFERTILITY, and HAIR LOSS might be compelling reasons to motivate a diet change.

Bulky, fibrous cellulose or HEMORRHOIDS, HERNIA, and APPENDICITIS? We have a choice.

Explore the digestive track first-hand, and witness the damage the wrong foods have on it directly, by way of ULCERS, CROHN'S disease, and DIVERTICULITIS.

What could cause one of Nature's greatest achievements— the immune system—to turn on us, resulting in more than 100 AUTOIMMUNE DISEASES?

The cause and cure for ASTHMA is very much a mystery. Who better to call on then, than Sherlock Holmes.

CHILDHOOD ILLNESSES are a tragedy, but they can also be an abomination. Learn the difference, and make our children's summers last forever.

Play the board game, FATIGUED, and see who can reach: The final square first, with a plant-based energy burst!

Do heredity and environment determine solely who we are, or is there a connection between FOOD AND BEHAVIOR, too?

60: Osteoporosis

OFFICER, SOMEONE IS STEALING MY BONES!

OFFICER: Your name, Ma'am?

WOMAN: Britt, Britt Tilbones.

OFFICER: Now what seems to be the problem, Ms. Tilbones?

WOMAN: Someone is stealing my bones. I mean, I've shrunk 2 inches in 2 years, and I've fractured a hip and my wrist in the last 6 months. I know I'm 65 years old, but should this be happening to me?

OFFICER: No, Ma'am. There is no flaw in your skeleton, either. It was meant to support you without any problems for 85 years or more.[1] You have a disease called osteoporosis and you're not alone. You see, 20 million American women suffer from it.[2] The disease causes someone to fracture a bone every 20 seconds, and a hip every 3 minutes, in the United States.[3] Ma'am, I'm sorry to break it to you, but the average American woman by your age has lost one-third of her skeleton.[4]

WOMAN: Sergeant, please don't say break.

OFFICER: Yes, Ma'am.

WOMAN: By the way, Sergeant, you may call me Britt.

OFFICER: Yes, Ma'am.

WOMAN: I drink a lot of milk, take calcium supplements, but apparently nothing is helping.

OFFICER: Yes, Ma'am, they won't. Osteoporosis is not a disease of too little calcium, it is a disease of too much protein. Animal protein, Ma'am.[5]

WOMAN: Excuse me?

OFFICER: Yes, Ma'am. If you are the average American you ingest at least twice the protein your body requires. It's 70 percent animal protein, and it's acidic.[6] This increases the pH of your blood requiring the alkaline calcium from your bones to neutralize it.[7]

WOMAN: I've never heard any of this before.

OFFICER: It's just the facts, Ma'am. We've known about it since 1930.[8]

WOMAN: So what do you mean milk and calcium supplements won't help. That doesn't make sense, Sergeant.

OFFICER: Yes, Ma'am. Studies show that the more milk that is drunk, the more calcium that is lost from the bones. The calcium isn't enough to compensate for the amount of animal protein present.[9] Studies also show that no matter how much extra calcium is added to the diet—if the diet is the American diet of meat and animal proteins—then there is more calcium leaving the bones than entering them.[10]

WOMAN: How much extra calcium are you talking about?

OFFICER: People in the study ingested 1,400 milligrams daily and still had a negative calcium balance. The group on low-protein diets taking 500 milligrams had a positive calcium balance.[11] It might interest you to know that the four countries with the highest intake of dairy products, Finland, Sweden, the United States, and England also are the four countries with the highest rates of osteoporosis and hip fractures.[12]

WOMAN: Amazing!

OFFICER: Yes Ma'am, it is, isn't it. Eskimos consume as much as 2,500 milligrams of calcium a day but lose 10 to12 percent of their skeleton per decade because their diets are high in animal-based foods.[13] The African Bantu women, on the other hand, take in about 350 milligrams of calcium a day, and osteoporosis is unknown. They subsist on grains, fruits, and vegetables.[14]

WOMAN: Doesn't heredity play a part in osteoporosis?

OFFICER: No, Ma'am. It doesn't appear to. When African blacks move to affluent countries and change their diets and lifestyles, osteoporosis becomes common among them also.[15]

WOMAN: Sergeant, it sounds like you are telling me vegetarians have a better chance of avoiding osteoporosis.

OFFICER: Studies have shown that while the average bone loss of an omnivore is 35 percent at age 65, the average herbivore woman has lost only 7 percent.[16] Studies have shown that 200 milligrams of calcium a day is adequate for those not eating meat, dairy, and eggs. Most of the world's people ingest 400 milligrams, and the American vegan ingests 600 milligrams, both without consuming animal-based foods.[17]

WOMAN: So where are vegetarians and vegans getting their calcium from?

OFFICER: The soil Ma'am. Calcium comes from the soil. Plants use it for varying needs, so vegetarians and vegans get their calcium from plants.[18]

WOMAN: Is that a fact. You're not just an average Joe, are you? How do you know so much about osteoporosis?

OFFICER: Ma'am, it's a big city. A lot of crime is obvious. The two-bit criminal, the dope pusher, the bank robber. Then there are crimes that aren't so obvious—like osteoporosis. I take this crime just as seriously, and I do my best to educate myself. When this kind of crime affects you, the average citizen, I go to work.

WOMAN: So who is pulling it over my eyes?

OFFICER: Ma'am?

WOMAN: The wool? It seems like I am being misled.

OFFICER: Osteoporosis is a multi-billion dollar industry. Dietary supplements, too.[19] That might have something to do with it. I don't know. We'll work on it, Ma'am. Two-thirds of the world's population doesn't drink milk and osteoporosis is not a problem for them.[20] That should tell you something, Ms. Tilbones.

WOMAN: You know what I think Sergeant?

OFFICER: Ma'am?

WOMAN: I think there are some folks out there profiting from my ignorance. I want you to catch them and lock them up. Maybe you could put out a dragnet for them. Say, by Friday?

OFFICER: Ma'am.

WOMAN: Yes, Sergeant?

OFFICER: I'll take care of the puns. You take care of your bones.

WOMAN: Right.

61: Endometriosis

THE RODNEY DANGERFIELD OF DISEASES

Endometriosis may well be the Rodney Dangerfield of diseases. It gets no respect.

In endometriosis, the cells that make up the inner lining of the uterus grow outside of it within the pelvic cavity attaching to the ovaries, intestinal tract, bladder, or elsewhere.[1]

Endometriosis affects 12 million American women, from all ethnic backgrounds, in the prime of their lives. The disease manifests itself by producing severe muscle cramps, pain during intercourse, chronic pelvic and lower back pain, heavy menstrual bleeding, nausea, vomiting, painful bowel movements, and constipation. Of those who suffer from it, 1 in 3 have difficulty conceiving.[2]

For a disease that is so debilitating, and causes the suffering of millions of women, we would expect that a good deal of attention has been paid to it, and our knowledge, diagnosis, and treatment of endometriosis is progressing.

To date, there is no known cause, no known cure, and it is misdiagnosed more than any other disease. The average woman can expect to visit the doctor five times before proper diagnosis and in 70 percent of first visits she can expect to be told there is no physical reason for the pain.[3] Surgery, short of a hysterectomy, doesn't solve the problem. Drugs are a temporary fix with side effects.[4] Research on the disease has apparently been sparse.[5] And genetics account for only 4 to 5 percent of cases.[6]

Mr. Dangerfield has some company.

Maybe we can make some progress ourselves. Oftentimes having a roundtable discussion to exchange ideas with the principals can be beneficial. With that in mind we have brought together an eclectic group to try and unravel the mystery of endometriosis.

They are: a woman, her husband, Dr. Dometri (her gynecologist), the woman's estrogen, the woman's immune system, and Dr. Endd (her second gynecologist). Let's listen in.

WOMAN: What the author just described sounds like *my* symptoms: severe muscle cramps, pain during intercourse, chronic pelvic and lower back pain, and occasionally nausea. Do you think I have endometriosis, Doctor?

DR. DOMETRI: We shouldn't be too quick to make a diagnosis. It could very well be nothing, or something more serious. We just don't know. I believe some tests are in order.

HUSBAND: Her symptoms are hard to pin down. But they sometimes occur at the most inopportune times, if you know what I mean.

DR. DOMETRI: Yes, I understand.

(Two months and three visits later.)

DR. DOMETRI: The results of the laparoscopic surgery of your abdominal cavity are in, and they confirm endometriosis.

WOMAN: What does it mean and what can you do?

DR. DOMETRI: Don't worry, it's a very common ailment that millions of women have. Your uterine cells are overflowing into areas where they don't belong. They take root and cause inflammation. We don't know why it happens, but there are...

WOMAN'S ESTROGEN: (interrupting) Well, I think I know why it happens.

WOMAN'S IMMUNE SYSTEM: Yeah, me too.

DR. DOMETRI: Did you say something?

WOMAN: No.

HUSBAND: No.

WOMAN: I believe the voices came from—me.

DR. DOMETRI: As I was saying, there are some steps we can take to relieve your symptoms. I want to start you off with some hormone-blocking medications.[7]

HUSBAND: Are you sure that's a good thing? I mean, aren't hormones necessary for, you know...

DR. DOMETRI: Oh, don't worry, this should eventually improve your sex life. If those medications don't work then we can try...

WOMAN'S ESTROGEN: ...a low-fat vegetarian diet? Did it ever occur to you, Doctor, *why* the uterine cells are spilling into other parts of her body, like root beer foam overflowing a frosty mug?

The fat in animal-based foods promote my production, increasing my levels by 50 percent in this woman here.[8] You do eat meat and dairy products, right?

WOMAN: Yes.

WOMAN'S ESTROGEN: It's no surprise then that I go into overdrive producing an excess of uterine cells. My vegetarian estrogen friends not only don't have this problem, they are very efficient in leaving the body as they are excreted in the feces at a rate of 2 to 3 times greater than us estrogens driven by a meat-based diet.[9] Plant-based foods because of fiber, isoflavins, and many other properties would maintain me at the proper levels.[10]

However, I won't take all the blame. My friend here, the Immune System, is indirectly at fault, too.

WOMAN'S IMMUNE SYSTEM: Thanks for squealing. Actually, if this woman would switch to a plant-based diet I would be much stronger and better able to knock out the maverick cells. I have a hard enough time fighting off her colds as it is.

Her dietary habits weaken me in a number of ways:

Contaminants, such as PCBs and pesticides, concentrate in muscle tissue and milk of the animals and fish she eats. Women with high blood levels of PCBs have a higher prevalence of endometriosis.[11]

Also fat, cholesterol, protein, and iron from these foods sap my strength.[12]

And she gives me little help from plant-based foods in the name of carotenoids, glucarates, tocotrienols, saponins, flavonoids, phytates, Vitamin C, Vitamin E, and beta-carotene that keep me strong.[13]

WOMAN: Could my estrogen and immune system be right, Doctor Dometri?

DR. DOMETRI: To my knowledge no studies have been conducted placing women with endometriosis on a vegetarian diet.[14] I doubt if there is much substance to their claims given the complex nature of this disease.

DR. ENDD: Doctor Dometri, if I may interrupt. I had a 24-year-old woman I treated. I suggested low-fat, purely vegetarian foods, and within 3 months she was noticeably better, and at 6 months her pain was gone! I then suggested this regimen to three other women and they told me the diet was helpful in reducing their pain. In fact, one woman said by having some dairy products or a bit of chicken, her pain came right back.[15]

WOMAN: That's impressive. I would try just about anything to get rid of this awful problem.

DR. DOMETRI: Well, if you are really that worried I can always do a hysterectomy. That will take care of the problem once and for all.

WOMAN: I think I might try a low-fat, vegetarian diet first.

HUSBAND: Does this mean no more Friday night meatloaf?

WOMAN'S ESTROGEN: Yes.

WOMAN'S IMMUNE SYSTEM: Yes.

62: Hearing Loss

AGE IS AN INNOCENT BYSTANDER

The loss of hearing might be the personification of old age. Maybe more than any other trait we have come to associate hearing loss with aging. When we see a hearing aid it is most often in the ear of an older individual. We *expect* the elderly to be hard of hearing.

When an elderly person is featured in a movie or television show, invariably they are depicted as hard of hearing because, sadly, hearing impairment is an easy target for humor. The following example of two elderly gentlemen conversing on a park bench illustrates the point.

FIRST MAN: Do you have a dime?

SECOND MAN: The time? I have 10:00.

FIRST MAN: Well, I only need *one* dime.

SECOND MAN: It's 1:00? My watch must have stopped.

FIRST MAN: Pop? Yes, I'm very thirsty. Could I borrow a dime?

SECOND MAN: Time? I don't know, I think my watch broke.

FIRST MAN: You're broke? I guess you don't have a dime, then.

There are 28 million Americans that have suffered some degree of hearing loss, and most of them are elderly. Of Americans older than 75, 40 percent are hard of hearing.[1]

Given our experiences and this data, who would suggest that hearing loss could be caused by anything other than aging?

We all should.

It doesn't necessarily follow that because we associate hearing loss with aging that it is also the cause—association and cause are not interchangeable words. The fact is, the biological basis of late-life hearing loss is unknown.[2] Aging may well be an innocent bystander mistaken for the criminal at the scene of the crime.

Who is the criminal, then?

Let's examine some different data, and a different pool of people, and see if we can identify the perpetrator.

LACK OF VITAMINS: Several micronutrients, including low levels of vitamins, could be involved in the development of many age-related hearing disorders in humans and animals.[3] (Antioxidants like vitamin C, vitamin E, and beta-carotene, and phytochemicals are predominately found in plants.)

BONE LOSS: In one study, 70 women ages 60 to 71 with impaired hearing were found to have 11 percent lower spinal bone density than their same-age counterparts with normal hearing.[4] (Studies have shown that while the average bone loss of an omnivore is 35 percent at age 65, the average herbivore woman has lost 7 percent.)[5]

ANIMAL PROTEIN: A high homocysteine blood concentration could interfere with the blood flow to the inner ear.[6] Homocysteine is converted from methionine, a protein 2 to 3 times more prevalent in meat.[7] Folic acid found in green leafy vegetables and whole grains prevents methionine from being converted to homocysteine.[8] (Alzheimer's patients also have high levels of the protein building block homocysteine.)[9]

IMMUNE SYSTEM REPAIR: There is evidence to suggest that hearing loss could be caused by the immune system being compromised since ongoing repair is a must in maintaining the moving parts involved in hearing.[10] (Given what we know about the plant kingdom, and its hand-in-glove relationship with the immune system, this wouldn't be a reach.)

The ear, like every other organ of the body, is dependent on sufficient blood flow and proper nutrients to operate at peak efficiency. Given the highly sensitive nature, and intricate design of the ear, these requirements become even more crucial.

The uniformity of our experience with older Americans and hearing impairment has the same consistency as something else:

the Self-Induced Carnivorous Killer (SICK) diet that most Americans share. With no contrasting condition—a Wholly Eating Leaves to Live (WELL) diet—it is understandable how we have come to assume aging equals hearing loss.

Let's see if we can find some contrast with other populations.

- When scientists compared the hearing of the African tribes people called Maabans, with the people in Wisconsin, they couldn't find any of the Africans, at any age, with hearing losses like those common in Wisconsin, the dairy capital of the United States.[11]

- When scientists studied the Finnish people, who eat a high-fat diet, and Yugoslavs who subsist on a low-fat plant-based diet, they found Finnish children with hearing losses at the age of 10. By the age of 19, those Finns had a marked inability to hear high-frequency sounds. Yugoslav children had no such hearing loss.[12]

- People in Third World countries eating their traditional diets, that don't include meat, have better hearing at the age of 70 than the average American has at 20.[13]

The connection between nutrition and hearing is not a new idea. Research dates back to the 1930s and 1940s.[14] But apparently few people have been listening.

The loss of any one of the senses diminishes the quality of life and is profoundly devastating. Losing our hearing is losing the birds chirping, trees rustling, and brooks gurgling. It's losing the loving words of a spouse, laughter of grandchildren, and favorite song on the radio. It's losing a piece of ourselves.

It appears we have identified the perpetrator who has taken our hearing from us. Catching and locking up the criminal is the next step. It's our choice to make.

When we make that choice, another loss will occur that won't hurt us at all— the loss of humorous subject matter for television and movies.

63: Vision Loss

Glaucoma, macular degeneration, and cataracts. Many people would recognize these as degenerative diseases of the eye. But given their dispassionate names, many people might not recognize that their result could be blindness.

To get our attention maybe these diseases should be given more expressive names to remind us of their devastating effects. Intraocular pressure, optic nerve damage, and blood vessel leakage might fit the bill. Blurry vision, clouded sight, and tunnel vision is even better. But maybe the most effective approach would be to name them by what we might be *missing* instead. Glaucoma, macular degeneration, and cataracts would change to: A Colorful Sunset. Our Child's Smile. A Good Movie.

Are these three diseases of the eye due to aging and heredity, consequently out of our hands? Or are the eyes like our other organs, influenced by the foods we eat, at the mercy of the health of the arteries that feed them, and the nutrients of the blood that bathes them?

This is an eye test we don't want to fail. To help with the answers, let's bring the evidence into focus.

CATARACTS: (aka: A Colorful Sunset.) Cataracts are characterized by opacity, or cloudiness, of the lens. They have been started, or prevented, by the following influences:

- Cataracts have been linked to diabetes, a disease virtually absent from populations consuming high-fiber diets of grains, vegetables, and fruits.[1]

- Another sugar related influence is the milk sugar, galactose, which as we age is more difficult to break down and passes into the lens of the eye. We find corroborating evidence by way of a genetic disorder where babies who can't break down the sugar from cows' milk can develop cataracts before the age of two.[2]

• Oxidation, due to the bombardment of free radicals from light, the environment, or excessive iron can lead to cataract development.[3] (The omnivore has 2 to 4 times more stored iron than the herbivore.)[4]

• People who eat less than 3.5 servings of fruits and vegetables a day have 6 times the risk of developing cataracts.[5]

MACULAR DEGENERATION: (aka: Our Child's Smile.) Macular degeneration is the leading cause of vision loss in those older than 55 due to the deterioration of the retina cells.[6] It has been started, or prevented, by the following influences:

• Oxidation of the rods and cones, the light sensitive receptor cells on the outer surface of the retina.[7]

• Fatty acid leakage and high cholesterol.[8]

• Nutritional intervention is effective at slowing, stopping, and even reversing this degenerative disease.[9]

• One survey showed that people who ate the most beta-carotene and other carotenoids, particularly as supplied by spinach and collard greens, had almost half the risk of macular degeneration as those eating fewer carotenoids.[10]

• People who consumed higher intakes of two antioxidants found in green leafy vegetables, lutein and zeaxanthin, were 70 percent less likely to develop macular degeneration.[11]

GLAUCOMA: (aka: A Good Movie.) Glaucoma is characterized by abnormally high intraocular fluid pressure in the eye. It has been started, or prevented, by the following influences:

- Reduced blood flow to the eye has been implicated as a possible cause.[12] This isn't too hard to understand given the influence that reduced blood flow has on other organs. Heart attack and stroke come to mind.

- People on fat-free intravenous fluids, for reasons not related to this disease, improved their intraocular pressure.[13]

- Research from the 1940s showed a significant and continuous improvement in intraocular pressure when subjects were placed on a low-fat rice diet.[14]

A different organ. The same story.

When we supply the wrong substances—fat, sugar, and excess iron—instead of the right substances—vitamins, antioxidants, phytochemicals, and complex carbohydrates—to our organs, in this case the eyes, the result is insufficient blood flow, oxidation, and other metabolic anomalies that can lead to impaired vision or blindness.

We have a couple of options. We can either pick fruits, vegetables, and whole grains from the grocery store, or pick surgery, implants, and medications—if those are even options —from the ophthalmologist. The choice seems as clear as 20/20 vision.

Eyesight would likely be the clear choice as the last sense we would want to lose. If we hesitate to agree, it might be a good exercise to close our eyes for 5 to 10 minutes and simulate the loss.

Walk around, get a drink of water, and go outside. Listen to the sounds and try to imagine the pictures that go with them. Walk inside, make a meal, and turn on the television. Sit quietly and imagine the experience as permanent.

A Colorful Sunset. Our Child's Smile. A Good Movie. We hope we will always see them; we hope we will never get them.

64: Impotence, Infertility, Hair Loss

THEY ONLY HAVE TO BE NIGHTMARES

If you're a man, this may be the first place you came to in the book. Maybe women, too.

Who can blame us given the toll that impotence, infertility, and hair loss, can take on our pleasure, our desire to have a family, and our vanity. Because even though these are not life-threatening events, they may well elicit similar anxiety.

So what do these disorders, most often associated with emotional troubles, bad luck, and hereditary factors, respectively, have to do with diet?

Quite a lot.

And given that the most universal response to any one of these three menaces is, "I'll do whatever it takes to overcome this," there won't be any problem getting an attentive audience to learn about the diet's role in them.

Let's start with the disorder most likely to take the wind out of our sails.

> We come home from work and our wife greets us wearing provocative nightwear. She informs us that the children are playing down the street, and she leads us by the hand to the bedroom. An hour later we turn to her and for the fourth time profusely apologize for what happened—or more precisely, what didn't happen—but we have no idea why. She sobs loudly. We bolt upright in bed in a profuse sweat. It's dark and our wife is asleep.

It was only a nightmare. And that's all it has to be.

The number one cause of impotence, responsible for 85 percent of occurrences, is not what is muddling the brain, but what is clogging the artery—specifically the one that feeds the penis.[1]

The fat and cholesterol of the SICK diet that leads to plaque and atherosclerosis, doesn't discriminate. The same reduced blood flow to the arteries that feed the heart and brain causing them to fail is the same reduced blood flow to the artery that feeds the penis causing it to, well, leave us hanging.[2]

Just 10 percent of erectile dysfunction is attributed to emotional troubles.[3] In this country, 34 percent of middle age men suffer from impotence. By the age of 60, 1 in 4 men is impotent.[4]

Men are capable of retaining their sexual vitality and activity well into their 80s and beyond.[5] It's their choice to do so with Viagra, vacuum pumps, and penile implants, or cauliflower, cashews, and corn.

> We find ourselves late to a meeting with our wife and her gynecologist. We open the door to his office and there they are, solemnly staring at us. The doctor hands us a lab report and informs us that the inability to start a family during the past year is a problem with *us*. We faint and hit our head on a desk. We startle, open our eyes, and it's dark. Our heart rate begins to slow.

It was only a nightmare. And that's all it has to be.

In 1 out of every 3 cases, infertility is due to a problem with the man, specifically a deficient sperm count.[6] Ironically, too much testosterone appears to be the culprit. How do we know that?

In one test, an injection of 200 milligrams of testosterone a day shut off sperm production in 70 percent of test subjects.[7]

Since animal fat is known to promote higher levels of testosterone in the bloodstream, the following study is no surprise.[8] When animal fat consumption was plotted against birth rate for 60 countries, a 77 percent inverse correlation was indicated.[9] Put another way, 3 of 4 couples eating the SICK diet, and having difficulty trying to start a family, might want to consider…

> Consuming products of wheat,
> instead of fatty meat.

We have just come home from work. We walk in the door and our wife gasps. The children stop in their tracks and stare. Even the dog cocks her head, as if perplexed. We turn to look in the mirror, and we turn pale. All our hair is gone! We scream. We wake up in bed, it's dark, and we are still screaming. We grab the top of our head, and breathe a sigh of relief.

It was only a nightmare.

Yes, heredity is the primary factor in hair loss. However, increased testosterone plays a secondary role, and can make a difference in the rate of hair loss.

It was first observed in 1942—and later studied—that men who had their testicles removed for medical reasons, and therefore weren't producing testosterone, also *weren't* losing their hair. Little consolation. Later when they were given testosterone shots to compensate for their unfortunate operation, their hair fell out.[10]

One study demonstrated that hair falls out at twice the rate in the fall (just like the trees), when testosterone levels are higher, compared to the lower spring levels.[11]

In Japan where more people are changing to a more Western diet, more baldness is occurring. Other research found that men with high cholesterol levels and heart problems are more likely to be bald.[12]

It might help to remember it this way…

> Eat a pear, save a hair.
> Eat some game, lose our mane.

The damage to our vanity, pride, and ego can be as destructive as physical damage. Fortunately we don't have to choose between them when it comes to diet. We can win on all fronts.

What it comes down to is this:

Do we want to build up our pride and have our ego stroked in the kitchen, by way of downing a 22-ounce porterhouse or consuming the most turkey at Thanksgiving? Or do we want to build up our pride and have our ego stroked in the bedroom, the nursery, and in the bathroom mirror?

65: Hemorrhoids, Hernia, Appendicitis

A TALE OF TWO FECES

It was the best of times on the WELL diet; it was the worst of times on the SICK diet.

The solid waste material that the body produces, transports, and excretes is not "waste" until it leaves the body. Up until then, it is still a functioning member of our anatomy where it can either perform valuable chores or cause great distress.

The waste byproducts of any process can reveal much about the nature of the raw materials that went into it, and the success of the process itself. Let's look at the human digestive process, and by way of comparing the feces from meat-based and plant-based diets, see what it reveals.

We hope the differences are appreciated. Certainly the fact none of us had to personally gather the data is.

FECES PROFILE: PLANT-BASED DIET[1]

- Life cycle and transit time: 35 hours
- Weight: 470 grams
- Best features: Contents of cellulose and water
- Worst features: None
- Description: Spongy, moist, fibrous, and agile
- Summary: Absorbs poisons, works fast, exits smoothly
- Non life-threatening conditions: None

FECES PROFILE: MEAT-BASED DIET[2]

- Life cycle and transit time: 83 hours
- Weight: 104 grams
- Best Features: None
- Worst features: Excessive bacteria and bile acids
- Description: Hard, dry, underweight, and putrid
- Summary: No initiative; must be forced into action
- Non life-threatening conditions: hemorrhoids, hernia, and appendicitis

The feces are as different as the diets themselves.

The meat-based feces is inefficient in waste gathering (weighs 4 times less), and slow moving (twice as slow), making it potentially toxic to the body. It becomes a liability instead of the asset it is supposed to be.[3]

A plant contains plenty of bulky, fibrous cellulose that isn't digestible for a good reason. It acts as a sponge, absorbing the body's poisons and holding water that helps propel it easily down the digestive tract. An animal is made of muscle, ligaments, and fat. It contains no cellulose.

Even at the end of its journey our meat-based fecal matter can cause us problems. We could say in one respect, but not in another, it is all pooped out. Unable to go the distance we have to step in and help it to daylight. Unfortunately, our effort can lead to hemorrhoids, hernia, and appendicitis.

HEMORRHOIDS: Straining, pushing, and forcing are the operative words, words not found—insofar as diet goes—in a vegetarian's vocabulary. The straining engorges the anus vessels with blood. The vessels are then pushed downward and out through the anal opening, rupturing them open.

Hemorrhoids are rare in Asia and Africa where the diets are predominately plant-based. In North America and Western Europe this is not the case.[4]

There is also a leg version of hemorrhoids. We know them as varicose veins. Same action, different result. Straining on a daily basis pushes blood back down the veins of the legs, destroying the valves, and creating the look that every woman can't wait to acquire. But it's more than vanity that can be harmed. As time passes the damaging of the veins can lead to blood clots and phlebitis.[5]

Hemorrhoids may be a good subject for humor, but if we are the butt of the butt jokes, hemorrhoids are anything but funny.

HERNIA: A hiatal hernia occurs when the stomach protrudes through the esophageal opening of the diaphragm. This can occur from abdominal pressure of daily straining. The symptoms are chest pains and indigestion. One out of 5 people in the United States has this problem. Some never feel any symptoms, the rest are taking heartburn medicines.[6]

APPENDICITIS: Although this disorder is not a result of straining, it is a result of the small, hard, concentrated feces. One of these can sometimes get stuck in the opening to the appendix, the fingerlike organ near the abdomen. There are 250,000 cases each year of appendicitis in this country.[7]

Appendectomies are the most frequent emergency operation in the United States and England.[8] In rural Africa where the diet is plant-based many surgeons have never seen a single case.[9] The message is clear: Unless a plant-based diet is on our itinerary, Africa probably shouldn't be.

We have heard the appendix serves no useful purpose, so we shouldn't worry about it. Aside from the serious nature of acute appendicitis, there *is* some evidence that the appendix may have an immune function, because certain cancers like Hodgkin's are more common among those who have had their appendix removed.[10]

Maybe we should defer to Nature when it comes to evaluating the necessity of our parts.

Most of the time, hemorrhoids, hernia, or appendicitis are not going to be life-threatening, but they might be indicative of conditions occurring during the digestive process that are. And most definitely they are indicative of a diet filled with meat, fish, dairy, and eggs.

Now that we know the tale, we can avoid the worst of times, and look forward to the best of times ahead.

66: Ulcers, Crohn's, Diverticulitis

NOT THE BRAIN — THE BOWELS

Which organ controls the body? The brain would be our most likely response. However, if we thought about it for a moment, we might have given a different answer.

Let's think back to our last episode, or bout with one of the following: stomachache, nausea, cramping, heartburn, vomiting, diarrhea, or abdominal pain. How did we feel? Did it immobilize us? Would we have written a substantial check to make the feeling go away? Were we able to think about anything else?

The bowels—not the brain—appear to be in charge.

Analogous to this might be our assumption that Mr. CEO is running his company when really it's his wife calling the shots.

For many of us, stomach and intestinal disorders, although they can hit hard, pass relatively quickly. But for those suffering from ulcers, Crohn's disease, or diverticulitis, or any other serious digestive track disorder, that may not be the case.

We know the effect the wrong foods have on the body's systems, but what effect do they have on the body's *parts* they come directly in contact with? Maybe the best way to find out is for us to take a tour of a human digestive system to see some of the damage first hand.

Let's put on our raingear—goggles if we have them—the environment could be pretty nasty.

*****

"Here we go. Hold on!

"Well, here we are in the stomach. Look, over there. See those three open sores that are bleeding slightly? Those are peptic ULCERS. See the liquid splashing up against them? Hydrochloric acid. Button up tight; we don't want to come in contact with that. The acid can dissolve a razor blade in less than a week, and digest the stomach itself if the problem is bad enough. This guy is probably not feeling too well right now.[1]

"Watch out! Milk and fried chicken comin' through. Well, that's no surprise. Both these foods are acid forming foods, as are other meats, cheese, and eggs, and have no fiber to boot. These upset the delicate balance between the protective mucus and stomach acid that can lead to ulcers.[2] Given that these foods are the standard American fare, it isn't surprising that 33 million Americans will sustain an ulcer at some point in their lives.[3]

"Most foods from the plant kingdom are base-forming, that is, alkaline, and contain plenty of fiber. In a study of 48,000 male health professionals, those that consumed 30 grams of fiber a day were half as likely to get ulcers as those who took in 13 grams a day.[4] An internist took his ulcer patients off dairy products for 2 weeks and it changed their lives.

"Let's move on before the acid makes an ulcer out of us.

"The last 8 feet of the intestine looked pretty good.

"Oh, oh. Look at all the lacerations there. And a complete hole! See the stitches there? It appears he has had part of the intestine removed. I'd bet this man has CROHN'S DISEASE. If so, he is one of 500,000 Americans who suffer from it.[5] This is one destructive disease: bloody diarrhea, stomach pain, nausea, vomiting, inflammation, holes in the intestines, fever, severe joint pain, weight loss, and lack of energy.[6]

"The disease is mostly found in the United States, Scandinavia, and United Kingdom, where meat and dairy consumption is the highest.[7] Some suspect it may be caused by a microorganism present in cows' milk not killed by pasteurization.[8] Other data suggests animal protein as the culprit. However, it appears that vegetable protein is associated with reduced incidence.[9]

"Feel that rumble? We better keep moving quickly forward, or we might find ourselves moving quickly backwards.

"It's a little roomier down here. We are in the large intestine now.

"Look over there. And there. And down there. Those small pouches that look like an inner tube pushing out a hole in a bicycle tire are diverticula. This man probably suffers from DIVERTICULI-TIS. It's inflammation and sometimes bleeding and infection can cause stomach pain, bloody stools, diarrhea, and anemia.[10]

"Look here. Feel that stool? Hard as a rock. No fiber in his diet. The result is constant pressure against the colon wall that forms these pockets.[11] This almost never happens in populations where the diet contains a high level of vegetable fiber and very little fat. But in the United States, 10 percent of those older than 40, and 35 percent older than 50, have evidence of this disease.[12]

"In one study, 70 diverticulitis patients were placed on a high-fiber diet. Before the diet they tallied 171 different symptoms. After a time on the diet, 88 percent of the symptoms disappeared, and the number of patients taking laxatives went from 49 to 7.[13]

"It looks like there's light at the end of the tunnel. We have traversed this man's complete digestive track.

"Hold on. Here we go!

*****

"That was some experience. If everyone could take a tour of a digestive tract like that one, we would see a lot of instantaneous diet changes from meat to plants—not unlike taking everyone on a prison tour and seeing a reduction in the crime rate.

"You have a couple of questions? How did we know that this particular man would have all these problems?

"Simple. The food in front of him gave it away—chicken, potato skins with cheese, and milk.

"And the second question? You want to know where you can take a nice, long shower."

67: Autoimmune Diseases

COLONEL OTTO M. YUNE HAS A CLUE

If Mother Nature's greatest artistic achievement is the human body, then her greatest scientific achievement has to be the immune system.

The immune system is an innate and adaptive interweaving mechanism of cells, molecules, and organs that fight and destroy invaders with precision and consistency, while memorizing all of its activities, and distinguishing between a *billion* foreign proteins. There are no words available to describe the system. Perfect, is the closest we can come.

Autoimmune diseases are illnesses that occur as a result of the immune system producing antibodies against normal parts of the body as if they were foreign substances.

More than 100 autoimmune diseases afflict 50 million Americans.[1] Some of the diseases are, rheumatoid arthritis, lupus, asthma, scleroderma, nephritis, multiple sclerosis, insulin-dependent diabetes, ankylosing spondylitis, Graves' disease, psoriasis, fibromyalgia, relapsing polychondritis, and myasthenia gravis.[2]

What happened! How could a *better* than perfect system go completely haywire, attacking the body, inflicting multiple diseases and suffering on millions of Americans?

No one knows. The cause of autoimmune disease is unknown.[3]

What could be the stimulus, then? Given that it affects so many individuals, the agent must be something many people are exposed to. Given its many locations of attack—namely many diseases—it must be something that enters the bloodstream. And given that it confuses our defenses the offender must be something that resembles *us*.

Could the cause in someway be related to food?

Everyone eats, so everyone is exposed to food. The components of food enter the bloodstream. But what about the third piece—something that resembles us?

Long amino acid chains make up proteins, and proteins make up humans, animals, and plants. The human immune system recognizes all 100 percent of its own protein chains. The plant proteins' amino acid sequences are 100 percent different than human proteins. However, animals and humans share many of the same amino acid segments.[4]

Is it possible that these shared amino acid sequences between animal and humans are in some way confusing our defenses, the immune system?

Who better to call on, and maybe shed light on this question, than a member of the armed forces. The military, like the immune system, also fights an enemy and provides defense. So we have asked Army Colonel, Otto M. Yune, to join us, and see if he can provide any insight into this enigma by way of his experience.

Let's welcome, Colonel Otto M. Yune.

"I'm not sure I can help, but I do have a story that might be of interest.

"Years ago on a classified mission overseas, I was walking sentry duty as a young private. The uniforms we wore on this mission required unique colors. They were a tri-color red, white, and blue. Our allies on this mission also had unique uniforms and colors. Their uniforms were a single, solid color, and *no* red, white or blue at all.

"A man approached me wearing a green uniform with orders to deliver drinking water. I knew he was an ally, so I let him through. Another man came to my gate with communication equipment. He was wearing a solid orange uniform. No problem. Then a man approached, and told me he was to deliver our rations. His uniform was a tri-color red, white, and blue. But the colors were in slightly different places, in slightly different proportions, than our uniforms. This meant he was most likely the enemy, so he was eliminated.

"It then occurred to me that some of our troops, or at least who I thought were our troops, had uniforms not unlike the man we just eliminated. Their uniforms, too, were slightly different than the uniform I was wearing. I didn't know what to think now. Were they our men, or not?

"If we eliminate these men, and they are our men, we commit a terrible act, not to mention we reduce and weaken our own forces. But if we don't, and they aren't our men, then we risk the lives of all the men, and probably a complete mission failure. There was no choice. We had to eliminate them.

"Unfortunately, they did turn out to be our men. But given a repeat of the same circumstances, we again would be forced to take the same action.

"Well, that's the story. I hope it was useful."

Thank you, Colonel. That was a most interesting story. A most relevant story.

Can animal proteins enter the bloodstream? Does the immune system consider them invaders, thus producing antibodies against them? Does our immune system then react to similar human proteins, and attack them—therefore us—instigating autoimmune disease?

Let's look at what we do know.

Autoimmune disease sufferers have an abnormality of the digestive tract called "leaky-gut syndrome" that allows incompletely digested foodstuffs to pass through the intestinal lining and enter the bloodstream.[5] It's hypothesized that this circumstance can lead to some of the following autoimmune reactions:

RHEUMATOID ARTHRITIS: A protein in cows' milk, bovine albumin, has shared sequences of amino acids with the collagen in our joints. It's theorized that antibodies synthesized to attack the foreign cows' milk proteins, end up attacking our joint tissues, causing this disease.[6]

Rheumatoid arthritis is rare in Africa, Japan, and China where meat is seldom eaten. As recently as 1957, no case of rheumatoid arthritis could be found in Africa. When Blacks move to America and adopt a meat-based diet, their incidence of rheuma-toid arthritis rises dramatically.[7]

LUPUS: Protein from beef and dairy that has produced antigen-anti-body complexes has been found in the blood of people with this disease.[8]

Lupus is less common in Chinese people in China who fol-low a traditional Eastern diet, than in Chinese people who have moved to Hawaii and adopted a Western diet.[9]

MULTIPLE SCLEROSIS: A long-term 34-year study tracked sur-vival rates of multiple sclerosis patients. Symptoms of those that followed a diet restricting red meat and milk were slowed or stopped; the group had a 95 percent survival rate. Those that failed to follow the restricted diet had a 20 percent survival rate.[10]

ASTHMA: A long-term trial of a vegan diet—elimination of all ani-mal-based foods—was tried on patients. The result was a signifi-cant improvement in 92 percent of the 25 patients who completed the study.[11]

RELAPSING POLYCHONDRITIS: A woman with a rare autoim-mune disease, which is progressive, incurable, and potentially fatal, was placed on a low-fat vegetarian diet. One month later her blood tests were normal and she was symptom-free.[12]

Given the compelling evidence that exists, how is it that the cause of autoimmune disease is considered to be unknown? Given the sophistication of the immune system how could it completely fall apart?

Could a complex spectrum of diseases all have a single root cause, and be something as simple as the food we eat? Does Colonel Otto M. Yune's story provide us a valuable analogy into the mechanism of autoimmune disease?

Maybe our next guest should be Mother Nature.

68: Asthma

IT'S ELEMENTARY MY DEAR AUTHOR

Asthma might be the most primal cruelty ever perpetrated on humanity. Any disease that taunts people, often children, by making them stare death in the face every episodic second they take a breath, deserves that label.

Asthma, a chronic lung disease in which bronchial muscles contract and the airways become inflamed, assails 17 million Americans, including 4.8 million children. That is a lot of labored breaths, each and everyone precious.

This translates annually to 500,000 hospitalizations, 10 million missed school days, 3 million lost workdays, 10.4 million doctor office visits, and $11.3 billion in costs.[1]

Given its horrific nature, one would think our motivation to identify a cause, and implement a cure, would have made asthma nothing but a bad memory by now. But neither is in sight. It is still a mystery.

A mystery? Who better to get to the bottom of a mystery than Sherlock Holmes.

With that in mind, we contacted Sir Arthur Conan Doyle in the hopes that Mr. Holmes might be available to help. He agreed to loan us Mr. Holmes for the duration of this segment. We are pleased to have in our presence, Mr. Sherlock Holmes.

THE AUTHOR: Mr. Holmes, thank you for coming. You've read the introduction. Asthma is a devastating disease with many unanswered questions as to its cause, prevention, and cure. Can you help?

MR. HOLMES: I am pleased to be challenged. I do enjoy a good mystery, you know. Would you mind telling me what is known about asthma?

THE AUTHOR: There seems to be a long list of varied triggers that bring on attacks. From pollens to fumes, exercising to emotions, colds to weather.[2]

It's predominately a disease of Western Culture. Poorer nations see little of it.[3]

About one-third of asthma sufferers are children. At age 15, one-half of children have no more symptoms.[4]

Foods play a part—some improve the symptoms and some make them worse.

The immune system also appears to play an important role. Where does one start?

MR. HOLMES: Always at the beginning. The basic pieces of the puzzle, if I may take the liberty of boiling down your description, are this: The Air, The Body's Physical and Emotional State, The Western Culture, Children, Food, and The Immune System.

Let's try a little deductive reasoning. Are any of these items peculiar to the Western Culture?

THE AUTHOR: Well, I guess one significant difference is the food. A Western diet is more meat-based. The other potential factors aren't significantly different from country to country, culture to culture.

MR. HOLMES: What can we say is unique to children?

THE AUTHOR: Well, they are growing and developing.

MR. HOLMES: Would this include their immune systems?

THE AUTHOR: Yes, the immune system is one system that learns, and becomes stronger with time.

MR. HOLMES: Do children eat differently than adults because they are growing and developing?

THE AUTHOR: They are encouraged to drink milk. I guess children drink more milk than adults.

MR. HOLMES: Is this true of children worldwide?

THE AUTHOR: Two-thirds of the world's population doesn't drink cows' milk.[5] It's predominately a Western practice.

MR. HOLMES: You stated that some foods improve symptoms, but others make it worse. Which foods aggravate the problem?

THE AUTHOR: I guess milk is one of the greatest offenders. Fifty percent of all children in the United States are allergic to cows' milk.[6]

Asthmatics can find a marked improvement in their condition by eliminating milk from their diets.[7]

One pediatrician recommended that all of his patients eliminate milk from their diets. After that, he did not have a single child with asthma.[8]

MR. HOLMES: What foods or vitamins improve the condition?

THE AUTHOR: In a study of 18,000 children, the subjects realized a lower risk of asthma when they ate more vegetables and fiber that included vitamin E, calcium, and magnesium.[9]

Another long-term study placed 25 patients on a vegan diet, which resulted in significant improvement for 92 percent of the subjects.[10]

A dozen asthmatics, given 500-milligram vitamin C supplements after exercise, had a reduction in their symptoms.[11]

One study showed that those with the highest vitamin E intake from food had only half the risk of asthma.[12]

And in yet one more study, 20 of 38 patients receiving natural beta-carotene were protected against exercise-induced asthma.[13]

MR. HOLMES: Do any of these substances—minerals that come from the soil, or vitamins that originate in plants—influence the immune system?

THE AUTHOR: Yes. Vitamin C, vitamin E, and beta-carotene are all known boosters of the immune system. In fact, fruits, vegetables, whole grains, and legumes contain many antioxidants and phyto-chemicals that strengthen immunity.[14]

MR. HOLMES: What can you tell me about the immune system as it relates to asthma?

THE AUTHOR: There is increasing evidence that asthmatics have an underlying immune-system dysfunction.[15] Possibly the immune system is overreacting or it is confused by something.

MR. HOLMES: Is it possible for milk, or other foods of the Western diet, such as meat, to get from the stomach to the lungs?

THE AUTHOR: Yes, there is something called leaky-gut syndrome that can allow irritating, foreign proteins into the bloodstream. They can lodge in sensitive tissues and create inflammatory condi-tions.[16]

Additionally, it has been theorized that the commonality of animal proteins to human proteins causes confusion to the immune system resulting in an autoimmune response where the immune system turns on the body it is defending.[17]

MR. HOLMES: Does the immune system turn on the body it is defending in places other than the lungs?

THE AUTHOR: Yes, in the joints it is rheumatoid arthritis. In the nervous system it is multiple sclerosis, nephritis in the kidneys, dia-betes in the pancreas, Crohn's disease in the intestines. I believe there are more than 100 autoimmune diseases.[18]

MR. HOLMES: I see. May I take a crack at solving this caper?

THE AUTHOR: By all means.

MR. HOLMES: It appears asthma is an autoimmune response in the lungs due to the consumption of animal proteins, with a hypersensitivity to cows' milk protein.

THE AUTHOR: Yes? Is that all?

MR. HOLMES: What else does one need to know? Identify the perpetrator and all the other suspects become good citizens again.

THE AUTHOR: What about children being more vulnerable? What about the apparent causes like exercise and emotion that have nothing to do with food? What about...

MR. HOLMES: (interrupting) If you must be indulged, very well. The lungs are unique organs and children are unique creatures. But these elements have little to do with asthma once you remove the catalyst.

The lungs touch the outside world every second with each breath, making them vulnerable to whatever the atmosphere brings to them.

The lungs move to the emotions of the mind; if the mind is excited they billow quickly.

The lungs move to the rhythms of the body; if the body is moving rapidly they have to keep up.

The lungs, then, are a dynamic and potentially volatile spark to the gasoline and kindling supplied by animal protein.

Children exhibit their emotions more freely, not having built their defenses as adults have, and the lungs mirror the difference.

Children are more active and regularly in motion, and the lungs mirror the difference.

Children in the Western Culture drink milk, probably more milk than adults.

Children are picky eaters, thus less likely to ingest foods from the plant kingdom that contain the vitamins, antioxidants, and phytochemicals required to strengthen their immune systems.

Children's immune systems have not fully developed.

THE AUTHOR: When you put it in those terms it all seems to make sense. Thank you for solving our mystery.

MR. HOLMES: I don't believe there *was* a mystery to solve.

THE AUTHOR: I'm still impressed.

MR. HOLMES: It's elementary my dear author, elementary to be sure.

69: Childhood Illnesses

MAKE THEIR SUMMERS LAST FOREVER

Childhood is a time of blushing innocence and pure happiness, where every day is a new adventure, and every summer seems to last forever.

Adulthood, in stark contrast, is a time of duty and obligation, where every day demands responsibility and every summer becomes, well, just another one of the four seasons.

Children deserve their childhood. They deserve to have it without tragedy—meaning a child contracts a disease or ailment, or abomination—meaning the disease or ailment could have been prevented.

The following diseases are either associated with, or have their beginnings, in childhood.

Ear infections, colds, diarrhea, big tonsils, rashes, leukemia, high blood pressure, insulin-dependent diabetes, cancer, learning disabilities, emotional disorders, asthma, retarded growth, Sudden Infant Death Syndrome (SIDS), food poisoning, atherosclerosis, toxoplasmosis, canker sores, skin conditions, post nasal drip, obesity, high cholesterol, anemia, and breast cancer.

Do any, or all, of these diseases or aliments have their roots in animal-based foods? If they do, then the conditions can be prevented and the tragedy becomes an abomination.

The following—most appropriately 21—exhibits might determine the odds of the correct word to use.

- CHILDHOOD OTITIS MEDIA (EAR INFECTION): This disease affects 10 million children and is linked to an allergy from cows' milk. Colds, diarrhea, big tonsils, and rashes have also been attributed to milk. These conditions have all shown improvement on a whole-foods diet.[1]

- LEUKEMIA: The highest rates of leukemia are found in children 3 to 13 who consume the most dairy products. It is estimated that 20 percent of the American dairy cattle are infected with the leukemia virus.[2]

- CHILDHOOD LEUKEMIA: The risk is shown to increase almost 10 times with the high consumption of hot dogs. Cancers in children were doubled with the consumption of hamburgers or hot dogs at least once a week.[3]

- HIGH BLOOD PRESSURE: We are led to believe this is a disease of the elderly, yet 1 in 8 American children have blood pressure that is too high.[4]

- INSULIN-DEPENDENT DIABETES MELLITUS (IDDM): Milk is suspected of triggering this disease due to an autoimmune response. Studies have shown that IDDM patients generate antibodies to bovine serum albumin *and* their own pancreatic cells, suggesting that the commonality of animal and human amino acid sequences confuses the immune system.[5]

- CANCER: In 1950, cancer was a rarity in children. Today, cancer is the second leading cause of death in children under 15. Pesticides could be one factor. Meat and dairy foods carry many more times the amount of pesticides than plant-based foods. And an omnivore mother exposes her unborn and newborn to the toxicity of pesticides by way of her placenta and breast milk, increasing her child's risk of developing cancer.[6]

- MENTAL AND PHYSICAL DISABILITIES: Pesticide exposure by way of an omnivore mother's placenta and breast milk may contribute to other more subtle disorders that present themselves as learning disabilities, attention-deficit hyperactivity disorder (ADHD), lower IQs, weakened immune systems, and emotional disorders.[7]

- INTELLIGENCE QUOTIENT (IQ): A study of vegetarian children showed that they had IQs of 116, well above average.[8]

- ASTHMA: A lower risk of asthma was achieved for youngsters who ate more vegetables and fiber that included vitamin E, calcium, and magnesium. The study included 18,000 children.[9]

- GROWTH: Clinical studies have shown that children on a diet of mostly vegetables, fruits, grains, and legumes, when consuming adequate calories, not only grow at normal rates, but also have been shown to attain greater height than omnivore children.[10]

- SIDS: Immune responses to milk proteins have been implicated in Sudden Infant Death Syndrome.[11]

- FOOD POISONING: Children are more susceptible to food poisoning, like E. coli, because of their underdeveloped immune systems.[12]

- ATHEROSCLEROSIS: Children show fatty streaks in their arteries at 9 months, signs of the disease at 3 years, and scar tissue formation in the teenage years. In a study of 2 to 15-year-old youngsters who died of trauma, 50 percent had fatty streaks and 8 percent had fibrous plaque in their coronary arteries.[13]

- EATING HABITS: Family history may be more environmental than genetic. Children generally eat the same foods as their parents for 18 years, and then carry those learned habits into adulthood.[14]

- TOXOPLASMOSIS: Approximately 30 percent of all pork products are contaminated by this parasite. A pregnant woman can transfer it to her unborn child causing serious consequences.[15]

- SKIN CONDITIONS: These, along with canker sores and postnasal drip can be caused by dairy products.[16]

- OBESITY: Of children 6 to 17 years old, 25 percent are overweight.[17]

- HIGH CHOLESTEROL: Of children 12 to 14 years of age, 17 percent have cholesterol levels greater than 180 milligrams per deciliter.[18]

- ANEMIA: Children who drink too much cows' milk run the risk of iron-deficiency anemia from intestinal bleeding and blood loss.[19]

- BREAST CANCER: This cancer is a hormone-dependent cancer. Menstruation starts 4 years earlier for girls, and menopause begins 4 years later for women, eating high-fat diets. Thus, for 8 additional years, women have higher levels of estrogen in their systems, which doubles their risk for contracting breast cancer during their life spans.[20]

- VEGETARIAN CHILDREN: Well-informed dietitians, doctors (including the late Dr. Benjamin Spock), and other health professionals accept vegetarianism as a healthy option for infants and children.[21]

Children deserve their childhood. Parents wouldn't knowingly allow an abomination to get in the way of that magical time.

Now that parents have the facts, and *know*, they can help make their children's summers last forever. At least until adulthood.

70: Fatigued

THE BOARD GAME THAT'S EASY TO WIN

Fatigue has a nondescript face, but a sinister underbelly.

Chronic fatigue is an elusive disorder. Is it a disease or a symptom? Is it one ailment or many? Does it have one cause or multiple causes? Is it an ailment, sickness, illness, or syndrome? Is it laziness or depression? Is it mental or is it physical? Or is it Chronic Fatigue Syndrome (CFS) and possibly caused by a virus?

Because fatigue is so vague, it's difficult to treat, often not taken seriously, and elicits little sympathy. Which is all very unfortunate. Because as benign as the perception of chronic fatigue *is*, the result of what it *does*, is anything but harmless.

Chronic fatigue takes a toll on productivity, colors judgment, saps strength, induces long hours of sleep, and can immobilize its sufferers for months at a time. Short of a life-threatening disease it may not get any worse than this.

Where do we go from here, then?

How about backwards.

Many years ago someone thought they had the cause and cure of chronic fatigue pegged. They took steps to publicize it, but unfortunately chose the wrong avenue. They thought turning the knowledge into a board game would make for the best media. They were wrong. Here's what they did.

They took their idea to the Triple "O" (Overworked, Overtaxed, and Overstrained) Toy Company. They produced the board game, then marketed it as a "bored" game, and called it, *Fatigued*. It didn't catch on. People who played it said it made them lethargic, weary, and tired. Production was discontinued after 1 day, and the information never reached the public.

We have obtained one of the rare copies, and after looking it over found the game might provide some relevant clues into the cause and cure of this malady. Here is an overview of the game, *Fatigued*.

OVERVIEW: Players have a game piece (different colored shopping carts) that they move forward with a roll of the dice. They land on squares that have street names like, Thyroid Street, Chronic Fatigue Syndrome Drive, Anemia Lane, Hypoglycemia Circle, and Fat Avenue.

Then they must answer correctly a true/false or multiple-choice question to have the right to roll again. Sometimes players can get slowed up by having to spend time in bed, or can leap ahead by answering bonus questions correctly.

The object of the game, as it says on the box is, "Reach the final square first, with a plant-food energy burst!"

Let's sample a few cards and see how we do.

1. True or False: A deficiency of thyroid hormones character-ized by lethargy could be due to inadequate consumption of foods rich in complex carbohydrates, such as rice, pasta, fruits, vegetables, and beans. (*Answer: True*)[1]

2. After an animal-based, fat-laden meal, one might go lie down on the couch to:

   a) escape from clearing the table.
   b) check for flaws in the ceiling plaster.
   c) overcome fatigue due to thickening of the blood.
   (*Answer: c*)[2]

3. Hypoglycemia, a condition of low blood sugar resulting in fatigue, can be caused by which of the following:

   a) Excess meat consumption.
   b) Excess dietary fat consumption.
   c) Incorrect ratio of proteins, carbohydrates, and fats.
   d) All of the above.
   (*Answer: d*)[3]

4. True or False: The remedy for hypoglycemia is to increase complex carbohydrates like vegetables, beans, and rice, as they blunt the insulin response allowing a more gradual absorption of glucose. (*Answer: True*)[4]

5. To overcome fatigue, Echinacea, Ginseng, and Ginkgo Biloba are often taken as energy boosters. They originate from:

   a) the animal kingdom.
   b) the plant kingdom.
   c) small containers with childproof caps.
   (*Answer: b*)[5]

6. True or False: Fatigue can be caused by lack of iron sometimes resulting in anemia from which herbivores suffer less often than do omnivores. (*Answer: True*)[6]

7. Which of the following problems resulting from a meat-based diet can cause iron to be lost from the body and fatigue to set in?

   a) Hemorrhoids.
   b) Intestinal bleeding from dairy products.
   c) Heavier menstrual periods.
   d) Ulcers.
   e) All of the above.
   (*Answer: e*)[7]

8. Fatigue is often caused by poor elimination. This is most likely due to:

   a) lack of bulky, fibrous cellulose found in plant-based foods.
   b) a diet of muscle, ligaments, and fat found in meat.
   c) both A and B.
   (*Answer: c*)[8]

9. True or False: The SICK diet can result in the intake of at least twice our protein requirement that can cause fatigue. (*Answer: True*)[9]

10. True or False: Chronic Fatigue Syndrome (CFS) is basically a weakened immune system causing chronic weakness. The immune system's killer T-cells can be strengthened by numerous plant-based foods including beta-carotene, and potentially weakened by animal protein. (*Answer: True*)[10]

11. Fibromyalgia, which is not technically classified as an autoimmune disorder, has as one of its symptoms chronic fatigue. In a study, 19 of 30 patients eating the following foods showed dramatic improvement in symptoms.

    a) Cheese Doodles.
    b) Milk Duds.
    c) Buttermilk and liver.
    d) A mostly raw, pure vegetarian diet.
       (*Answer: d*)[11]

12. True or False: The lack of proper nutrients and the build-up of free radicals and cellular wastes can occur from a meat-based diet. Both interfere with the body's ability to access and break down energy stores, subsequently causing feelings of lethargy. (*Answer: True*)[12]

13. True or False: Toxicity from an animal-based diet can result in fatigue. This could be due to meat and dairy products that contain 14 and 5.5 times, respectively, the amount of pesticides as do plant-based foods. (*Answer: True*)[13]

14. Hypertension is quite often an instigator of fatigue. Which two choices are true about high blood pressure:

   a) The disease is incurable.
   b) Hypertension is 13 times more likely in meat-eaters.
   c) Diet plays little role in the disease.
   d) In one study, after changing to a vegetarian diet 58 percent of people came off their medication.
   (*Answer: b and d*)[14]

We have gotten a pretty good feel for the game, so why don't we stop at this point.

It appears the people who originally purchased the game were right. It is predictable and easy to win, thus boring, because all of the answers lead to the WELL diet. It's simple to see why people got weary and tired playing the game.

Changing to a plant-based diet may not eliminate all cases of chronic fatigue, but playing and winning this game on the large game board—life—would be an excellent place to start. A place where we don't want to gamble with a bad roll of the dice.

71: Food and Behavior

HEREDITY, ENVIRONMENT — AND FOOD?

Nature versus Nurture. The ongoing debate of which has the greater influence on our behavior—if either does—will probably never be settled.

The genes are the blueprint and our design. Prior to our first breath we are predisposed with genetic material that has been programmed through the centuries. Many believe that this factor, Nature, is the overriding influence of our behavior.

If the genes are the blueprint, then the environment builds our structure. After our first breath we are put together by such builders as parents, friends, teachers, siblings, and significant emotional events. Many have the opinion that this factor, Nurture, is the overriding influence of our behavior.

Whether it's a 50-50, 60-40, or 40-60 split, it all adds up to 100 percent. Nature and Nurture are the two components that make us who we are—the genes on the inside and the environment on the outside. But is that all? Is it possible there is a third influence? A factor that starts on the outside and ends on the inside?

There is something we consume on average 5 pounds per day, 140,000 pounds in a lifetime.[1] We call it food. We generally view food as a requirement for life support, but should we expand our perception of its role? Is it possible that foods, depending on which foods we consume, influence behavior?

The following data might provide some food for thought.

- SEX OFFENSES: When daily animal fat consumption was plotted against sex offenses for 54 countries a correlation of 50 percent was found. Put another way: 1 of every 2 men convicted of a sex offense should have to switch from the SICK to the WELL diet. Dietary fat and lack of fiber increases testosterone levels in men making them more violent.[2]

- DIVORCE: When daily animal fat consumption was plotted against divorce for 65 countries a correlation of 54 percent was found. Put another way: For every 1 of 2 couples on the brink of divorce a diet switch might do some good.

    Dietary fat and lack of fiber increases hormone levels in both men and women. This further increases the sex differences that already exist; women become more nurturing and men more sexually aggressive.[3]

- WARS AND CIVIL WARS: When daily animal protein consumption was plotted against the number of wars and civil wars for 58 countries, a correlation of 35 percent was found.[4] Put another way: Possibly the *Third* World War could be avoided with a global switch to a vegetarian diet.

    Animal protein reduces tryptophan in the brain, which in turn increases aggression. Certain tribes in Africa, groups of Indians in northwest Brazil, and the Piaroa Indians in Venezuela, have built very peaceful societies based on cooperation without a trace of aggression. Hatred is unknown. It is common knowledge that these people are vegetarians.[5]

- VIOLENT CRIME / SUICIDE: High-fat diets inhibit the uptake of magnesium. A magnesium deficiency increases irritability, belligerence, and depression, and thus the rate of violent crime and suicide. Magnesium also reduces the level of serotonin.[6]

- HARMFUL BEHAVIOR: Serotonin has been shown to suppress harmful behavior impulses. Serotonin levels were found to be low in children who tortured animals and were hostile to their parents. Serotonin levels are low in many depressed or suicidal patients.[7]

- MALE VIOLENCE: Omega-6 fatty acids from meat were found in significantly higher levels in 34 habitually violent, impulsive male criminals when compared against the prison staff. In addition, men who had attempted suicide had roughly 20 per cent higher omega-6 concentrations, compared to men who had never tried to take their own lives.[8]

- VIOLENT CRIMINALS: Seven studies have demonstrated that steroids, pesticides, antibiotics, and other toxic chemicals often contained in meat have been found at elevated levels in violent criminals compared with prisoners who are not violent. A diet filled with high-fiber food leads to a greater excretion of pollutants.[9]

- VIOLENT BEHAVIOR: Adrenal hormones and uric acid remain in the muscle and fat of meat at slaughter. These strong chemicals can instigate violent behavior in human beings.[10]

- DOMINEERING BEHAVIOR: Triglyceride levels, raised by meat eating, have been linked to hostile acts and domineering behavior, according to a study in the British medical journal, *The Lancet*.[11]

- DEPRESSION: Cheese, chicken, eggs, and other animal-based foods can cause hypoglycemia (low blood sugar), which can cause depression.[12]

On the other side of the behavior scale are these examples:

- LESS DEPRESSION: Omega-3 fatty acids, predominately from the plant kingdom, can raise concentrations of serotonin in the brain. Three separate studies show that in societies with a high dietary intake of omega-3 fatty acids such as Japan, China, and Taiwan, rates of depression are lower than in countries with a low intake of these fats.[13]

- EVEN-TEMPERAMENT: Whole grains, beans, and vegetables rich in complex carbohydrates increase the brain's supply of serotonin making people calm and even-tempered.[14]

- CALMNESS: A plant-based diet can change hormone levels and check aggressive tendencies.[15]

- RELAXATION: A vegetarian diet induces alpha waves, which indicate a state of neuromuscular relaxation, not just of the brain but also of the whole body as shown by electroencephalograms (EEGs).[16] Complex carbohydrates better regulate the release of insulin and in turn improve metabolic efficiency.[17]

The factors that influence human behavior are multiple and complex. To suggest that food plays a dominant role in our behavior is to over-emphasize its importance. However, to assume food plays no role at all is to greatly underestimate its power.

Each form of life, every species, is programmed for behavior that will sustain it, rather than destroy it. There are no doubt sound evolutionary reasons for carnivorous animals to be fierce and aggressive, and non-carnivorous animals to be peaceful and sociable.[18] One might conclude that violence is not innate in humans, that it is being kindled by an unnatural influence. If animal-based foods do damage to our bodies, why couldn't they do the same to our minds, thus negatively affecting our behavior?

As we continue to debate the influences of human behavior, of Nature versus Nurture, we should expand the discussion to include food. And maybe from here on out refer to the debate as: Nature versus Nurture versus Nutrition.

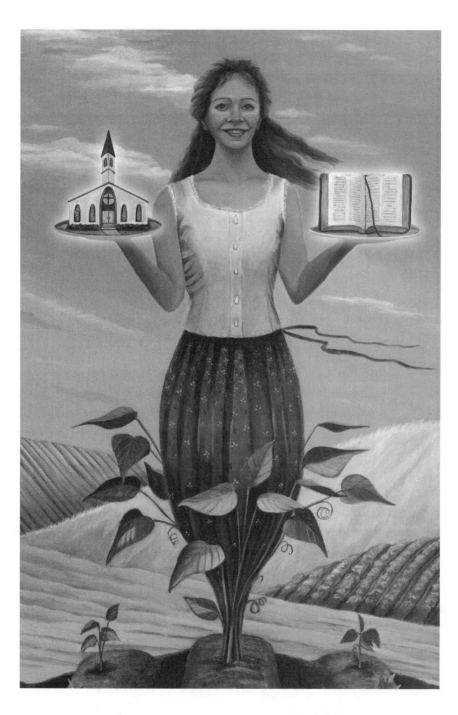

We Can Reason or Rationalize

∼ 9 ∼
Religion
A PERFECT MARRIAGE

Can we find in the vast sea of theology by way of commandments from a supreme being, teachings from a spiritual leader, or language from scriptures, any direction or clues to the nature of humankind's diet? Assuming we found something relevant, if we can't apply scientific methods to it, interview eyewitnesses, or corroborate the discovery, do we have anything of value?

For people whose life is centered on religion an insight might carry more weight than knowledge acquired scientifically. For people who do not practice a religion, but believe in a supreme being, i.e. God, an insight might have a degree of influence. And for those who are atheist, agnostic, positivist, etc., an insight, if profound, might inspire them toward a more spiritual life.

Ahead in this chapter...

Did God intend for humankind's DOMINION over animals to mean absolute authority or benevolent guardianship? It appears to be ambiguous instruction. Find out why it is not.

Does THE BIBLE teach about our diet? Given diet's importance to the success of humankind shouldn't we be able to find a clue—maybe on the first page?

We all complain about the world, but do we think we could design a better one than GOD? Take on the job of Planet Architect and be prepared to see a different perspective.

Is there evidence to support the possibility that JESUS was a vegetarian? If he was, would Christians—whose religion is named for *him*—be compelled to reconsider their dietary choices?

Logically, religious principles and vegetarianism are a perfect marriage, yet there's no sign a religious person is more apt to be vegetarian. How do various RELIGIONS address the issue?

What does religion have to do with GLOBAL HUNGER? Listen in to a radio talk show and hear what a special call-in guest has to say on the subject.

72: Dominion

Not Ambiguous at All

A 5-year-old boy was sitting in Sunday school at the First Methodist Church, a large brick building where it seemed the steeple bells were always ringing. His mother had packed him a baloney sandwich for a snack. While the boy nibbled at his sandwich, the Sunday school teacher told the class how God made everything on the earth: the flowers, the trees, the animals. She said that God loved all his creations, and he wanted everyone to love them, too. She told the class that God wanted all the boys and girls to treat others as they would want to be treated. "Love your neighbor as yourself," she told them. She made a special point to explain that God wanted people to shepherd and take care of God's creatures.

As the young boy continued to eat his sandwich, he recalled that baloney was also called meat, and that meat came from animals. He raised his hand and asked his teacher if baloney was an animal. The teacher said something like, "Well no, not anymore." The little boy thought about it, and then put his sandwich down. The teacher seeing this told the youngster that he needed to finish his sandwich because his mother would want him to grow up big and strong.

With that, the boy began to cry. He told his teacher, as only a little boy could, that he had not taken good care of the creatures. An animal was now in his sandwich, and he was afraid of what God would do to him.

Later in life the little boy became a vegetarian; the teacher may have become one that day.

*****

God tells us by way of the Bible, *Genesis 1:26*, that we have dominion over animals. The passage reads:

"Let them (man) have dominion over the fish of the sea, the birds of the air, and the cattle, and over all the wild animals and all the creatures that crawl on the ground."

Given the variation of diets, and treatment toward animals throughout the world, there seems to be two different and distinct interpretations of the word, dominion.

Some believe the passage says to use our power and authority over animals to serve our best interests. This would presumably include for food, clothing, labor, entertainment, and scientific research. Others believe the passage means to shepherd and take responsibility for the animals, as parents would for their child. This would presumably include *not* for food, clothing, labor, entertainment, and scientific research.

It might strike us as incredibly ironic that the Bible—the word of God—containing instructions crucial to the success of humankind would be so ambiguous, open to interpretation.

But maybe *Genesis 1:26* is not ambiguous at all.

Is it possible there is nothing to reconcile between the two interpretations, meaning the word dominion is crystal clear? That using animals to serve our best interests, *and* to care for and shepherd them, are one and the same and not in conflict?

Let's explore the possibility.

FURTHERING TECHNOLOGY:

- Observing birds take flight gave our forefathers the knowledge and provided the inspiration to build the airplane. If the observers had been hunters, we might still be traveling cross-country by train.

- The ideas and prototypes for navigation, jet propulsion, and hydraulics came from the animal kingdom.[1] Technology that presumably would never have been developed, if we chose to exploit or eat the animals, instead of learning from them.

- Hedgehog spines inspired space-station design.[2]

- The water spider gave us the idea for the first diving bell.[3]

- Bees, ants, and beavers gave us insights into advanced construction methods.

We have advanced technologically and enjoy a better quality of life because of our respect for, and stewardship with, animals.

IMPROVING CHARACTER:

Three of the most honorable traits are loyalty, patience, and sacrifice. If each and every person embodied these traits, would the world not be a better place?

- Look to the chicken for fierce loyalty.
- Look to the cow for incredible patience.
- Look to the pig to learn what sacrifice is.

These traits cannot be obtained by way of digestion.

MAINTAINING THE EARTH:

Even if we desire not to be directly involved with the earth's creatures, we still benefit from their presence by letting nature take its course. The more than 1 million species on this planet make life possible for us by maintaining and sustaining our water, climate, soil, and air.[4]

Technology to advance, character to grow, and maintenance of the earth to survive. Taking care of the animals—having dominion over them—is the equivalent of taking care of ourselves. Eating, wearing, and exploiting animals not only takes away the gain, but adds to the loss, in the form of our health, environment, and food supply.

The meaning of dominion appears to be clear given the products of its differing interpretations. Therefore, as we would expect and count on, there is no ambiguity of the words in the Bible.

But this isn't news to the 5-year-old boy in the Sunday school class. He knew by way of his teacher's words exactly what God meant. He wasn't confused at all.

Maybe this is what *Isaiah 11:6* is all about: ...and a little child shall lead them.

73: The Bible

For some the Bible is a daily source of inspiration. For others, it doesn't play a part in their lives. But whether one is Christian, Jewish, or Islam, Buddhist, Hindu, or Muslim, atheist, agnostic, or positivist, or perhaps some other data point along the religious-non-religious spectrum, the Bible evokes some level of curiosity. After all, it is offered as the word of God.

The extraordinary books of the Bible, or the sacred writings of any religion, would be expected to put forth the fundamental guidelines and rules for humankind to abide by. To convey right from wrong. To provide the basic truths necessary for success and happiness.

Given that food is our lifeblood, a necessity for the survival of humankind and all living organisms, wouldn't we expect food to be a subject addressed somewhere in the 66 books of Bible? If not in the first book?

Let's open a Holy Bible to see if we can find any reference to food. We will use the King James Version. Look here. On the first page, of the first book, second to last verse from the bottom, *Genesis 1:29.* It reads:

> "And God said, Behold, I have given you every herb
> bearing seed, which is upon the face of all of the
> earth, and every tree which is the fruit of a tree
> yielding seed; to you it shall be for meat."

The guideline for the human diet appears clear. Herbs, seeds, and fruit all come from the plant kingdom. It would be hard to rationalize this passage into a sanction to eat animals. However, one word does seem out of place. Meat. According to scholars, the English translations of the Bible used the word "meat" to simplify all the variations of food used in the original Greek scriptures.[1] (Broma means "food," phago means "to eat," trophe means "nourishment," and so on.)

Are there other passages on the first page that might shed additional light on the subject of food?

The passage right before *Genesis 1:29*, although not referring directly to food, may give us additional insight. *Genesis 1:28* reads:

> "Be fruitful, and multiply, and replenish the earth, and subdue it; and have dominion over the fish of the sea, and over the fowl of the air, and over every living thing that moveth upon the earth."

If dominion was interpreted as giving us the discretion to do with animals as we saw fit, including killing and eating them, it wouldn't seem logical that in the very next passage we would be directed to obtain our sustenance from plants. It's almost as if God wrote *Genesis 1:28*, and as an afterthought said to himself, "Gee, I hope they don't interpret dominion as a license to kill and make animals their food. I know! I'll make it clear in the very next verse that they are only to eat plants. Seeds, herbs, and fruits are the words I will use."

Is there other front-page news that might reinforce the notion that God intended the human diet to be exclusively plants?

There are five full verses on the first page of the book of Genesis dedicated to the creation of animals, ending with, "It was good."

Although we are often told we can't take the verses of the Bible literally, it would seem a stretch to suggest that God would go to great lengths to create the animals and creatures (five verses), admire them ("It was good"), and then serve them up as food.

Yet, despite what would appear to be clear direction coming from God by way of these three examples from the first page of Genesis, the fact is, the majority of people whose religion is based on the Bible subscribe to the Self-Induced Carnivorous Killer (SICK) diet. Not even the sixth commandment that tells us not to kill mitigates the choice for them.

The magnitude of the apparent contradiction looks irreconcilable. But the Bible is more than one page; it is a thousand pages. And in those pages are many references to the consumption of meat, fish, and lamb, which is hardly rousing testimony supporting the argument for a vegetarian diet. Even Jesus is witnessed as eating fish and lamb.

However there are biblical scholars who put forth cogent arguments bringing into question the many references used as arguments for a meat-based diet. For example:

- English translations of the Bible used one word, "meat" to cover all the variations of food in the original Greek scriptures.

- The references to "fish" may well be fish plant rolls, a popular delicacy in Jesus' time, which are still eaten today.[2]

- Reasonable evidence suggests Jesus did not partake of the Paschal Lamb.[3]

- Evidence suggests that Jesus was a vegetarian. His brother James was a practicing vegetarian.[4] Certainly Jesus' actions and what he stood for would be consistent with vegetarianism.

- Some scholars assert that in the fourth century, priests and politicians completely altered original Christian documents to make them acceptable to Emperor Constantine, and to make them the accepted creed of the Roman Empire. Among the alterations were certain teachings they did not propose to follow—such as those against the eating of flesh.[5]

There are those who argue that food is a trivial matter in comparison to the deeper and more consequential issues the Bible addresses. But what could be more consequential than a food choice that is injurious to us, our planet, and potentially to our survival?

There are those who argue that the sixth commandment, *Thou shall not kill*, applies only to humankind. But would God create millions of living organisms, and then selectively apply this command to only one of them?

There are those who argue that the language of the Bible is largely symbolic. But how can we faithfully carry out God's plan if there are contrasting interpretations for any given passage?

There are newspaper editors who argue that the most important news stories go on the front page, because they are the issues that affect our lives most.

Maybe that's what our Editor-in-Chief had in mind.

74: God

PLANET ARCHITECT — A NEW PERSPECTIVE

Complaining. We all love to do it. We can let off steam, feel noble thinking we can do better, and make conversation, all in one verbal swoop. Complaining has become a habit for many, and made into a fine art by others.

People complain about war, poverty, crime, sickness, their life, and the world they live in. Just about anything that isn't working well is a target. But after a while complaining gets old and monotonous, and it's time to step up to the plate and see if we can really do better. The only problem is, nobody has ever given us the opportunity to make a better world.

Well now somebody has. If we think we can do better, we will be given an uncultivated planet in the galaxy to populate and develop. We will be in charge of design and production. Let's go.

JOB TITLE: To get us started it's important to have a job title that reflects our important assignment. Maker? Not enough pizzazz. Supreme Being? Too showy. God? Already taken. What about, Planet Architect – Apprentice? It commands respect, but at the same time it's honest.

JOB TRAINING: We are on our own, however the author will make some suggestions.

FIRST TASK — POPULATING THE PLANET: Unfortunately we can't start from scratch because we have a deadline to meet, but we do have some options.

- We could create a single species. However, that might get boring.

- We could have multiple species, with one being superior

and in charge. But that might lead the superior species to abuse its role, which could lead to problems.

- We could have multiple species, with one species further evolved—a principal species. Each species would have a purpose and supporting role, and each life form would be reliant on each other for survival.

  For example, the supporting species could maintain the planet's natural resources, inspire creativity and technology for the principal species, and provide variety, interest, and beauty for the planet. We could call the principal species, womankind.

SECOND TASK – PROVIDE NOURISHMENT: Womankind will need a daily food source to sustain life. The nourishment should probably include the following features:

- Variety, simplicity, and accessibility
- Potential to be produced anywhere on the planet
- Ability to absorb nutrients already placed into the planet
- Species to spread seed around the planet for replenishment
- Immobile—inability to run away
- Compatible with womankind's anatomy

THIRD TASK – INSTRUCTION MANUAL: Provide guidelines and mechanisms to minimize risk of failure, and thus increase the planet's chance of success. There are two different and distinct paths we could take.

- FIRST PATH — Write it all down and put it in a book. This would appear at first glance to be the proper route. But as the planet evolved and the people and language changed, the book could become less understood and muddled. This could leave the instructions open to interpretation, potentially leading to confusion, discord, and alienation. The result being that we would have been better off not producing a book at all.

- SECOND PATH — A system of free will with built-in self-correction and 10 guidelines to live by. Womankind would be equipped with free will and unlimited potential. A closed feedback loop would provide consequences for every action—good or bad—signaling the principal species as to what was right and wrong. Adding 10 high-level guidelines would complete the system, furthering the chances of success. Something like:

  - Don't kill.
  - Don't steal.
  - Treat others as we would want to be treated.
  - Do good work.
  - Play fair.
  - Give to others less fortunate.
  - Develop unions to populate the planet.
  - Take care of the planet's natural resources.
  - Support all species in their purposes.
  - Treat the body well.

If for example there was massive hunger, degenerative sickness, or damaged and depleted natural resources, that would be a signal for the principal species to find the cause and take action to correct it.

FOURTH TASK — RESOURCES AND BACKUP: We might want to consider some kind of all-purpose resource for climate control, recreation, medicines, and a backup resource for nourishment and drinking water. Maybe some very large bodies of water to cover the planet. And maybe we should add something to the water so it isn't prematurely depleted.

That's it. That should be enough to get us started with our new planet. Are we ready to start work and create a better world?

What? We have changed our mind? We realize our planet already contains the raw materials and potential to flourish. That the ideas we suggested, with some minor exceptions, are not new ideas, but devices already incorporated in the planet.

The architect did its job, now it's up to the operators to do theirs. They have every opportunity to self-correct and fulfill the planet's potential.

75: Jesus

WHAT IF HE WAS A VEGETARIAN?

The majority of Christians in America consume meat, fish, dairy, and eggs. If the man their religion was named after *didn't*, and was a vegetarian, would Christian meat-eaters be compelled to reconsider their dietary choices?

Do Christians ever consider the issue? Or do some of the following reasons distance them from the thought?

- The Bible's many references to fish and meat.
- The reality that we can never know, so why consider it.
- The idea that food is not an overriding religious issue.
- The relevance of biblical diets and habits to modern times.
- The meat-eating habits of a Christian's peers and role models: the congregation, minister, and church hierarchy.

Given who Jesus was, and what he stood for, it wouldn't be a stretch to conclude that Jesus did not eat animal flesh. And let's imagine, if only for a moment, that he was a vegetarian. Would Jesus, and his Father, not have some issues with those who ate meat, fish, dairy, and eggs, given the horrific treatment that the animals must endure?

It might not be a bad investment of our time to take a few minutes and review some evidence. Evidence that suggests Jesus may well have been a vegetarian.

- Was Jesus from Nazareth or was Jesus a Nazarene? Early Greek manuscripts and references in The New Testament indicate that Jesus was a Nazarene, rather than coming from the city of Nazareth. The Nazarenes were a vegetarian sect.[1]

- James, Jesus brother, was a practicing vegetarian. Granted, all family members don't necessarily practice the same food choices, but would it not be easy to imagine that Jesus could have influenced his brother, just as he influenced many others?[2]

- Was Jesus condemned to die for cleansing the temple of the moneychangers by overturning their tables, or for disrupting the moneychangers' business: selling animals for sacrifice. The following words from Jesus as he drove the sacrificial animals outdoors, might provide a clue. "Stop making my father's house into a meat market!"[3]

- It would seem out of character that a man who preached simplicity and frugality would have dined on meat, a scarce and luxurious food for his time. And how could a religious and moral figure slit the throat of an animal and then relish its flesh?

- Could a man who said the following be more likely to be a meat-eater or a vegetarian? "And the flesh of slain beasts in his body will become his own tomb. For I tell you truly, he who kills, kills himself, and he who so eats the flesh of slain beasts, eats the body of death."[4] These are the words of Jesus according to the early Aramaic texts.

- The idea that Jesus was a vegetarian is not a conspiracy perpetrated by non-Christian vegetarians. There are a number of current sects of Christianity—The Order of the Cross, the Ebionites, and the Seventh-day Adventists—who believe that Christ was most likely a vegetarian and so follow a vegetarian regimen. A Christian vegetarian worth noting is John Wesley. Mr. Wesley founded the Methodists.

- Christians who eat meat could cite many examples from The New Testament of Jesus asking for meat and be satisfied that their diets were not in conflict with Christ's principles. However, the original Greek scriptures used a number of words for food (broma, brosimos, brosis, trophe, prosphagion, and phago). To simplify things, the English translations of the Bible substituted one word in their place: meat.[5]

- Did Jesus feed the multitudes with five loaves and two fishes, or five loaves and something else? According to John's Gospel, Jesus multiplied the two *opsaria*, which comes from the Greek word, *opson* (relish). A common accompaniment to bread at that time was a relish of olive and sesame paste.[6]

- Did Jesus eat the sacrificial lamb for the Passover meal at the Last Supper, or were these gatherings two separate events as John's Gospel suggests. The lamb is never mentioned in connection with the Last Supper. If Jesus were a meat-eater he would have used lamb, and not bread, as the symbol of the Divine Passion. His use of bread and wine in place of flesh and blood is indeed food for thought.[7]

We just came home from a party where we spent an hour or so talking to a nice man we had not met before. He struck us as a very loving and compassionate man. He touched on some issues that gave us the idea he was also a very moral and principled individual.

At one point we were talking about diet and he said, "He who so eats the flesh of slain beasts, eats the body of death."

Toward the end of the evening he told us he had gone to a slaughterhouse and at the risk of his own life, freed some of the animals. Although we didn't understand the remark he told us he had made as he left there, "Stop making my father's house into a meat market!" we knew there was no mistaking where he was coming from.

We enjoyed this person's company. In fact, we are having a dinner party in the next couple of weeks and we will definitely invite him and his wife. We just have to remember where our vegetarian cookbook is.

76: Religions

WE CAN BOTH REASON *AND* RATIONALIZE

Religion is defined as "A set of beliefs, values, and practices based on the teachings of a spiritual leader." The majority of humankind belongs to a religion, or if not, at least subscribes to some of religion's fundamental principles, such as:

- Love, mercy, and compassion
- A reverence for life
- Do unto others (as you would have done unto you)
- A moral code of conduct and ethical principles
- Condemnation of hate, violence, and prejudice

To eat meat—cause the death of an animal—encroaches on each of these fundamental religious principles. (If we think we can distance ourselves from the blade, consider that if we all stopped eating meat tomorrow, the demand, the supply—and the blade—all come to a screeching halt.)

Can we conclude, then, that a meat-eater cannot be a religious person?

The answer would most likely come back that they can be religious, because these principles were intended to only apply to our fellow human beings. Thus, even though religion addresses the search for truth, the meaning of life, and the creation of the universe making it all-inclusive, we have chosen to selectively apply religion only to our fellow human beings, making it all-exclusive.

Today, many people from many different faiths have no problem reconciling their meat-eating habits with their religious values. But long ago it might have been different.

- The earliest Jewish religious group, the Essenes, were vegetarian.[1]

- The Jewish Christians, the Ebionites, the first Christian community after the death of Jesus, were vegetarian.[2]

- The first Christians, the Nazarenes, were vegetarian.[3]

- The early Roman Catholicism orders—the Augustinians, the Franciscans, and the Benedictines—began as vegetarian.[4]

- Many of the outstanding masters of the major spiritual traditions were vegetarian.[5]

Between early religion and modern times is it possible a spin was put on religion's absolute and eternal laws that made meat-eating and religion reconcilable?

- Were Christian documents altered by "Correctores" in the fourth century to bring them in line with the interests of the Roman Empire? And did this include certain teachings that prevented the eating of flesh?[6]

- Was reincarnation—a widely held belief among Christians—abolished by the Second Ecumenical Council in Constantinople due to the fear people would live loosely knowing they would get another chance? This belief would have prevented the slaughter of animals and meat-eating.[7]

- Did the Talmud suggest that early rabbis, in order not to lose followers and ensure the survival of the Jewish tradition, dispense with the law prohibiting the eating of flesh?[8]

- Have "meatatarian" clergy tampered with Buddhist and Christian scriptures?[9]

- Did the Church of Rome suppress the original spirit of Christ's teachings, that animals possessed souls?[10]

- Did the priesthood of early Judaism encourage meat-eating, not as an end in itself, but to suppress sects that practiced vegetarianism so as to maintain spiritual authority and power?[11]

In essence, did authoritarian, political, and economic motivations bend the absolute and eternal laws of religious doctrine? There is some evidence to suggest they did.

Does this then mean that today vegetarianism and religion are no longer connected? Can we no longer find what would appear to be a perfect marriage of religious principles and diet—vegetarianism?

To the contrary, although they may not be perfect marriages, plenty of them abound.

BUDDHISM: Buddhism's first precept is not to kill any living being. Because eating meat involves killing animals, it would seem that vegetarianism is a consequence of the first precept. Not all Buddhists practice the tradition though, and many Buddhists today eat meat, but the tradition handed down indicates that Buddha intended the road to selflessness to include relinquishing the killing of animals.[12]

HINDU: The Hindu tradition advocates vegetarianism, and Hindu teachers have prescribed vegetarianism for hundreds of years. The religion grew out of the sensitivity to animals and the relationship between ecology and human prosperity. Mahatma Gandhi, the modern Hindu leader, was a vegetarian and viewed vegetarianism and the respect for the sacred cow as part of nonviolence.[13]

ISLAM: Islam does not prescribe a particular diet. But there is respect for animals and a contingent of vegetarians among those who practice Islam. Many of the Sufis, a sect of Islam, practiced vegetarianism in ancient times and still subscribe to the dietary practice today.[14]

BAHA'I: The Baha'i religion emphasizes spiritual unity of all humankind, and states, "Our natural food is that which grows out of the ground."[15]

JAINISM: Jainism requires its followers to be vegetarian. The practice of harmlessness and protection of all living beings is the very first vow of all Jains. Their motto is simply to respect all life in the world.[16]

JUDAISM: Judaism lays claim to many vegetarians. Compassion to animals is part of Jewish teaching, and one has an obligation to relieve the suffering of animals. Many Jews believe, however, that God has sanctioned the eating of meat by virtue of dietary laws governing their consumption—if the slaughter is humane and all blood is drained from the animal. But the Jewish vegetarian argues that "humane slaughter" is an oxymoron and that there is no way to completely drain the blood from an animal. Therefore, God was trying to show—albeit roundabout—that eating meat wasn't kosher.[17]

CHRISTIANITY: Christianity boasts many sects that follow a vegetarian regime. The Trappist monks of the Catholic Church are vegetarian. The Seventh-day Adventists recommend vegetarianism to their members, of which at least one-half follow the diet. The Friends Vegetarian Society of North America (Quaker) supports a plant-based diet. And the Mormons have a meatless contingent.[18]

TAOISM: One of the 3 main religions of China, Taoism, has always required a vegetarian diet.[19]

There are a number of major religions. And each of the religions has splinter sects. Each religion has a different leader, and each religion subscribes to a different set of beliefs, traditions, and rituals.

But there is also a common thread that runs through all religions; a thread that weaves a few fundamental principles through each one's fabric.

It is everyone's choice to pick his or her religion. It is everyone's choice to interpret the religion's values. It is everyone's choice to reason or rationalize.

77: Global Hunger

WHAT DOES IT HAVE TO DO WITH RELIGION?

"I'm dying for food," said the overweight American after his third day of dieting. "I'm dying for food," said a human being before he died of starvation.

The words are the same; the experiences are entirely different. Does one have anything to do with the other? Could the dieter have given the food that made him overweight to the human being that died from lack of food, solving both their problems? It would seem rather silly to think so, however...

There are 1.2 billion people in the world who are underfed and as a result are sick and die prematurely. There are 1.2 billion people in the world who are overfed and as a result are sick and die prematurely.[1]

Is it just a coincidence there are an equal number of sufferers on both sides of the equation? Maybe the following conversation can catalyze the issue:

STARVING PERSON: I see you have a cup of grain in your hand.

CATTLE FARMER: Yes, it is for my cattle.

STARVING PERSON: If you would give it to me, I could stay alive for a while longer.

CATTLE FARMER: I'm sorry. The grain is for my animals to produce meat for people.

(Sometime Later.)

OMNIVORE: That steak was yummy, but I need to go on a diet.

STARVING PERSON: Good-bye.

It takes 16 pounds of grain to produce 1 pound of beef.[2] If that grain was fed to human beings, instead of cattle for beef, we could feed

2 to 3 times the current population.[3] Instead, 15 million people die annually of malnourishment and starvation.[4] Could the scenario be that simple? Isn't there a whole web of social inequities and political realities that contribute to global hunger? Maybe. Maybe not.

The simplicity of the solution is often inversely proportional to the complexity of the problem. Combine this maxim with the applied logic of Newton's third law of motion—for every action there is an equal and opposite reaction—and maybe the remedy is as we have identified it.

But what do underfed people and overfed people have to do with religion? Is this God's way of controlling the population, weeding out the weak, or punishing the sinful?

Let's listen in to a local radio talk show. A special call-in guest may be able to help answer the question.

HOST: This is radio station KATL, and I'm your host, Steve Stevens. Today we will be discussing global hunger. We have as our in-studio guests, Pastor John Smith, from the Main Street Church, and a parishioner from his church, Bob Jones. Gentlemen, welcome. Pastor Smith, can you tell us what your church is doing to help with the problem of global hunger?

PASTOR SMITH: Yes. I have asked each member of our congregation to add an additional one dollar to the collection plate each week. This money will be used to buy a variety of canned foods to send to hungry people overseas.

HOST: Which countries will be receiving the foods?

PASTOR SMITH: I don't recall. But Bob Jones is in charge of our canned food drive. I'll let him speak.

HOST: Bob, tell us what you're doing.

BOB JONES: Yes, Mr. Stevens. With the extra money from the collection plates we will buy a wide variety of canned foods, which will go to a selection of third world countries. Let's see…I seemed to have misplaced the list of the countries.

Anyway, I want to stress for those members who are buying the canned food themselves, please don't. We will do that after we collect the money. Last week, Mrs. Johnson, bless her heart, brought in a can of sauerkraut. I tried to tell her that…well…I just told her we would buy the food and thanked her.

HOST: Well it sounds like your church is really stepping up to the plate, trying to do its part to solve the world hunger crisis. Why don't we take some calls from our listening audience to find out what others might be doing.

Our first caller on the line tonight is…what is this Debby? Debby is our screener, folks. Ok, I'll play along. Our first caller tonight is, *God*. What's on your mind?

GOD: It's usually not my place to interfere, however I must make exceptions from time-to-time.

You may recall me saying that I have given you all that you need, or words to that effect. Meaning that no one should go hungry. I also encouraged you to be fruitful and multiply, with no stipulations. Meaning that no matter how many of you there became, no one would go hungry. And I thought I was pretty clear on how to sustain yourselves with herb-bearing seeds, tree-yielding fruit, and so forth.

I also provided what I thought to be a clever system of checks and balances. So when things did go wrong, especially something as catastrophic as global hunger, the solution would be easy to identify and implement.

I appreciate your compassion and your desire to help, however let me suggest that you reassess your approach to the problem. Thank you for taking my call.

HOST: Ahhh, yes. Stay with us for a moment if you would, Sir. Our guests might have some questions for you. Anybody?

BOB JONES: You have some nerve, whoever you are. How disrespectful! Down right blasphemous representing yourself...

PASTOR SMITH: Mr. Caller, what's your name? (pause) OK, then. What you just said has piqued my interest. I've never heard it put quite that way before. Would you be willing to come to our service this coming Sunday and speak to us about it?

GOD: I'll be there. As always.

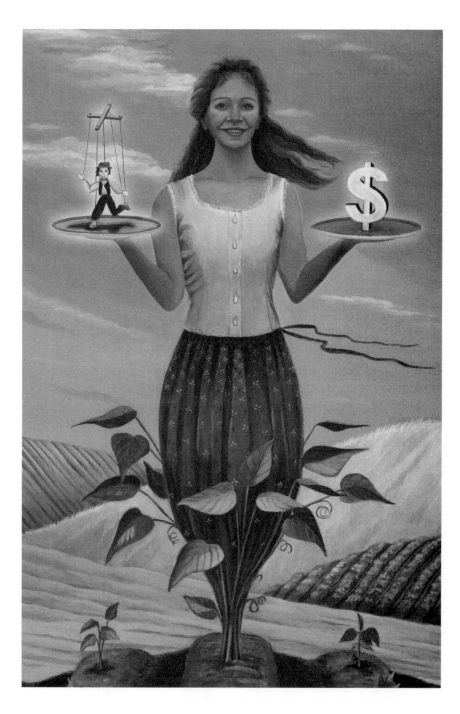

One Green Undermining Another

~ 10 ~
Manipulation
CAUTION: ECONOMIC FORCES AT WORK

Have our meat and dairy habits, and the perception of their effect on our health, been influenced by powerful economic forces?

Ahead in this chapter...

Have the peddlers of PROTEIN—the producers of animal-based foods—put a tiger in our closet?

Should the FOOD GUIDE PYRAMID instead be shaped like a wedge—a wedge of Swiss cheese: smelly with lots of holes?

How have the BEEF TRADE ASSOCIATIONS prevented their dam from bursting, washing away $60 billion in annual revenue?[1]

Is the DAIRY COUNCIL a distributor of honest promotion, or a peddler of dishonest propaganda?

Are SCHOOL DONATIONS—educational materials and food commodities—philanthropic gestures or psychological and physiological conditioning?

Are GOVERNMENT SUBSIDIES that lower the prices of animal-based foods, leapfrogging the free-market system, in our best interest?

Why do millions of ADVERTISING dollars go to promote the potato chip, but few go to promote the potato?

We call it healthcare, but the system is not designed to keep us healthy, therefore wouldn't ILLNESS-CARE be a better label?

Is it possible the power and wealth of the PHARMACEUTI-CAL INDUSTRY is a direct result of our failure to utilize the foods and immune system that Nature provided?

Does the history of the MEDICAL PROFESSION indicate it to be a humanitarian endeavor, or a profit-directed business?

Could the success of fighting cancer be compromised due to the CANCER BUSINESS being the second largest industry in the United States?[2]

Is MENOPAUSE a natural event in a woman's life, or a medical condition requiring intervention and drugs?

78: Protein

IS THERE A TIGER IN OUR CLOSET?

Once upon a time there was a 4-year-old boy who had a very cruel father. When the boy's dad tucked him in at night he warned him that if he didn't stay in bed a ferocious tiger would come out of his bedroom closet and get him. The ploy worked. The boy never left his bed for fear of the tiger. Why take a chance, he thought. Besides, he trusted his father and had no reason to doubt or question his motives.

Have the producers of animal-based foods put a tiger in our closet? Is the fear of not getting enough protein *our* tiger, placed there by the producers of animal-based foods to ensure we buy their goods? Is our reasoning, why take a chance? Have we trusted them, not doubting or questioning their motives?

The most important question though is this: Do humans need to consume animal-based foods to get enough—or the right kind of—protein?

Let's begin to work our way toward the closet door.

How much protein do humans need as a percentage of calories?

- 2.5 percent: In 1945 the *Annual Review of Biochemistry* suggested that many populations have lived in excellent health on this amount.[1]

- 2.5 percent: The minimal protein requirement reported in 1968 in the *American Journal of American Nutrition* was this amount.[2]

- 2.5 percent: In 1987, Dr. John McDougall, whose work in the field of medicine focuses on the prevention of disease, based on his and other's scientific research, reported that humans require this amount.[3]

- 3.0 percent: Research done in the 1940s and published in 1952 by research scientist Dr. William Rose, showed that humans stay in nitrogen balance with this amount.[4]

- 5.0 percent: The World Health Organization recommends this amount as a minimum requirement.[5]

- 5.0 percent: Human breast milk, at a time of critical growth, contains this amount of protein.[6]

- 6.0 percent: The Food and Nutrition Board, after adding a safety margin of 30 percent to cover 98 percent of the U.S. population, has this as their figure for the Recommended Daily Allowance (RDA).[7]

- 10.0 percent: The U.S. RDA for protein.[8]

How much protein do Americans consume?

- 16.5 percent: The average omnivore American gets this amount of protein of which 11.0 percent comes from meat and dairy products.[9]

- 13.0 percent: The average lacto-ovo vegetarian who consumes dairy products takes in this amount.[10]

- 11.0 percent: The pure vegetarian who only eats from the plant kingdom consumes this amount.[11]

How much protein, as a percentage of calories, do plant and animal-based foods contain?[12]

PLANTS:*	ANIMALS:
- 8.0 percent in Fruits	- 25.0 percent in Dairy
- 15.0 percent in Nuts / Seeds	- 38.0 percent in Eggs
- 15.0 percent in Grains	- 47.0 percent in Meats
- 26.0 percent in Vegetables	- 49.0 percent in Poultry
- 30.0 percent in Legumes	- 68.0 percent in Fish

* Examples of protein percentages from the plant kingdom:

> FRUITS: cantaloupe 9.0, orange 8.0, grape 8.0
> NUTS / SEEDS: peanuts 18.0, sunflowers 17.0, cashews 12.0
> GRAINS: wheat 17.0, oats 15.0, barley 11.0
> VEGETABLES: spinach 49.0, mushrooms 38.0, tomatoes 18.0
> LEGUMES: soybeans 35.0, lentils 29.0, kidney beans 26.0

Note: Vegetable protein on average is 60 percent usable by the body. Animal protein 70 percent.

Is plant protein of sufficient quality for human nutrition?

- Of the 22 amino acids that the human body requires, 9 must come from foods to manufacture all the necessary proteins.[13]

- Plants contain all 9 essential amino acids, and with few exceptions, are in the right proportions for the body to absorb.[14]

- Experiments have shown that subjects eating only plant sources of protein have maintained nitrogen equilibrium.[15]

- According to the American Dietetic Association, if we get enough calories and eat a reasonable variety of plant-based foods, it is virtually impossible not to meet protein needs.[16]

Can consuming too much protein be harmful?

> Too much protein, especially animal protein, has been implicated in the cause and promotion of the following: kidney disease, osteoporosis, heart disease, cancer, and the autoimmune diseases: Crohn's disease, multiple sclerosis, insulin-dependent diabetes, lupus, and rheumatoid arthritis.[17]

On average, individuals in the United States who subscribe to the Self-Induced Carnivorous Killer (SICK) diet are acquiring animal protein by consuming the following amount of animal-based foods a year:[18]

- 200 pounds of red meat
- 50 pounds of chicken and turkey
- 10 pounds of fish
- 586 pounds of dairy products
- 300 eggs

Are American vegetarians, who number 12 million, suffering ill health by consuming only plant proteins?

- The primary disease of a protein deficiency is Kwashiorkor. There are virtually no cases of this disorder in the United States.[19]

Given the answers to all the previous questions, how did animal-based foods become a requirement to meet human protein needs?

To determine how to make their *animals* grow the biggest, in the shortest time, for the most profit, livestock producers initiated the first studies of protein needs. Osborne and Mendel conducted the research in 1914. They used rats and determined that rats grew faster on animal protein than they did on plant protein.[20] In the 1940s further research found that the amino acid patterns of animal protein were more "complete" than plant protein. A pattern close to the egg was found to optimize growth in the rat.[21]

This data was used by the meat, dairy, and egg industries to promote animal protein, and thus their products, as a superior form of nutrition for humans. No mention was made that the experimental subjects were rats; that rats' breast milk contained 49 percent protein in calories to a human's 5 percent; that rats consuming animal protein died earlier and were sicker than rats consuming plant protein.[22] And that fast growth was translated to mean optimal health!

Before anyone noticed, these industries had grabbed the ball and were off running. It wasn't long before the concept of complete and superior protein from meat and dairy, versus the incomplete and inferior protein of plants, was taught in school science and health education.[23]

These conclusions were wholly accepted as fact, and went unchallenged for many years. Ultimately the studies, as applied to humans, were determined to be unfounded, and modern nutritionists have abandoned the theory. Net Protein Utilization is now used as a basis to determine how much protein we derive from various foods.[24]

Over the years, the quantity of protein a person needs has been pushed around by political and economic forces rather than by science. The most overt example occurred in 1958, when the Minimal Daily Requirement (MDR) became the Recommended Daily Allowance (RDA). Where an MDR is more likely to be based on a scientific number, an RDA lends itself, by virtue of its definition, to greater subjectivity.[25]

It is going to take time to undo a half-century or more of falsehoods, conditioning, and brainwashing. However, we are moving toward the closet and getting closer to the door. Eventually we will put aside our fears, allow rational thought to prevail, and fling open the door.

And just as the little boy grew up to find no tiger in his closet, we will do the same, and find none in ours.

79: Food Guide Pyramid

MORE LIKE A WEDGE — OF SWISS CHEESE

We have been eating poorly and we know it. We have gained weight and realize we must change our eating habits. What better place to start, we surmise, than the U.S. Department of Agriculture (USDA) Food Guide Pyramid.

It's time for lunch so we pick our food choices from the various Pyramid nutrition groups. After a surprisingly satisfying lunch, we lean back in our chair and think to ourselves: *This wasn't so bad, I just might be able to handle this diet.*

In fact, we're rather cocky because we covered at least 1 item from each of the 6 food groups at one meal. Our lunch consisted of a cheeseburger with mayonnaise, french fries, chocolate cake, milk, and an apple. And even though we are not too terribly found of apples, we made the sacrifice in the name of good health.

No doubt we can make better choices from the food groups, but our lunch did stay within the Pyramid guidelines. French fries from the vegetable group. Cake from the grains, breads, and cereals group. And the rest of the meal covered the meat, dairy, oils-sweets, and fruit groups.[1]

The Food Guide Pyramid is guiding us all right—straight toward ill health. Granted this is a hypothetical example. Surely if we undertook a study with a large sampling of the population following the Pyramid guidelines, we would see some measurable improvement in their health compared to the general population.

More than 51,000 men and 67,000 women participated for 8 and 12 years, respectively, in a Harvard study that monitored food choices against the Pyramid. Women who followed the guidelines were no less likely to develop a chronic disease than those who didn't. The men were no less likely to develop cancer, but did show a modest, 11 percent, risk reduction in cardiovascular disease.[2]

Essentially, the Food Guide Pyramid made little difference to the benefit of one's health. But in a country where the USDA Food Guide Pyramid represents the official nutrition model, and there are 100 million Americans that have a chronic disease with conservatively 2 out of every 3 attributable to diet, then maybe we shouldn't expect too much from the Pyramid.[3] In fact, maybe the pyramid shape should be a wedge shape instead. Like a wedge of Swiss cheese—smelly with a lot of holes in it.

What is the history of the USDA Food Guide Pyramid and why is it letting us down?

- 1862: Congress created the USDA to educate the public on agricultural matters, provide a reliable and consistent food supply, and promote farmers' interests.[4]

- 1916: The USDA published its first food guidelines.[5]

- 1943: The concept of "food groups" was developed. The Twelve Food Groups was published. Eight of the 12 groups were plant-based foods. Twelve groups proved to be cumbersome, so they were condensed down to the Basic Seven. This scheme also emphasized fruits and vegetables.[6]

- 1955: The nutritional model was completely overhauled, with some new contributors, and some new results. The Basic Four Food Group model was born. Developed at the Harvard University Department of Nutrition, it was largely funded by animal agriculture: cattlemen and dairy farmers.[7]

  Meat and milk now represented 2 of the 4 food groups, and as a consequence, the future foundation of our meal planning in this country. Some refer to this model as a marketing campaign masquerading as nutritional necessities.[8]

- 1956 to 1974: Evidence mounted that maybe the Basic Four's nutritional guidance left a lot to be desired.[9]

- 1975: A U.S. Senate subcommittee suggested that the Basic Four Food Groups be revised to reduce the intake of cholesterol and saturated fat and increase the consumption of fruits, grains, and vegetables.

The Basic Four Food Groups didn't get changed, but the subcommittee's report did. From "consume less meat and milk" to "choose lean meat and nonfat milk." [10]

- 1988: In the face of mounting nutrition research, the USDA began to redraw the Basic Four food chart. The new design depicted a foundation of whole grains, fruits, and vegetables. [11]

- 1989 - 1991: The new plan was developed, but not received well by certain interests, and its release was delayed for more than a year. [12]

- 1992: The new USDA Food Guide Pyramid was released. It contained 6 groups with a foundation of whole grains, fruits, and vegetables. The guide was a step forward, however it still recommended four plus servings a day of animal-based foods: meat, fish, dairy, and eggs. [13]

- 2000: The Physicians Committee for Responsible Medicine (PCRM) filled a lawsuit charging that the agency's guidelines were unhealthy and catered to the food industry. It stated that 6 of the 11 advisory members who devised the guidelines had explicit links to the National Dairy Board, the National Dairy Council, the American Egg Board, the National Cattlemen's Beef Association, the American Meat Institute, and the Dannon Research Institute. [14]

- 2001: A ruling found that the USDA violated federal law by keeping documents secret used in setting federal nutrition policies, and by hiding financial conflicts of interest among members of a diet advisory committee. [15]

The Food Guide Pyramid model released in 1992 is still the standard today. Although it reduced the emphasis on meat and dairy products from 2 of 4 groups, to 2 of 6 groups, the cattlemen and dairy farmers couldn't have been too unhappy as their products were still players in the nutritional game. And the 37-year run that animal-based foods had at the top of the charts, conditioning our desire and forming our buying habits, continues to influence us.

The Food Guide Pyramid is still a far cry from ideal nutritional guidance. The defenders say it presents an appropriate compromise between "what is realistic and what is optimal."[16] Which is much like saying: Even though eggs and bacon can initiate atherosclerosis and cancer, people will continue to eat them, so they should try to keep the servings down to two or three times a week. If we took this approach to parenting our reasoning would be: We know our kids are going to run into traffic anyway, so we should advise them not to do so more than two or three times a week.

Those that develop the next version of the USDA Food Guide Pyramid, in addition to depicting a more accurate reflection of nutritional research, might also consider a change to its shape. From a pyramid to a spinach leaf perhaps? Or better yet, what about the profile of Abraham Lincoln. Honest Abe.

80: Beef Trade Associations

PLUGGING THE HOLES IN THE DAM

Beef consumption has declined every year since 1977.[1] This is frankly a surprise. Not because most Americans still consider beef to be a nutritional necessity, but because the beef trade associations have done such a thorough job in creating a positive image, while suppressing unfavorable coverage for their product. A job not unlike trying to keep up the maintenance on a badly leaking dam.

Organizations such as the National Cattlemen's Beef Association (NCBA), American Meat Institute (AMI), and National Livestock and Meat Board (NLMB) have a full-time job plugging up the holes in the dam, caused by the very shaky ground the dam was built on. And although it continues to leak and lose water every year, the dam is still plenty full, with $60 billion in annual beef revenue.[2]

Education, government, science, medicine, and the media have all been employed to keep the dam intact. The following materials have been used to repair and maintain the barrier, but it's anybody's guess how long they can keep it from bursting.

EDUCATIONAL AIDS: The NCBA had planned to reach 10.5 million school children with "educational" kits during a 5-year period, beginning in 1997.[3] Based on the material of past kits an example might have included, "The Story of Beef," a cartooned story directed at young children portraying a calf apparently tickled to death to become their future meal.[4] Well, maybe not *tickled*.

NUTRITION LABELS: We find them on all packaged and processed foods. We don't find them on beef and other fresh meats. Packaged foods are regulated by the Food and Drug Administration (FDA); Fresh meats and beef are regulated by the Department of Agriculture (USDA).[5] Should the governing organization make a difference in what food gets labeled and what food doesn't? Are there good reasons for beef not to have nutrition labels? Maybe the amount of calories, cholesterol, and saturated fat, along with other questionable ingredients might discourage sales. Or maybe the label would just be too big to fit on the package.

MAGAZINE ARTICLES: In 1997 the NCBA visited food editors and writers of some of the nation's largest magazines to provide recent information on beef. (Although one has to wonder how dead flesh changes.) These visits paid off handsomely, resulting in more than 7,000 positive beef stories—stories that carry far greater credibility than paid advertising.[6]

MEDICAL PRINT ADVERTISING: The NLMB has taken out full-page color ads in the *Journal of the American Medical Association*. Gaining the allegiance of the medical profession is a critical gear in the public image machine.[7]

SCIENCE: Research conducted on rats in 1914 to determine how to get livestock to grow faster (answer: animal protein), is still used today as the basis of the claim that animal protein is superior for humans.[8]

POLITICAL CONTRIBUTIONS: From 1987 to 1996 the NCBA gave $1.4 million to Congress in campaign contributions. The meat industry gave House Speaker Newt Gingrich $232,239, Kay Hutchinson $409,178, and Phil Gramm $611,484. Although these are lawful contributions, are they ethical contributions if they produce favorable laws and regulations for the beef industry?[9]

FOOD SLANDER LAWS: Laws have been enacted to prevent citizens and the media from speaking out against food products. No, not by an oppressive regime in a foreign land. In America. Thirteen states currently have laws making it a civil crime to disparage foods without reasonable and reliable scientific inquiry, facts, or data. Promoted by agriculture, chemical, and biotechnology industry lobbyists, these laws have been legislated only in the early 1990s. Most likely they were not enacted to protect the sales of apples and oranges.[10]

TV MEDIA: Oprah Winfrey was sued for $20 million under food disparagement laws for remarks made on her show about beef and Mad Cow Disease by *Mad Cowboy* author Howard Lyman. She won the suit, however the Beef Promotion Council pulled $600,000 in advertising from the network. Given that most media outlets generate significant advertising revenue from the meat and dairy industries, how often are we going to get unbiased information about beef from TV news.[11]

INTERNET PROPAGANDA: Former U.S. Surgeon General, C. Everett Koop, M.D., who once wrote that 68 percent of all deaths in the United States are diet-related, signed a deal in 1999 with the American Council of Science and Health (ACSH) to supply nutrition and health articles for his web site.

One such article was titled "Red Meat Can Come Off the Forbidden List." It enthusiastically proclaimed that "new research" suggests Americans do not have to avoid red meat for fear of raising cholesterol and increasing heart disease risk. Food and chemical companies fund ACSH. The study touting new research was funded by the NCBA.[12]

MEDIA POLICE: In 1999, the Texas and Southwestern Cattle Raisers Association set up a hotline so those in the industry could report any media-generated negative publicity about beef. A task force would then be dispatched to re-educate the uninformed party.[13]

The challenge of representing, promoting, and defending beef might run a close second to the challenge of doing the same for tobacco.

Whether we should fault members of trade associations for representing beef is a tough call to make. They, too, have to make a living. They also have a mortgage, car insurance payments, and their children's braces to pay for. One could almost feel sorry for them given the job they must perform.

But if we don't feel sorry for all of their members, certainly we might for one of them, David Stroud, of the American Meat Institute. That is, assuming he still has a job there. He stated, "Some people are still going to want to eat meat...we do agree though that vegetarianism is a healthier diet." [14]

81: Dairy Council

EDUCATOR OR PEDDLER?

The National Dairy Council was founded in 1915 with a charter to increase the demand for U.S. produced dairy products on behalf of America's dairy farmers.[1] Back in the early 1900s its job had to have been easy in comparison to today with the barrage of criticism now leveled at milk. Despite the bad publicity, the Dairy Council, with chapters in 128 cities, has risen to the challenge with perseverance and skill to help generate revenue of $19 billion annually.[2]

Some argue the Dairy Council crosses the line from honest promotion to dishonest propaganda. That by using unethical methods and money to influence government, education, and the medical and scientific communities, it has subverted institutions that we trust to be unbiased to favor its products. Others, including the Dairy Council itself, would argue it is carrying out the job it is paid to perform and is breaking no laws in the process.

Both sides have reasonable arguments it seems. Who is in the right? Has the Dairy Council crossed the line? Do we really care if and how milk is promoted?

Let's see if we can shake out the argument, condense the issues, crystallize the answer, and thereby evaporate any doubts we have by staging a hypothetical debate between a concerned citizen and a Dairy Council member.

CONCERNED CITIZEN: The Dairy Council spends more than $300 million annually just at the national level to influence the nutrition industry by paying doctors, researchers, and dieticians to advance dairy products.[3] This occurs despite evidence that milk can increase the risk of prostate cancer, and increase hip fractures among women.[4]

COUNCIL MEMBER: The nutrition industry is well aware that calcium is an important nutrient and that dairy products are an important source of calcium. The well-respected professionals that work with the Dairy Council are more than willing to assist in spreading that word.

CONCERNED CITIZEN: The National Dairy Council is the single largest supplier of nutritional education materials to U.S. public schools. Rather than providing an "education" of views on nutrition, the materials present a biased means of getting children hooked early on dairy products.[5] This occurs despite evidence that milk can contribute to the cause of ear infections, anemia, asthma, and insulin-dependent diabetes.[6]

COUNCIL MEMBER: It's well-known that children have an important need for calcium to build strong bones. It is also well-known that children, being the picky eaters that they are, run an increased risk of not meeting their daily calcium requirement without milk.

CONCERNED CITIZEN: The Dairy Council tries to give the appearance of being an impartial group of educators and scientists concerned with the public health, when its charter is to sell dairy products.[7]

COUNCIL MEMBER: The Dairy Council IS concerned with the public health, that's why it promotes dairy products. These are not mutually exclusive objectives. Because members conduct themselves with the utmost dignity and integrity, they certainly could be mistaken for educators and scientists.

CONCERNED CITIZEN: By law, public schools are required to serve milk *and* more than 60 congressional leaders in Washington receive campaign contributions from the National Dairy Council.[8] Is there any connection? This occurs despite evidence that milk is deficient for human nutrients in essential fatty acids, iron, fiber, vitamin B_1, and vitamin C, and may increase the risk of childhood leukemia.[9]

COUNCIL MEMBER: Potential legislation must go through many

hoops before it can become law. The risk of a law ultimately being enacted without a sound basis could rarely, if ever, happen. Besides, it is highly doubtful that any legislator, many of whom have children, would knowingly allow *any* law to be passed that might harm the youth of this nation.

CONCERNED CITIZEN: To ostensibly elicit outcomes favorable to the dairy industry, the Dairy Council is known to pay for studies and research conducted under the guise of impartial science.[10] However, one clinical study it conducted didn't come out as expected. It showed that drinking three glasses of milk a day resulted in a negative calcium balance and an *increased* risk of osteoporosis.[11]

COUNCIL MEMBER: Obviously, the research isn't being conducted with partiality toward the dairy industry if the results obtained are unfavorable to us, correct? One study does not provide a conclusive argument anyway. There are many variables that can degrade the credibility of any study. It's not wise to risk a calcium deficiency because calcium is necessary for blood clotting. We need to think about that the next time we are bleeding.

CONCERNED CITIZEN: Both the American Dietetic Association and the Osteoporosis Foundation receive money from the dairy industry.[12] Might that color their judgment?

COUNCIL MEMBER: Both these highly professional organizations need funding to carry out their work and research. How much have *you* given lately? These organizations and the dairy industry are all working toward the same goals and if we are to be castigated for trying to further the cause of human health and welfare, then it is a very sad circumstance indeed.

CONCERNED CITIZEN: The Dairy Council sponsored an event called the Calcium Summit in Washington, D.C. to provide strategies on how to increase calcium consumption among Americans. More than 250 people representing government, health, and non-profit groups attended the event that was free to the public. USDA

Under-Secretary Eileen Kennedy was the keynote speaker. Given that many leafy green vegetables contain more calcium per calorie, with greater absorption than milk, how come these foods weren't mentioned?[13]

COUNCIL MEMBER: A vegetable growers' union wouldn't sponsor an event and talk about milk, would it? It wasn't a government-supported event anyway. The Under-Secretary was there only to lend support.

CONCERNED CITIZEN: The dairy industry succeeded in getting the USDA to raise the Recommended Daily Allowance (RDA) for calcium to 1,000 milligrams per day for obvious reasons.[14] Vegans, vegetarians, and cultures that don't subsist on high-protein diets that include meat and dairy, do fine on 500 milligrams of calcium a day.[15]

COUNCIL MEMBER: It's not possible to say one way or the other how people on fringe diets, and other cultures do on less calcium. The diet most Americans subscribe to requires the RDA that has been set to take care of their body's needs—teeth and bone health, muscle contraction, transmission of nerve impulses, and much more. These are critical functions of the body that shouldn't be left to chance. And if we overshot it a little, well maybe that's a good thing. A little insurance doesn't hurt.

That concludes our hypothetical debate. After hearing both sides of the argument what conclusion have we come to?

Is the Dairy Council operating in the public interest selling milk and doing so responsibly, thereby acting as an educator? Or is the Dairy Council operating solely in the dairy industry's behalf and doing so irresponsibly, thereby acting as a peddler?

Either way, does it ultimately matter to us? Can the Dairy Council do us any harm? Probably not—but its products may be another story.

82: School Donations

BOTH ARE TRUE, ONLY ONE IS TRUTHFUL

Food commodities are donated to schools by meat and dairy wholesalers, and the government. Educational materials are supplied to schools by meat and dairy trade associations, and by food retailers. From a distance it appears to be an innocent, philanthropic gesture, benefiting all parties.

> School budgets are tight and teachers are overworked. Private industry donates educational materials to help relieve the burden of teacher preparation and ease budget overruns. The government donates millions of dollars of food to the school lunch programs. Food producers are relieved of food they are unable to sell. Children from lower class or impoverished families get a hot lunch at little or no cost.

However, when we view the situation close up, the gestures look quite different—economic interests are the motives and not all parties benefit.

> The wholesale suppliers of meat and dairy products, and the commercial producers like Oscar Mayer and McDonald's, indoctrinate impressionable children through both psychological (educational materials), and physiological (donated food) conditioning.[1] The truth about the foods is shaded or ignored. The government subsidizes the private sector with taxpayer's money. Poor business practices of wholesale producers are rewarded. Schools compromise their purpose by dispensing advertising rather than education. And the health of children is jeopardized with the potential for lifelong chronic illness.

Which portrayal is the truth? They both are. But only one is truthful.

The following are examples of the educational materials provided to schools in both early and later grades.

In early elementary school the teacher is a child's most trusted friend. As a result, the teachings are accepted and absorbed without question.

- In preschool, children are first introduced to Dairy Council materials by way of food pictures. They are asked to identify a multitude of dairy products. It is then that a subtle but powerful conditioning begins.[2]

- A movie is shown called, "Uncle Jim's Dairy Farm." It portrays a happy cow giving milk so children will be assured of proper nutrition.[3]

- A coloring book portrays a chicken clucking and singing, proud and happy to be laying eggs for us.[4]

- The "Story of Pork" has as its main character a happy-go-lucky pig. But the unhappy, and not so lucky ending, is not part of the story.[5]

- Posters, puzzles, playing cards, and records are other materials used to convey their nutritional message.[6]

As school children move up in grades, their focus switches from their teachers to themselves. The messages provided by the meat and dairy industries also make the adjustment.

- "Hooray for the Hot Dog," a material once issued by Oscar Mayer touts the hot dog as having just 30 percent fat. However, if measured against calories rather than weight, it contains 80 percent fat. Either way the benefit stands as Oscar Mayer states, "Fats supply essential fatty acids, help the body use other nutrients, and supply energy."[7]

- The dairy industry also has a convoluted approach to fat. For losing weight it recommends a stay-slim sundae that is fruit instead of chocolate syrup on top of *ice cream*. When it comes to a balanced diet it recommends a good balance— of dairy products only. It includes milk with every meal and some foods like cheese, ice cream, custard, and cream-of-tomato soup with butter on top.[8]

- A poster on the cafeteria door reads, The Healthy School Lunch Program. The poster shows photos of trim athletes and pictures of foods, including a cheeseburger, hot dog, pepperoni pizza, and whole milk.[9]

- For those who miss seeing the poster, the National Livestock and Meat Board has provided science classroom material that suggests eating too little meat could result in stunted growth.[10]

A close step behind the education, are the foods.

Presently, more than one-half of youths in the United States consume close to 27 million lunches provided each day by the National School Lunch Program (NSLP).[11] Government commodities make up 20 percent of foods used by schools.

Commodities like cheese, butter, fatty beef, and whole milk are high in fat and cholesterol.[12] A USDA report reveals that school meals from commodity programs have 85 percent more sodium, 50 percent more saturated fat, and 25 percent more fat than amounts recommended for a healthy diet.[13] Of the 111 foods on the list of USDA commodity foods that were available in school fiscal year 2002, only 5 were fresh fruits and vegetables.[14]

The educational message, combined with the commodity foods, provides a one-two punch of psychological and physiological conditioning that gets children off to the perfect start in life. The perfect start toward degenerative diseases.

- Close to 5 million children between the ages of 6 and 17 are overweight, a number that has more than doubled since 1970.[15]

- Increasing numbers of children, often as young as 10 years old, are being diagnosed with Type II diabetes.[16]

- Milk is suspected of triggering juvenile diabetes. The highest rates of leukemia are found in children ages 3 to 13 who consume the most dairy products.[17]

- Nearly 1 in 5 (17 percent) of sixth-to-eighth graders have cholesterol levels greater than 180 milligrams per deciliter.[18] By the end of their teen years, 90 percent already have clear evidence of atherosclerosis.[19]

Long ago milk was an icon of childhood and innocence. Today it is safe to say that it is no longer true—which is a good thing—but in other ways it is a little bit sad. The following stories illustrate the point.

Long ago a 5-year-old boy in kindergarten was called upon to be milk monitor for his class. This required a special trip to the cafeteria to carry milk back to the classroom for mid-morning snack time. The little boy took his responsibility very seriously, and struggled to carry the heavy tray filled with individual cartons back to the classroom so his classmates would get their milk. He made it without incident and was so very proud of himself.

The same boy now in third grade helped with a project to layout a dairy farm on the classroom floor. Complete with grass (green painted floor), fences, barns, and plastic cows. A field trip to a real dairy farm followed shortly after the completion of the classroom replica. The smell of hay, the sound of milking machines, and the good feelings toward the cows that provided his milk, stayed forever in his memory, even as an adult.

The boy, now a father, and very aware of the potential health consequences of milk, found himself writing a letter to his son's pediatrician. The note requested a prescription, required by law, for his son to take to school allowing him to substitute another beverage for milk.

Times have changed a lot. They need to change a lot more.

83: Government Subsidies

THIRTY-FIVE DOLLARS A POUND

What if we walked into the grocery store tomorrow and hamburger cost $35 a pound.[1] What if all other meats ran in amounts equal or greater than this. And milk and cheese also ran 10 times their current costs. Would we still purchase them?

Our first reaction might be to go looking for the store manager to strangle him. Then if he was still conscious after roughing him up, ask him what was going on because it wasn't April Fools' Day. He would inform us that the government no longer provides agricultural subsidies in support of meat and dairy products; we now have to pay their real costs. Dumbfounded, we pass on the animal-based foods—at least until we hit a lottery jackpot—and pick up some pasta and vegetables for dinner.

Decades later, a week before our 102nd birthday, we are daydreaming about the time in the grocery store that changed our food buying habits and diet forever. Our husband now 105 years old yells out to us, "Hey, wake up. Is it 30-40 or 40-30?"

"YOU wake up. That was game, set, and match," you correct. "How about we stop off on the way home and get a pasta salad. My treat."

The government, or more accurately our tax dollars, foot the bill for a large share of animal agriculture costs through subsidies, loans, buyouts, and tax breaks, while fruits, vegetables, and organic farming are not subsidized.[2] If a free market was allowed to prevail, meat and dairy products would be cost prohibitive for most people.

The government began to subsidize animal agriculture after World War I when profits started to sag.[3] Initially, subsidies were promoted with honorable intentions to shield small farmers from market forces, and to ensure that Americans received the foods that were then considered necessary for proper nutrition.[4] As time passed, a different animal emerged—or maybe two animals—donkeys and elephants.

As meat and dairy producers grew into economic juggernauts so did their ability to influence the political machine. Formidable lobbies and substantial campaign contributions translated into formidable and substantial subsidies, such as:

- WATER: About one-half of water needed to grow feed grains is subsidized. The total value of subsidized irrigation water used by animal feed growers is $500 million to $1 billion each year. It takes nearly 50 times more water to produce a calorie from beef, than a calorie from potatoes.[5]

- LAND: Ranchers on public lands, mostly in Western states, enjoy grazing fees at roughly one-quarter their value. The cost to U.S. taxpayers is about $50 million annually, with about $10 million of it used to subsidize predator control.[6]

- FEED: Feed grains are subsidized at a rate of $16 billion a year. And cheap grain translates into cheap meat.[7]

- ENERGY: Commercial fishermen are exempt from a 20-cent-a-gallon federal diesel fuel tax, a subsidy worth about $250 million a year.[8]

- ADVERTISING: Advertising and nutritional education kits are tax deductible, in essence a subsidy.[9]

- PROMOTION — OVERSEAS: The Market Promotion Program provides taxpayer money to private companies and their trade associations for overseas promotional activities such as advertising and market research. For example, McDonald's has been paid nearly $2 million to promote Chicken McNuggets to the developing world. Tyson Foods, a chicken producer, has received $800,000 for overseas promotion.[10]

- BUYOUTS: In 1998 the USDA purchased $30 million of beef, $30 million of pork, $8 million of lamb, $18 million of poultry, and $10 million of salmon for school lunch and food assistance programs. They also purchased $141 million of beef for the 1997 school lunch program. Although the gestures appear philanthropic, it amounts to our tax dollars being used to pay for poor business practices. Then the products are dumped on those who are least able to choose what they will eat—the children and poor.[11]

- LOANS: Farmers can't lose on government-backed non-recourse loans. If they have a good year they pay back the loan and pocket the difference. If they have a bad year and are unable to sell their crop, defaulting on the loan, they don't have to pay it back, and their goods are unloaded into food programs.[12]

- HEALTHCARE: It is estimated that $123 billion a year is paid in medical costs to treat the diseases caused by poor diet. Roughly half, $61 billion, is being subsidized by tax dollars.[13]

If we consume meat and dairy products we probably aren't too upset that the government is subsidizing these foods. Given all the taxes we pay it's nice to see a tangible benefit coming back to us for a change. And keeping hamburger meat from costing $35 a pound is definitely tangible.

But for every action, there is an equal and opposite reaction.

Meat and dairy producers, and politicians have leapfrogged the free market system and colluded in enticing us to purchase animal-based foods to serve their interests, rather than our interests. Our interests would be to have a choice of what foods we consume based on a free market—the free market system of capitalism that made America great.

Instead the government uses our tax dollars to artificially lower prices on foods that are a drain on the economy, negatively impact the environment, and damage our health. Not to mention the 12 million tax-paying vegetarians who are paying for foods they don't eat.

If someday government subsidizing of animal agricultural products ceases, causing their prices to skyrocket, we will have a decision to make. But why wait until then. Why not make our decision now.

We could start by purchasing a pasta salad, giving ourselves every opportunity to finish *life's* game, set, and match.

84: Advertising

WHY THE POTATO CHIP AND NOT THE POTATO?

The dictionary definition of advertising is: "An entity that influences behavior, as it deadens, paralyzes, benumbs, anesthetizes, and dopes."[1] Actually this is not the definition of advertising, it's the definition of *drugs*.

The dictionary definition of advertising is: "The application of a concentrated means of persuasion, or repeated suggestion, in order to develop a specific belief or motivation."[2] Nope. This isn't the definition of advertising either; this is the definition of *brainwashing*.

Advertising is one of the most powerful legal influences on earth—although some would suggest that it shouldn't be lawful. More than $150 billion—that's with a B—is spent every year on advertising.[3] Included in that is $5 billion spent on pharmaceutical ads and $2 billion on food ads.[4] One food producer spent $20 million just to promote *one* new sugared cereal.[5] These are pretty good indicators of just how influential those that are paying for advertising think it is. Are they getting a return on their investment?

- When meat consumption was sagging during an 18-year period (1938-1956), the American Meat Institute (AMI) spent $30 million to get meat back in our diets. Meat consumption doubled.[6]

- The Dairy Council spent $190 million on the "milk moustache" campaign in 1998. The advertising helped contribute to raising milk sales by 1 billion pounds in 1 year alone.[7]

- A child will see 1,000 ads every week on TV promoting processed and junk food; adults almost as many.[8] So while those on traditional diets worldwide are getting 75 to 80 percent of their total dietary energy from whole grains, the American SICK diet is getting 1 percent from them.[9]

So what. We said advertising was legal. A food maker, for that matter any American, has the freedom to inform the marketplace about its legal products. And we have the freedom to reject them. A greater awareness of the dynamics taking place might motivate us to do so.

Most Americans receive their information about foods from television. And let's not fool ourselves. Television doesn't exist to entertain us; it exists to sell us products. The shows are only made because no one would watch television if it ran commercials 24/7.

What kind of food information do we get from TV?

Seen an advertisement extolling the virtues of the potato lately? Say within the last 5 years? The potato is an amazing food, full of our basic fuel source, complex carbohydrates, with 11 percent protein, 1 percent fat, and full of the vitamins B_1, niacin, and C.[10] The cost of a 5-pound bag is less than $3.00.

Seen an advertisement extolling the virtues of the potato chip lately? Say within the last 10 minutes? Potato chips are an amazing food, too. A defilement of the potato that has 5 times the calories, 60 times the fat, 80 times the sodium, and all of it for only 8 times the cost of potatoes.[11]

Potato chip makers spend more than $50 million yearly to convince us to buy their products.[12] Would we buy them if they didn't? After all, they have to convince us to buy a questionable nutriment, and pay for the packaging, processing, and advertising, at many times the cost of its parent food.

Why don't we see advertising for the potato? Because we already know what a wonderful food it is. Don't we?

Most food advertised has been processed for profits, not for the nutritional benefit of the buyer. Most likely we would find a high indirect correlation between a food's advertising budget and its food value. Despite the fact that 80 percent of the public believes advertising to be dishonest and degrading, producers still spend $150 billion each year on promotion.[13] *That's* the power of advertising.

That brings us to animal-based foods advertising.

How do the producers and commercial enterprises promote foods unnecessary for human nutrition, which also contribute to chronic disease? Easy. They promote them as foods *necessary* for human nutrition, and put lots of money behind the message to make sure it is heard clearly and often.

They flood schools with educational materials and free samples in the form of commodities. They generate TV and radio public service messages and conventional advertising. They create scientific-like press releases. They advertise in newspapers, magazines, and medical journals. They make political contributions, hire lobbyists, and form trade associations.

With little or no promotion of fresh fruits, vegetables, and whole grains to balance the advertising message, animal-based foods stand out as what appears to be the only choice. And the unbiased news media can't do much to balance the message either because, well, you don't bite the hand that feeds you—that is risk losing millions of dollars in revenue from animal-based food ads.[14]

One of the greatest advertising success stories in American history has as its primary product, animal flesh. A commercial enterprise by the name of McDonald's. How do they do it? Here is one example:

In one of their booklets, McDonald's touted one of their more popular meals: cheeseburger, fries, chocolate shake, and cookies as fitting within the recommendations of a healthier heart, at 33.5 percent fat. That was true. Nutritionists recommended we reduce our fat intake from between 40 to 45 percent, down to 30 to 35 percent of calories.

The meal started at 44 percent with the burger and fries, which the booklet stated was much too high. The remedy? Add in plenty of white flour and sugar from the cookies and shake, and presto! We have a healthier heart.[15]

The booklet had all the elements of great promotion: some truth, meeting an impartial positive standard, and avoidance of contrary information—in this case, the Physicians Committee for Responsible Medicine (PCRM) recommending a whole foods diet that runs at 10 percent fat—none saturated—for optimal health.[16]

McDonald's promotional success is so powerful that even vegetarians patronize them. With locations at almost every major interstate off-ramp, restrooms 10 minutes apart, the golden arch has a whole different meaning for them.

85: Illness-Care

A HEALTHCARE SYSTEM ALREADY EXISTS

We don't have a healthcare system in this country. We have a sickness-care, illness-care, disease-care, call-it-what-we-want-care system, but *not* a healthcare system. What's the difference? Sounds like semantics.

An illness-care system is a system where the medical profession treats our illnesses with the goal of making us healthy. A healthcare system implies a system that cares for and maintains our health, keeping us from getting sick—presumably the state we would all prefer.

The language is subtle but meaningful. If we called it illness-care, wouldn't we be more motivated to stay well? Who wants to participate in *illness-care*? And if we referred to a physician as a mechanic, might it be a better reminder about the state we are in— broken. Physician means "teacher," but they're not there to teach us anything—they're there to fix us. When we talk about mammograms we call it healthcare *prevention*, but mammograms don't prevent anything, they detect illness.

Our heathcare system is not designed to keep us healthy. But should it be? Does the medical profession have an ethical responsibility to keep us in good health, so we don't return to their business? Let's explore this.

Doctors sacrifice 6 to 8 years of their lives and tens of thousands of dollars to educate themselves on how to diagnose illness, prescribe medicine, and cut disease out of us. They didn't make this commitment, nor were they trained, to discuss with us the multiple attributes of fiber, and the differences between heme iron and non-heme iron, in the hope that we'll spend the rest of our lives on the tennis courts, in good health, never to patronize them again.

The pharmaceutical companies don't invest millions of dollars in research and development on drugs, so they can produce a pamphlet informing us about the 1,000 active compounds in plants such as tocotrienols, limonoids, and glucarates that fight disease, neutralize carcinogens, and strengthen the immune system.[1]

The medical system is not in the business of health. The fact is there is no money to be made from health. They are in the business of illness.

Many argue the medical system should be in the business of health, along the lines of managed care (HMOs), prevention focus, and fee incentives for healthy patients. But this hasn't worked and it never will. Why? Because we are bucking fundamental human nature, and a system not built on that premise.

When we get sick, we want every test and diagnostic procedure known to humankind to be performed no matter what the cost. And medical personnel are trained to do everything they can to make us well and to succeed financially in a capitalistic society. All the players in the illness-care system are in unison. From this standpoint the illness-care system works perfectly.

But from another standpoint—the only one that really counts—it fails miserably.

- According to *Nutrition Action* (June 1999) heart bypass surgery will extend life in 2 percent of cases with a 25 to 50 percent chance that after 6 months blood vessels will again become blocked if patients' diets haven't changed.[2]

- According to the National Cancer Institute in Bethesda, MD (2000), chemotherapy success rate is 5.8 percent. It appears cancer patients are living longer, but this is a function of earlier diagnosis due to improved diagnostic technology that starts the clock earlier. A person dies from cancer in America every 1 minute.[3]

- According to the *Journal of the American Medical Association* (1983) one study showed that among those with mild hypertension on drug therapy, the number of deaths was reduced by just 1 percent. Has this figure changed in 20 years? If it has, it isn't apparent by the heart attack rate: a person dies from a heart attack every 1 minute in this country.[4]

- According to the *Journal of the National Cancer Institute* (2000), adding an annual mammogram to a careful physical examination of the breasts does not improve breast cancer survival rates compared to getting the examination alone.[5]

- According to the *New England Journal of Medicine* (1995) taking estrogen therapy to reduce the risk of osteoporosis and heart disease for more than 5 years will increase the risk of hormone-dependent ovarian and breast cancer by 30 to 40 percent.[6]

- According to *The Growing Epidemic of Disease* (David M. Homer), in 1900, a 55-year-old male could expect to live to age 72. In 1990, a 55-year-old male could expect to live to age 75. A modest 3-year improvement during a 90-year period.[7]

- According to the World Health Organization (2000), the United States ranks 24th of 191 countries in Healthy Life Expectancy (HALE). The rank would be even lower if not for the heavy toll that infectious disease and malnutrition takes in Third World countries.[8]

This country has the most highly skilled doctors and the best technology in the world. This combination has been successful in reducing our chances of dying from an infectious disease down to 2 percent. However, our chances of dying from a degenerative disease is 80 percent.[9] The illness-care system, no matter how sophisticated, can do little to change this number. A healthcare system is necessary to do that.

Many would argue the United States has the makings of a healthcare system. On the fringe, but somewhat splintered, are chiropractic, homeopathy, osteopathy, naturopathy, massage therapy, biofeedback, and other specialties with a strong focus on prevention. They do achieve some measure of success, however they are businesses too, out to make profits like any other enterprise. And like the illness-care system they, too, are beaten before they get started.

Is it possible then to develop a true healthcare system? What would be the methodology and infrastructure? Who would the players be? How would it be paid for?

A healthcare system is already in place, but most of us have failed to use it. The technology is advanced beyond our understanding. It is on call 24/7, maintaining our health and addressing threats immediately as they arise. There are no plans, costs, or co-payments. Everyone has his or her own personal team of specialists. There are no office visits, long waits, or lost time from work. The system is nearly flawless.

The only responsibility we have to the system is to perform some minor daily maintenance with the proper tools: A Wholly Eating Leaves to Live (WELL) diet.

86: Pharmaceutical Industry

A SAFETY NET WITH VERY LARGE HOLES

It's a perfect system. Who could argue with it. We get sick and go to the doctor. The doctor can either write a prescription, open us up, or give out advice. Getting cut open is too drastic, getting advice is not drastic enough, but getting a drug prescription is just right. The doctor writes a prescription and gets job satisfaction. The pharmaceutical company makes a profit. The insurance company covers much of the cost. We go home content that we are on the road to recovery.

Pharmaceuticals are like a large safety net. But we need to be careful each time we fall because the net has some very large holes in it. Let's see where the weak spots are.

LIFE EXPECTANCY: We have assumed that our life expectancy has increased significantly during the last century, and that medicines are the primary reason, but statistics show otherwise.

Life expectancy, according to Mckinlay and Mckinlay (*Health and Society*, Summer 1977), during the past century is due mostly to improved sanitation and better food distribution, with only 3.5 percent, or about 1 year of added life due to medical and drug advances.[1]

DEATHS: According to the American Medical Association, prescription drugs *properly* used cause 90,000 to 160,000 deaths a year. No doubt the practice of feeding antibiotics to animals contributes to the problem.[2]

SIDE EFFECTS: We know most every drug has the potential of multiple side effects because more print is devoted to them than to the description, instructions, and benefits all put together. Aside from the possibility that the remedy might be worse than the illness, could this phenomenon tell us something about drugs being the answer to the maintenance and repair of the human body?

NATURE'S WAY / TECHNOLOGY: We look at the world around us and can't help but be impressed by our progress and all the benefits of technology. We naturally assume that pharmaceuticals is one of its many examples. But can drugs, no matter how technologically advanced, rise to a level to affect the greatest technological achievement—the human body?

BIG BUSINESS: Pharmaceutical companies grossed $141 billion on prescription drugs in the year 2000.[3] They have a big stake in making sure we have no doubts that prescription drugs are the only answer to preventing, healing, and controlling disease.

The companies assist doctors by providing medical journal articles, scientific research, conferences, patient handouts, lectures, publications, free samples, and drug advertisements to ensure the doctor knows how best to treat our family—that is, with the proper drugs.[4]

The companies spend 2.5 times more on marketing and lobbying (they have 1 paid lobbyist for every 2 congressmen), than on research and development.[5]

The companies make sure we don't miss the message. When was the last time we turned on the television or opened a magazine and didn't see an advertisement for a drug that would take care of our woes, such as acid reflux, menopausal estrogen therapy, high cholesterol, and hypertension?

Since we aren't presented other alternatives we naturally presume pharmaceuticals are the only solution.

EFFECTIVENESS AND ALTERNATIVES: Are pharmaceutical drugs doing the job we are led to believe they are doing? If not, what is there to take their place? To help answer the questions let's use as examples the following diseases/disorders: hypertension, diabetes, attention deficit hyperactivity disorder (ADHD), cancer, menopause, and high cholesterol.

- HYPERTENSION: Prescriptions are written 9 out of 10 times for the disease. For mild hypertension (diastolic of under 105), from which the majority of the 50 million people suffer, there is little evidence that drugs will improve survival rates and reduce the risk of stroke and heart attack.[6]

  Conversely, 58 percent of people can come off their medication after changing to a vegetarian diet.[7] In Third World societies where strokes and heart attacks are unheard of, those in their 80s have the same blood pressure as teenagers.[8]

- DIABETES: Adult-onset diabetes, of which more than 15 million people suffer is perceived as a disease of too little insulin, when it's more precisely a disease of consuming too much fat.

  It's no surprise then that in three separate studies, 60, 75, and 90 percent of the subjects switching to the WELL diet were able to stop taking insulin.[9] Diabetes is rare among Africans, Asians, and Polynesians who subsist on plant-based diets.[10]

- ADHD: Ritalin is prescribed for 3 to 5 percent of American school children. But one has to wonder given that medication is rarely prescribed in Western Europe, if hyperactive children are only born in the United States.[11]

- CANCER: Chemotherapy drugs are an $8.6 billion a year business.[12] They have a success rate of about 1 in 20 cases, and they destroy the immune system.[13] Conversely, Essiac, an herbal preparation that has shown success in treating cancer, does so by strengthening the body's immune system.[14]

  In one study, vegetarians had more than double the ability to destroy cancer cells.[15]

According to the National Cancer Institute, 8 of 10 incidents of cancer are due to factors that have been identified as within our control (diet/smoking).[16]

- MENOPAUSE: Estrogen is prescribed for menopause—a natural part of life, not a disease—to reduce the risk of osteoporosis and heart disease; both diseases of the SICK diet. As of 1995, more than 8 million women were on ERT, making menopause a billion dollar business for the health-care and pharmaceutical industries.[17]

  Michael Klaper, MD, has watched many of his patients who eat a strictly plant-based diet go through menopause largely unfazed.[18]

- HIGH CHOLESTEROL: There are drugs that will lower cholesterol but with many side effects. Plants have no side effects. A pure vegetarian diet will maintain cholesterol levels at or below 150 mg/dL, virtually assuring no coronary artery disease. With little effort, populations that eat only vegetables, fruits, grains, and legumes—like those in rural China—maintain cholesterol levels below 150 mg/dL, and have little or no coronary artery disease.[19]

There are a lot of holes in the safety net. A safety net we would not want to rely on to save our lives if we were on a high wire and should fall. Yet on the ground, in our everyday lives, we rely on pharmaceutical drugs to do just that.

However, there is a clear alternative to the pharmaceutical safety net: the potent combination of plants and immune system. They don't initiate revenue, prescriptions, or advertisements; instead they initiate protection, maintenance, and healing.

The human body was built not to fall, but on the rare occasion when it does, prescription drugs do have their place and can be a welcome safety net—and this particular net has no holes.

87: Medical Profession

HYPOCRISY IN THE HIPPOCRATIC OATH?

Is the medical profession doing a good job? Is there a way to quantify its performance? How about how much money we spend on healthcare as a nation? If the medical profession is striving to care for our health—after all it is called healthcare—it should follow that the *less* money we spend on healthcare, the better job its doing.

The cost of U.S. healthcare in 1995 was more than $1 trillion, 14 percent of the gross national product (GNP), and it was projected to reach $1.5 trillion by 2002.[1] By this measurement we can conclude there is plenty of room for improvement.

Is there another way to measure its success?

In 1847 a trade lobby was formed. One of its first charter goals was to eliminate the competition, with the objective of gaining economic proprietorship, and looking after the economic interests of its members. The organization was the American Medical Association (AMA).[2] If we use this as a measurement for success, then we can conclude the medical profession has succeeded with flying colors.

Although these two analyses of the medical profession's success could be considered gross generalizations, in other ways they might be the quintessence. This leads us to the question: Is the medical profession a profit-directed business, or a humanitarian endeavor?

Let's review the history and actions of medical doctors, and the AMA, and see if we find hypocrisy anywhere in the Hippocratic Oath. This discussion has three sections: Competition and Profits, Nutrition and Medicine, and Tobacco and the AMA.

COMPETITION AND PROFITS: In 1850 the AMA set out to eliminate its competition.

- FEMALE HEALERS: Since they were the primary providers of abortion, what better way to undermine them than to make abortion illegal. Under the guise of sanctity of life the AMA lobbied successfully. Abortion didn't become legal again for more than 100 years, and when it did, abortion-related maternal deaths in the United States dropped 5 times.[3]

- MIDWIVES: In 1847 midwives were present at almost 100 percent of the nation's births. By 1960 that number had dropped to less than 1 percent.[4] The unrelenting campaign by organized medicine to eliminate midwifery and turn birthing from a natural event into a lucrative business was successful. While the AMA claimed home birth was child abuse, comprehensive studies were done in 1916 and 1977. Both concluded that non-intervening management of home-attended births by midwives was far safer for baby and mother than hospital births.[5]

- CANCER TREATMENT: In 1950 Harry Hoxsey operated cancer clinics in 17 states treating cancer with a formula of herbs. Although his regimen was far more successful than conventional treatments, the AMA set out to discredit him. He sued and the courts ruled that a conspiracy existed among the AMA, National Cancer Institute, and FDA to suppress his treatments. Although the AMA admitted under oath that his treatment had cured melanoma and other skin cancers, the FDA was able to close down all his clinics by 1960.[6]

- HOMEOPATHY: The practice of homeopathy had much greater success in treating epidemics of the nineteenth century than conventional medicine.[7] The AMA responded by placing a clause in its Code of Ethics that any AMA member consulting with a homeopath would be dismissed from the AMA.[8]

- CHIROPRACTIC: Although chiropractic had been proven to be safe and of value, the AMA waged an all-out war on the profession to put it out of business on the basis that it was dangerous and fraudulent.[9] The attack lasted from 1963 through 1976, until three chiropractors filled suit against the AMA. Eleven years later, in 1987, the court found the AMA guilty of attempting to eliminate the chiropractic profession.[10]

NUTRITION AND MEDICINE: Apparently they don't mix.

- NUTRITION ADVICE: It is not uncommon for doctors to shun giving nutrition advice to their patients for a number of reasons.

    Doctors aren't educated on the subject because of the lack of nutrition education provided in medical school.[11] But given the impact diet has on health, shouldn't nutrition education be mandatory?

    Doctors argue that nutrition education is the job of the dietician. But how often do people visit dieticians in comparison to their doctors?

    Doctors believe advising a radical diet change would not be accepted by their patients.[12] But shouldn't they give the advice and let the patients make that decision?

    Although a physician's motive may not be to increase his or her income by declining nutrition advice, and thereby increase the patient's risk of disease, his or her actions produce that result.

- HEART BYPASS SURGERY: Bypass surgery is a cash cow for the medical profession. Research has shown that diet can reverse heart disease. In cases where this might be an option for patients, doesn't the doctor have an ethical responsibility to discuss it with them?[13]

- ITS BELIEF: In 1979 the AMA was quoted as saying, "A strictly vegetarian diet can lead to deformities and even death."[14] Was this statement made out of ignorance or economics?

- NEW FOOD GROUPS: In 1991 the Physicians Committee for Responsible Medicine (PCRM) issued its New Four Food Groups, which included no meat or dairy products. The AMA issued a press release criticizing the plan. What could be the motive?[15]

- MCDONALD'S: We can find McDonald's restaurants in hospitals. Although we can excuse the restaurant's motive, can we excuse the medical profession's consent? Is it innocent circumstance or symbolic commentary?

TOBACCO AND THE AMA: Friends or foes?

- ENDORSEMENTS: In 1925 evidence indicated that cigarette tar caused cancer.[16] In 1938 a major study showed that smoking reduced life expectancy.[17] Nonetheless, the AMA continued to run cigarette ads in its journal and endorse cigarettes.[18]

- INTEGRITY: In 1950 it was revealed that 97 percent of patients with lung cancer had been smokers.[19] In 1957 the U.S. Surgeon General reported the evidence was conclusive that cigarettes caused lung cancer. While *Reader's Digest* was running articles on the dangers of smoking, *The AMA Journal* was touting its favorite brand, Kent, manufactured by the P. Lorillard Company, which was also paying a hefty retainer to the editor of the journal.[20]

- ENIGMA: By 1964 the Surgeon General issued an emphatic report condemning smoking, as it caused lung cancer, heart disease, and emphysema, and was costing the country billions of dollars in healthcare.[21] The AMA's response, to at least the tobacco growing state of Kentucky was, "The AMA is not opposed to smoking and tobacco."[22]

- EXPLANATION: The explanation given for the indirect endorsement of smoking and tobacco in the state of Kentucky was confirmed in 1981 by the AMA president. It was to gain the support of tobacco state lawmakers to help fend off Medicare and proposals for national healthcare, both of which would impact its fees.[23]

- WARNING LABELS: The AMA was opposed to warning labels on cigarette packages. It defended its position by saying, "Who are we to destroy an $8 billion industry on the extreme theory that the American people need to be protected from themselves."[24]

In 1995, PCRM published an analysis in *Preventive Medicine*. It stated, "The combined medical costs attributed to smoking and meat consumption exceed the predicted costs of providing health coverage for all currently uninsured Americans."

An AMA spokesman responded: "We have very serious reservations about the report."[25]

Maybe a more appropriate response would have been: Send us the bill, it's our obligation to pay it.

88: Cancer Business

A LOT OF PEOPLE OUT OF WORK

If tomorrow we eradicated cancer forever, everyone would be dancing in the streets. Maybe not everyone. Given that more people now make a living from cancer, than die from cancer, we might find a significant number of people with mixed emotions staying home.[1] And since they won't have jobs now, they might be staying home for some time.

One out of 4 Americans will die of cancer.[2] But before that happens it will cost each one, and his or her insurance company, roughly $100,000.[3] Cancer generates $55 billion a year.[4] The cancer industry is now the second largest industry in the United States. Only the petrochemical industry is larger.[5]

Winning the battle would mean the loss of $8.6 billion a year for the pharmaceutical companies in chemotherapy drugs.[6] Cancer hospitals would all but disappear. Many oncologists, radiologists, surgeons, nurses, and medical support personnel would be looking for new work or collecting unemployment. The Cancer Institute would close its doors. The American Cancer Society (ACS), taking in more than $6 million annually, with cash reserves of more than $1 billion, would be going door-to-door issuing refunds.[7]

There would be a lot of people out of work. A lot of people with substantial loss of income. A lot of people with considerable loss of prestige. A lot of people wondering what happened.

Does this mean then there would be a lot of people, consciously or subconsciously, working to protect the status quo? Could we be so cynical to suggest such a thing? Is there any way to know? Any or all of the following behaviors or stances might serve as signs.

- Always the appearance of PROGRESS AND HOPE.
- Only the CURRENT REGIMEN has a chance to work.

- The disease can't be PREVENTED, only cured after detection.
- Financial CONFLICTS OF INTEREST among the participants.

PROGRESS AND HOPE: As long as the public at large sees headway being made, then there is no pressure to change the established approach.

- RELATIVITY: We are told by the cancer industry that in the early 1900s there was no hope of survival, but today 49 percent will live 5 years after diagnosis. The ACS touts that "cancer is the most curable chronic disease."[8]

  However, in the early 1900s, a tumor the size of an orange was considered a small cancer of the breast. People often died shortly after detection. Today, the cancer can be diagnosed much earlier when it is one-half centimeter. Thus, the appearance of longer survival is more often a function of an earlier start date (detection), than a later end date (death).[9]

- CREATIVE ACCOUNTING: Doctors speak of a 75 percent "response rate" from chemotherapy. However, tumor shrinkage does not often correlate with increased survival or improved quality of life.[10]

  The success rate of chemotherapy today is about 5 percent. The death rates of the more common cancers have stayed the same or increased during the last half century.[11]

- APPEARANCES: The ACS social-support programs seem more devoted to maintaining the appearance of success than healing support, by encouraging support volunteers who have gone through cancer treatment to downplay their physical and emotional scars.[12]

CURRENT REGIMEN: We have been led to believe that surgery, radiation, and chemotherapy are the only treatments that can combat cancer.

- ECONOMICS: Essiac, an herbal preparation, has been shown to shrink tumors, relieve pain, and prolong life, and with no toxicity. It is inexpensive and works by strengthening the immune system. President John F. Kennedy's personal physician, Dr. Charles Brusch stated, "I endorse the therapy as it has cured my lower bowel cancer." It is not approved for use as treatment in the United States, even though it has never been disproved through scientific trials. As an herb it can't be patented.[13]

- IMMUNE SYSTEM: Dr. Linus Pauling, a Nobel Prize winner in chemistry has shown that high doses of vitamin C have had remarkable success in treating cancer patients, extending lives from 10 to 21 times longer than those not taking the vitamin. It works by strengthening the immune system. The National Cancer Institute conducted its own study and showed the regimen had no value since it didn't kill cancer cells *directly*.[14]

- FAIRNESS: The ACS publishes *Unproven Methods of Cancer Management*. Three out of 4 methods have never been shown to be ineffective by solid scientific evidence. Even where alternative cancer treatments have shown promise, often the cancer establishment will not objectively evaluate them. Even if doctors believe in an unapproved therapy, they can have their licenses revoked if they participate in its use.[15]

- ONCOLOGISTS: What would oncologists do if they got cancer? In one poll, 75 percent said they would avoid chemotherapy due to its ineffectiveness and unacceptable degree of toxicity.[16]

PREVENTION: We are led to believe early detection is the key to addressing cancer.

- A BETTER KEY? More than one authority has claimed that anywhere from 70 to 90 percent of cancers are caused by personal habits, that is, smoking and diet.[17] If we address cancer *this* way we won't have to worry about early detection.

- DOUBLE-TALK? The ACS provides little information on the causes of cancer or ways we might prevent it. The literature discusses prevention by way of early detection. But if it has been detected, it hasn't been prevented.[18]

- COMMON SENSE? Each of us has hundreds of thousands of body cells that regenerate each day. Statistics have shown that one or more of these new cells will be cancerous. So every day, each one of us has cancer.[19] Therefore, those with properly maintained immune systems must be destroying cancer cells before they can multiply.

CONFLICTS OF INTEREST: If we accept the possibility that any business is potentially vulnerable to financial conflicts among its participants, why wouldn't we accept the possibility the cancer business could be too? Especially given the magnitude of its worth.

- Diet is not the focus of prevention by the ACS.

  DuPont provides financial support for ACS Breast Health Awareness Program; they manufacture mammogram-imaging equipment.[20] Zeneca Pharmaceuticals does the same for ACS Breast Cancer Awareness Month; they manufacture Tamoxifen, the world's top selling anticancer and breast cancer-prevention drug with $400 million in annual sales.[21]

- Memorial Sloan-Kettering Cancer Center is a strong advocate of chemotherapy.

  In 1995, three executives of Bristol-Myers Squibb—including the chairman of the board—responsible for half of the chemotherapy sales in the world, were directors of the cancer center.[22]

- The ACS continually refuses to take a stand against environmental carcinogens.

  The ACS accepts significant contributions from the pesticide industries.[23]

Is there an organized conspiracy to maintain the cancer status quo? No.

Is cancer a very profitable business trying to maintain its economic wealth? Most likely. That's human nature. We all want to have profitable businesses, and be well off financially. However, most of us aren't faced with a moral or ethical dilemma when we draw a paycheck.

Whether we patronize the cancer business by way of contracting cancer is predominately up to us by the way we live and eat. Will cancer ever be eradicated? It will when we come to recognize our personal power to do so.

And once we do, those in the cancer business will go on to find new and rewarding work, and then everyone can dance in the streets.

89: Menopause

BUSINESS HAS BEEN A LITTLE SLOW

At one time menopause was defined and perceived in the following way:

> The period marked by the natural and permanent cessation of menstruation, legislated by Nature, experienced by all women. A process that transitions women to the next stage of their lives.

Then at some time, in some place, a conversation like this must have taken place:

FIRST DOCTOR: Hey, business has been a little slow lately. What can we do to pick it up?

SECOND DOCTOR: Maybe we can invent a new disease.

FIRST DOCTOR: How about menopause?

SECOND DOCTOR: That's not a disease.

FIRST DOCTOR: No, but half of the population will have it for 25 years. That's a big market.

SECOND DOCTOR: Well, it's worth a try. What have we got to lose?

PHARMACEUTICAL REP: Do you mind if we participate?

FIRST DOCTOR: Sure, why not.

SECOND DOCTOR: We are going to have to change the public's perception, though.

Now menopause is represented and perceived in the following way:

> A *condition* requiring medical intervention, most often estrogen replacement therapy (ERT). "Deterioration and living decay" as described in one medical textbook. "The death of womanhood" as depicted by one doctor's book. "Dry, brittle, parched, and devoid of life" as portrayed by one drug company. "A promoter of serious illnesses like osteoporosis and heart disease" as characterized by the medical profession.[1]

The result? As of 1995, 8 million women were on ERT, making menopause a billion-dollar business for the healthcare and pharmaceutical industries.[2] A 1993 Gallup poll revealed that when physicians discussed menopausal symptoms with their patients, 84 percent of them discussed only ERT. Just 2 percent discussed alternatives like diet, exercise, or relaxation techniques.[3]

Despite the economic motives that gave birth to ERT, the regimen can reduce the risk of osteoporosis and heart disease, alleviate symptoms of menopause, and slow the downslide of womanhood.

What is wrong with intervening in Nature's business, then? Let's address these three issues, one by one.

If the risk of osteoporosis and heart disease is helped by ERT, then why not take advantage of it?

> Because it's more likely to take advantage of us. Converting to the WELL diet would have a far greater impact on reducing the risk of these diseases than ERT. Even if this wasn't the case, the health risks of ERT probably outweigh its benefits.
>
> • ERT has been shown to increase a woman's risk of breast cancer by 30 to 40 percent after she has been on the therapy for more than 5 years.[4]

- Long-term use increases the risks of ovarian cancer, and liver and gallbladder disease.[5]

- The risk of endometriosis is typically reduced when menopause is handled without intervention.[6]

- When only estrogen is prescribed, an increase of 10 times the risk of uterine cancer is realized. The addition of synthetic progesterone reduces this risk, but induces side effects—bloating and migraines among them.[7]

If hot flashes, vaginal dryness, and depression are relieved with ERT, why wouldn't women avail themselves of it?

Is it possible, even likely, that these symptoms don't have to accompany menopause? Why would Nature attach these burdens to menopause if it's a natural occurrence?

- Hot flashes are unknown in populations that subsist on plant-based diets.[8] In Japan, where the diet is near vegetarian, there is no term for hot flashes.[9]

- Dr. Michael Klaper, MD, has watched many of his patients who eat a strictly plant-based diet go through menopause with few or no problems.[10]

- Studies have shown that vitamin C and E, and bioflavonoids—all which are found abundantly in plants—significantly reduce, or eliminate hot flashes.[11]

- Vaginal dryness can be reduced by remaining sexually active.[12]

- Depression can be caused by factors other than estrogen depletion. Studies have shown that younger women suffer from depression in greater numbers than menopausal women. Studies have also shown that personality improvements promised with ERT are likely to make women "less overtly aggressive, but more inwardly hostile."[13]

If ERT helps a woman retain her youth and stay attractive to her husband—in essence maintaining her membership in womanhood—what could be lost in receiving the therapy? Maybe the question can best be answered with more questions.

- Is this our idea of what is youthful, attractive, and woman-like, or is this someone else's idea? Specifically, someone in the name of the beauty industry—cosmetics, fashion, clothing, hair design, jewelry, and so on that have a few dollars riding on *their* definition.

- Can women not live on past their ovaries with a purpose? Are women only sex objects without other values?

- Might menopause be a time of liberation? Not having to worry about pregnancy? Not having to worry about one's looks, and the energy and time that goes into maintaining them?

- Might staying youthful have something to do with attitude? Are there any more powerful aphrodisiacs than intelligence, self-confidence, and sense of humor? Is it possible that to remain a woman only requires her not to have a sex change?

- Could the native Celtic and Muslim cultures, where menopause is honored, respected, and seen as a positive event marked by celebratory ceremonies, inspire us to change our perspective?[14]

No doubt Mother Nature is shaking her head ruefully. She thought she was doing women a favor by relieving them of a lifelong responsibility of bearing children, and the distraction and discomfort of preparing for pregnancy each month. Instead, she inadvertently made life more difficult, anxious, and complicated for them.

There is little doubt that Mother Nature will correct her mistake the next time around and do away with menopause. That is, unless women figure it out before then, and realize all the gifts it has to offer.

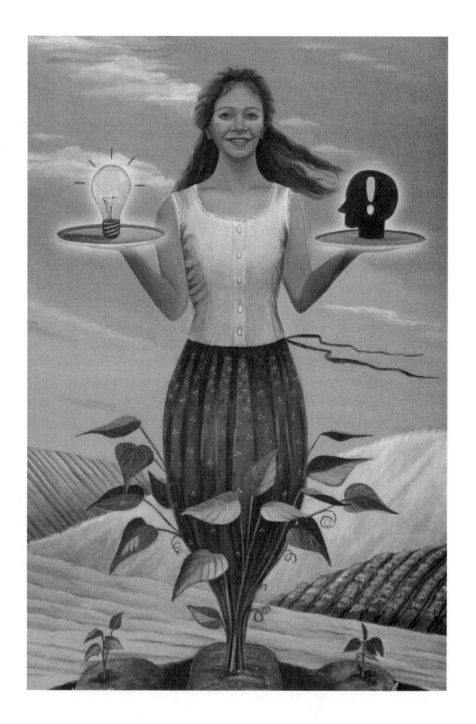

Food for Thought

∾ 11 ∾
Insight
OFTEN THE CATALYST FOR UNDERSTANDING

Sometimes a spontaneous insight can provide the missing catalyst, bringing instant understanding to a point of view foreign to us before. Sometimes spontaneity needs a little push.

Ahead in this chapter…

Almost as momentous as sacrificing our lives for OUR CHILDREN, would be *saving* our lives for our children.

Listen in as Herbert Vore clarifies the meaning of FREEDOM for his brother Carnahan, while they dine out one night.

Discover how pigeons and a dog can explain our food habits, and how the practical principles of PSYCHOLOGY can help change them.

Learn who SOCIETY is, why it disapproves of vegetarians, and why vegetarians are willing to pay the price.

MEAT AND TOBACCO have a history of remarkable parallels that could give the meat-eater a glimpse of the future.

Find out why we should see in the official cause of DEATH STATISTICS—Died Peacefully In Sleep—with 85 percent of deaths in the category.

Hear from two DOCTORS with very different perspectives on their profession, Dr. Phil Theerich and Dr. Dee Sent.

Until we look in a mirror, we can't improve our looks; until we look at U.S. RANKINGS in health statistics, we can't improve our position.

Benjamin Franklin's adage on PREVENTION has been taken to heart by Americans—except in one important area.

CELEBRITY vegetarians who we admire might subtly change our image of the vegetarian and the practice.

QUALITY OF LIFE is an impotent term until people and faces are put with it.

Nearly 300 pieces of the jigsaw puzzle have been assembled and THE PICTURE is unmistakable.

90: Our Children

WOULD WE SAVE *OUR LIVES* FOR THEM?

The boy was 8 years old when his father died of a massive heart attack—his third attack. Apparently the third time is not always a charm. His father ate the Self-Induced Carnivorous Killer (SICK) diet. No doubt it made a significant contribution to his premature death. His father paid the ultimate price; the boy paid a price that was priceless.

His father was a part of the boy's life for slightly more than 3,000 days, but the boy could only remember a handful of them: The time his father brought home a catcher's mitt so he could pitch to his father. The time his father took him to his office and introduced him around. The time his father scolded him for not brushing his teeth when it turned out he had. The time his father died.

The boy's father is buried in Forest Lawn Cemetery in California, about 75 yards from Stan Laurel of Laurel and Hardy. Oliver Hardy isn't buried next to his partner, but he ought to be. The boy, now a man, always stops by Mr. Laurel's grave to laugh before visiting his father's grave to cry. It helps to take the solemn edge off, because even in the cemetery one can't help but chuckle in the presence of Stan Laurel.

The father has been in the same place for many years. He doesn't move, he doesn't say a word. The time his son went 4 for 4 in a little league baseball game he didn't notice. The time his son had a straight-A report card he showed no interest. The time his son went on his first date and could have used some advice, he had nothing to say. The time his son graduated from college he couldn't make it.

There were other painful moments when not having a father profoundly mattered to the boy: father-son outings, YMCA campouts, getting in a fight and not being able to threaten the other kid with, "I'm going to tell my dad on you." Undoubtedly, there were many more, but they were too painful to remember.

When the boy stands over his father's grave, he sometimes wonders what kind of father his dad would have been. The kind of father who when shown a good report card would say nothing more than, "not bad," or the kind who would buy him a new bike? The kind of father who could give a barely perceptible look to show great dissatisfaction, or the kind who would lecture ad nauseam to leave no doubt? It doesn't really matter, the boy would have just settled for a father.

*****

If we are parents—then by virtue of reading this—we are parents who are alive and available to our children. If we are mothers of boys, we will be there to soften their rough edges; if mothers of girls, to listen carefully and often. If we are fathers of boys, we will be there to turn them into men just by the way we conduct ourselves; if fathers of girls, to protect them from all that is menacing.

As parents we would do just about anything for our children, including sacrificing our lives for them if need be. If they were drowning in a raging river, we wouldn't hesitate to rush in to keep them afloat. If an automobile was bearing down on them, we wouldn't consider the consequences before racing into traffic to push them out of harm's way.

Without question, we would do everything in our power for our children, even sacrificing our lives for them. But would we do everything in our power to *save* our lives for them? These situations may not be so different.

Maybe we never thought about it quite like that. Maybe life insurance was the only thing we thought about when we considered the welfare of our children and our deaths in the same thought. Maybe it's time to link the welfare of our children and our lives in the same thought.

When a vegetarian challenges a meat-eater on the adverse consequences of his or her diet choice, a common retort is, "It's my body, and my life, so why shouldn't I be able to eat what I please?" Because our children have a lot riding on that body and that life, would be one answer.

If we're willing to make the ultimate sacrifice for our children, by sacrificing our lives for them, then why wouldn't we be willing to make a trivial sacrifice, by way of our diets, to *keep* our lives for them?

*****

The boy often wonders if these thoughts ever crossed his father's mind. After two heart attacks did he consider eating differently? Did he consider taking steps to reduce the risk of another heart attack? Did he consider the profound impact his death would have on his child's life?

Standing on the perfectly manicured grass looking down on the brass placard that carries his father's name, the boy tells his father about all the things he missed—and about all the things he himself missed. The boy tells his father about the book he is writing, and wishes that it had been written many years ago for him to read. The boy tells his father that maybe it will be in time for other parents. The father says nothing and it makes his now-grown son sad.

Today the boy might need to stop by Mr. Laurel's grave before going home.

91: Freedom

H<small>ERBERT AND</small> C<small>ARNAHAN</small> V<small>ORE</small>

Herbert and Carnahan Vore, better known as "Herbie" and "Carney" to friends and family are brothers. Their relationship has forever been a tumultuous one. To portray the friction between them as a sibling rivalry would be far too great an understatement. Continuous feuding, arguing, and bickering would be much closer to characterizing their interaction.

The brothers haven't spoken for more than 5 years. Those who know them best say there is one fundamental issue at the heart of their contempt for each other. Herbie is a vegetarian and Carney, well, Carney is definitely not.

The story would end here, with the brothers never speaking to each other again, if it weren't for one thing. The brothers were married. Married to women, Meg and Peg, who were the best of friends. Married to women who were tired of their husbands' childish behavior. Married to women who were eternal optimists.

Like most wives, Meg and Peg wanted their husbands to bury the hatchet so they could all socialize together. They knew if they could bring their husbands together for a nice evening out, they could start the mending and eventually get them to be friends. This started the wives on a campaign of cajoling and nagging that wouldn't let up until the brothers agreed to go out for a nice dinner. And of course Herbie and Carney gave in. It may have been the last time Meg and Peg ever cajoled or nagged.

The following is an account of their dinner at *Chez Regret*, a family eatery out on the highway.

MEG: Isn't this nice.

PEG: Yes, isn't it.

HERBIE: Yeah.

CARNEY: Yeah. Let's order.

(The waiter asks for their orders.)

HERBIE: I'll have the pasta. No meat sauce, please. Dinner salad and bean soup to start. There's no meat in the soup, is there? OK.

CARNEY: *I'll* have the meat. I mean, an appetizer please. Buffalo wings. Then I'll have the Chateaubriand, rare. Baked potato with a salad. Antipasto. *Extra* ham.

HERBIE: You know Carney, you probably think you have the freedom to eat meat, don't you?

CARNEY: Last time I looked America was still free and eating meat was still legal. Has something changed since yesterday?

HERBIE: When you choose to eat meat you hurt others on a scale you probably never imagined.

CARNEY: Imagine this: The Declaration of Independence, The Constitution, The Bill of Rights. I have the right to life, liberty, and the pursuit of happiness. And believe me, meat brings me happiness.

HERBIE: Yes, but liberty means you have the right to act without restraint as long as your actions don't interfere with the equivalent rights of others.

CARNEY: I won't interfere with your rights. I promise not to make you eat any of my dinner. OK?

HERBIE: What I mean is, when you eat meat you directly influence global hunger and starvation, the suffering and death of billions of animals, government subsidies and higher taxes, water pollution and soil erosion, energy costs, deforestation, and our nation's health bill. Many paid for your meal tonight—some with their wallets, and some with their lives.

(The food is served.)

MEG: Isn't this nice.

PEG: Yes, isn't it.

CARNEY: Well Herbie, they *all* did a fine job. This is the best Chateaubriand I think I've ever tasted.

HERBIE: Do you know how much you would have to pay for that piece of meat if the government didn't subsidize the land, water, and energy costs to produce it? Fifty dollars, maybe more. Everyone who pays taxes is paying for your steak, including me.[1]

CARNEY: Thank you for contributing. I'll remember to spend a little more on your gift at Christmas.

HERBIE: Fifty percent of our water consumption goes into meat production.[2] Producing 1 pound of meat generates 17 times the water pollution as producing 1 pound of pasta.[3] Who do you think is paying for the increased cost of water and cleanup to support your meat-eating habits?

CARNEY: My water bill is peanuts, and clean water is still running from my tap. (Reaches into his pocket.) Here's a buck and a half. Are we square now?

HERBIE: Due to the carnivorous ways of you and others, our nation's health bill runs an additional $123 billion a year.[4] Who do you think pays for that?

CARNEY: My insurance company does. And they're doing a fine job, I might add.

HERBIE: No, we all do. In higher insurance premiums, higher taxes for Medicare, and higher product costs. About $2,000 a year per family.[5]

And what about the impact meat production has on our earth—the earth we all live on. Because of livestock agriculture the topsoil is being depleted at 7 to 13 times the sustainable rate.[6] If we continue at that pace it will all be gone in the not too distant future. Then we are left with deserts where nothing can grow.

We have cleared more than half the world's forests to accommodate livestock grazing.[7] The forests are the earth's filtering system and temperature regulator. Their destruction might mean our destruction.

CARNEY: Well, I'm not seeing any indication of these problems. But I am seeing a lot of satisfaction from this meal.

HERBIE: Your car runs fine right up until the moment you run out of gas. Then it is too late to do anything about it.

CARNEY: Speaking of too late, your pasta is getting cold.

HERBIE: OK, maybe you can rationalize the adverse impact your meat habits have on people's bank accounts or on their environment, but how can you ignore the fact that people suffer and starve to death, and animals suffer and die?

CARNEY: Look, I never said I was perfect. I don't claim to know or understand why people starve to death. I work hard for my money and I give some to charity including the hungry. I don't beat my wife or break the law. Is it too much to ask to get a little pleasure in life from food?

HERBIE: Is it too much to ask to consider what I have said?

CARNEY: You know, I'm surprised your tirade hasn't included a lecture on what this meal is doing to my health. What gives? Or are you not finished with me yet.

HERBIE: Frankly, if eating meat affected no one other than yourself, in any way, shape or form, meaning it didn't cause animals or people to suffer or die. It didn't require others to contribute one cent to your medical bills. It didn't deplete or pollute our natural resources or create higher taxes. And you had no family or children who would suffer due to your sickness or death. Only then would I agree you have the freedom to chow down and enjoy your Chateaubriand, even if it contributed to your demise.

CARNEY: Don't mind if I do. Sounds like we agree on something.

MEG: Isn't that nice, they have something in common.

PEG: Yes, isn't it.

92: Psychology

A DOG AND PIGEONS

The study of psychology conjures up a variety of impressions. For some, the science evokes visions of Freud, couches, and sexual symbolism. For others, psychology is a mysterious force capable of exposing our deepest secrets. And for still others psychology looks like a morass of gobbledygook.

All three impressions have some truth, but if a dog and pigeons don't come to mind when we think of psychology, then we will fail to realize that the discipline is also an elegant science that has practical value for our everyday lives. This is because the basic principles that drive human behavior can be explained by the results of two simple experiments: Pavlov and his dog, and B.F. Skinner and his pigeons.

Ivan Pavlov, a Russian physiologist, was able to get his dog to salivate with only the sound of a bell after pairing the sound repeatedly with the introduction of food (classical conditioning). B.F. Skinner, an American psychologist, was able to get his pigeons to perform the action he wanted by providing food rewards (instrumental learning).

CLASSICAL CONDITIONING: Let's use our love of the all-American hot dog as an example of how classical conditioning works.

Attending a sporting event is a pleasurable experience for us, just like salivating at the sight of food was for Pavlov's dog. When we repeatedly associate the bell and the hot dog with the pleasurable experience (the hot dog with the sporting event; the bell with salivation) the hot dog and the bell eventually by themselves elicit pleasure. The hot dog becomes an enjoyable food anywhere, anytime! More examples demonstrate this phenomenon.

- Hamburgers with cookouts.
- Barbecued chicken or ribs with picnics.

- Turkey and ham at the holidays with family and tradition when joyful times abound.
- Fast-food hamburgers with happy children and families in television advertising. (An indirect association but an equally powerful influence.)
- Corn-on-the-cob might well be America's favorite vegetable. It's associated with picnics, cookouts, and camping. Is corn *off* the cob just as desired? Why not? They are the same food.
- Cake with birthdays, weddings, and celebrations. Classic good times. After a few of these pairings, cake becomes a treat anytime.

Negative associations work on the same principle.

- Seeing on TV a malnourished person from a Third World country eating rice.
- Eating a food with getting sick creating an adverse association to the food.
- Onions with crying.
- Beans with flatulence.

INSTRUMENTAL LEARNING: We may resent being likened to Skinner's pigeons—our actions influenced by the outside forces of positive and negative rewards—nevertheless the mechanism has proven to be a simple but powerful force in shaping human behavior. The following positive reinforcements are subtle but powerful.

- "If you are a good boy, I will take you to *McDonald's*."
- "Eat all of your vegetables and you can have *dessert*."
- "Wow, you ate two 16-ounce *steaks* at one sitting!"
- "Drink all your *milk* so your bones will be strong."
- "Eat all your *roast beef* so you will have strong muscles."
- "Congratulations, you won first prize in the *chili* cook-off." (Or *fishing* contest, *hunting* contest, *dessert* bake-off.)
- "Beautiful *turkey*, Melba. I bet you slaved all day over it."

And negative reinforcement too:

- *"Nuts and seeds*? You eat like a bird."
- "A *salad*, Frank? That's all you're having? Really now."
- "Don't plan on leaving the table until you finish your *peas*."
- *"Beans and rice*? Isn't that some kind of foreign dish?"

Food by itself is like a blank slate or empty bucket. From our very first meal in life we gather experiences in the form of conditioning, associations, rewards, and customs that fill up the bucket, shaping our likes and dislikes for foods.

Have we ever wondered why children have such strong food likes and dislikes? With very few food experiences, any bad experience—or good experience—is magnified. As time passes more associations are added along the like-dislike spectrum, blunting its intensity, and moving the perception toward the center. No doubt we can all think of at least one food we hated as a child, that we can now tolerate, maybe even enjoy.

Music can work on the same principle. We hear a song on the radio we haven't heard in a long time and it brings back a very intense memory of a past experience or special time. We like the feeling so much we go out and buy the record. However, what we find is the more we play it, the more the intensity of the past memory is diminished. This is because we are blunting and eclipsing the initial association with new ones.

In essence what we are trying to say is: Our want of meat is not the result of a nutritional need the body is demanding, or a real desire, it's simply a function of the repetition of positive reinforcements, rewards, and associations that have their roots in our culture.

Can we prove this argument? If we are able to redirect our wants toward plant-based foods by simply unlearning the old behaviors and learning new behaviors, then this should validate our claim.

Behavior modification, desensitization, and aversion therapy are three proven ways to change our habits. They can help us get over our fear of snakes or flying, and they can help us to quit smoking or drinking. They can also help us to alter our food habits.

BEHAVIOR MODIFICATION: Behavior modification is nothing more than replacing foods we don't want to eat with the foods we do, and building new, positive associations.

Just about every meat—hot dogs, hamburgers, sausage—now has a vegetable equivalent made from vegetables, soy, or grains. They are excellent transition foods to move us away from meat and closer to a Wholly Eating Leaves to Live (WELL) diet. Eat these at cookouts, picnics, and special events to form new associations.

We can substitute meat lasagna with vegetable lasagna, meat burritos with vegetable burritos, meat stews with vegetable stews. Outdoor grilling? It's nothing more than having an outside heat source. Try vegetable shish kebabs, grilled potatoes, and the meat equivalents. More new positive pairings.

We will unlearn, relearn, and eventually never look back.

DESENSITIZATION: Desensitization is successful in helping people to dispose of their fears. Although food is not a fear, the method's principles apply.

This approach is nothing more than proceeding one step at a time by easing into new foods and relinquishing old foods. Getting comfortable at each step before moving on. Comparable to getting slowly into a cold pool in the shallow end, instead of jumping into the deep end.

Start with one meal without meat a week. One new vegetarian entrée a week. Smaller and smaller portions of meat per meal. One less egg or glass of milk per week. The idea is to progress at a pace that makes the transition as smooth and painless as possible.

AVERSION THERAPY: Unconventional, but nevertheless effective, this method instead of paring positive associations, pairs negative associations with foods.

For example, while eating meat we could listen to awful music, read a book about slaughterhouses, or watch a videotape of open-heart surgery. We could also overcook our meat, eat it without seasonings, or prepare it in a way we don't like. The possibilities are endless.

We may want to resist the idea that humans develop behavior and habits by such simple means, manipulated by outside forces like Pavlov's dog and Skinner's pigeons. However, what makes us human, and different from animals, is our capability to understand the mechanisms at work and thus steer our habits in a direction that will best serve our interests.

As we begin to use our power to change food habits the best positive reinforcements of all will kick in—how we look, how we feel, and how less frequent we make doctors' appointments.

93: Society

THE PRICE IS HIGH, THE GOODS A BARGAIN

There is a profound struggle we all face throughout our lives. For some it is infrequent, mild, and perhaps below the surface of awareness. For others it's a continuous and intense fight that defines their existence. The profound struggle is between the individual and society. We battle to honor our principles and beliefs, while society pushes back with its standards and conformity.

Society is a powerful force. When we choose to exercise behavior that is in conflict with the customs, traditions, and expectations of the majority, we choose a path of determined resistance. This resistance can bring us criticism, hostility, and alienation. But it can also bring us empowerment, growth, and liberation. When we choose to conform to society's standards, instead of being true to our principles, we have chosen the proverbial path of least resistance. A path with no obstacles and easy sailing, but also a path of stagnation and weakness.

Either choice we make exacts a price. However, one choice costs a great deal more. The following are examples of behaviors that might meet with disapproval or resistance from our society.

- Being in an interracial marriage or never getting married at all.
- Voting as an Independent or belonging to the Libertarian Party.
- Growing long hair (man) or cutting it to an inch short (woman).
- Choosing to give birth at home or do home schooling.
- Choosing to watch only public television or not own a TV at all.
- Being an agnostic or an atheist.
- Being an Apple-Macintosh user or not a computer user at all.
- Being an animal rights activist or a vegetarian.

Society appears to be quite judgmental. What is society, and why does it care what people choose to do with their lives?

A society is a set of common assumptions, beliefs, and behaviors that provide stability, order, and direction for a group of people. Those who conform to established standards often feel threatened by people who don't. Here are a few reasons why.

- Fear of the unknown.
- Feeling like they are being contradicted.
- Having to address new information and the potential for change.
- Being embarrassed by lacking knowledge of a subject.
- Happy, comfortable, and content with the status quo.

When an individual decides to become a vegetarian in a society where eating meat is the rule, all of these issues kick in. The meat-eating custom in our society is built on some of the following assumptions.

- Meat and dairy foods are necessary for good nutrition.
- Animals are inferior to humans.
- Animals don't experience emotion and pain the way humans do.
- Most chronic diseases are the result of the aging process.
- Diseases have their roots in heredity.
- Doctors will make us well if we get sick.
- The media is unbiased and would inform us if meat was bad.
- Natural resources are for our unbridled use.
- The environment will eventually regenerate even if we abuse it.
- The government ultimately has our best interests at heart.
- World hunger is mostly beyond our control.

Most vegetarians have questioned some or all of these assumptions. Society has responded by labeling the vegetarian as: misguided and rebellious, weak and overly sensitive, arrogant and presumptuous, critical and judgmental, and ignorant and out-of-touch. Consequently, vegetarians are often criticized and ostracized.

Why, then, are vegetarians willing to pay such a high price for their convictions? Maybe it's because they believe:

- their health will be better for it.
- the animals will be better for it.
- the earth will be better for it.
- humanity will be better for it.
- they must to be true to themselves.
- the evidence substantiates their choice.

Although the price is high, the goods appear to be a bargain.

We are all faced at some point in our lives of having to decide whether to follow our hearts or follow the crowd. Sometimes the issues are minor and inconsequential, and sometimes they are far-reaching and life-defining.

How do we know what decision to make when faced with these two paths? Asking ourselves the following questions might provide the answer.

- When we followed the crowd in the past what rewards did we receive?
- Name 10 people we admire most in life. How many of them made the list because they conformed to society's expectations?
- Are there people we are not fond of, but still respect them for following their principles?
- Do we have a purpose to fulfill on earth? If so, will we get there by taking the path of least resistance?

Next time we come in contact with a vegetarian we might see him or her differently.

Next time we have a choice to make we might see it differently.

Next time we look in the mirror we might see ourselves differently.

94: Meat and Tobacco

"NO MEAT EATING" SECTIONS

In the early 1920s evidence showed that this consumable was a health hazard. The substance, however, continued to grow in popularity. It was promoted by athletes and recommended by doctors. Most everyone used it. Those who did not were considered antisocial or odd. It was touted as healthful and certainly harmless. It became associated with man's virility and machismo.

As time passed, there was growing evidence that the substance may not be all that good for us. But it was heavily advertised, the government was supporting it with subsidies, and the producers assured us that it was safe. The hazards were only theories, the industry stated. There was much conflicting evidence, and more time was needed for study, they said. So people kept using it with little concern.

Americans enjoyed the substance immensely, looked forward to it regularly, and couldn't imagine living without it. As time passed, people began to get sick from it. Cancer and heart disease were among the illnesses attributed to it. In the late 1950s, early 1960s, the evidence had grown to be irrefutable. Official word went out to the American people that it was hazardous to their health.[1]

Some people stopped buying the substance, but most didn't. Those that didn't claimed it was legal, and being an American citizen gave them every right to exercise their freedom and avail themselves of it if they so desired. People began to cut back on their consumption. Products came to the market to help people transition off the emotionally and physically addicting substance, and these substitutes helped. However, people were still succumbing to disease, and dying by the thousands from using it.

As more time passed it became apparent that the substance was affecting the health of people *not* using it, and the health of the planet as well. As recently as 1990 at least 50 percent of the American people using it doubted whether it was unhealthy.[2]

The product referred to in the narrative is:

a) Tobacco
b) Meat
c) Tobacco and Meat

The correct answer is C—both tobacco and meat. Although meat and tobacco are very different, they both have much in common including their infamous histories. Some of the parallels are:

- In 1925, evidence indicated that cigarette tar caused cancer.[3] In the 1920s, due to World War I food shortages, the Danish government switched people from a less-efficient meat-based diet, to a more-efficient grain diet, and saw the mortality rate drop significantly.[4]

- At one time those that didn't smoke were labeled antisocial or odd. The same labels are often applied to those who do not eat meat.

- Both substances were touted for their health benefits: meat to ensure enough protein, and smoking to relax and overcome social nervousness.[5]

- Both substances were promoted as boosters of a man's masculinity.

- In 1957, and again in 1964, the Surgeon General of the United States issued formal reports condemning tobacco as a health-harming substance.[6] In 1961, the American Heart Association first publicly denounced saturated fat as a health hazard.[7]

- As time passed it became more apparent that those who ate meat and smoked cigarettes by claiming individual freedom were violating others' freedom: Second-hand smoke was shown to be hazardous, and meat production was shown to contribute to world hunger, environmental deterioration, and economic drain.

- The use of both substances caused disease, and consequently billions of dollars in medical costs.

- Both substances showed themselves to be physically and psychologically addicting, deeply rooted in our conditioning and social fabric.

- When the addiction was combined with massive advertising, government subsidies, and political leverage that the industry's economic clout generated, the perfect prescription for denial was created.

    Thus after 70-plus years of accumulating evidence (as of the early 1990s), implicating both these substances in the horrific toll on our health, 50 percent of smokers, and 95 percent of Americans (who still included meat in their diets), weren't convinced either substance was harmful.[8]

- New markets have flourished to assist in breaking the stronghold meat and tobacco have on our psyches. Smokers have patches and gum, and meat-eaters have analogs to help break the respective habits.

- At one time smoking was considered a healthy, socially acceptable habit. If not so many years ago people suggested otherwise, we would have laughed in their faces. Today, the consumption of meat is still considered by most Americans to be a healthy, socially acceptable habit. No doubt, many would laugh at the suggestion that it isn't.

Meat eating is a few steps behind smoking in its fall from grace. Given the similar path that meat consumption is on, it appears to be just a matter of time before the laughing stops. And not much longer after the laughing stops, meat and tobacco may only be a part of our lives—in the history books. No doubt under the chapter heading: American Calamities.

Between now and then though, is it possible we might see any of the following?

- "No Meat Eating" sections in restaurants.
- People sneaking off to fast-food joints for a hamburger.
- People being asked to eat their meat hors d'oeuvres outside at parties.
- The meat and dairy industries sued in court.
- People secretly flossing animal tissue from their teeth to hide a meat-laden meal.
- Taxes on meat and dairy to fund medical costs and educational programs.

Hard to believe? It happened to smoking. And who would have believed *that* not so long ago.

95: Death Statistics

We probably don't spend a great deal of the day pondering our death. What's there to ponder? We don't know how, when, or where it will happen. Our only thought might be: We hope we live a long life and then die peacefully—past the age of 100 and in our sleep comes to mind. We have no control over our death so why waste time contemplating it. At least we think we have no control.

The fact is we have a lot more say about how our life ends than we think. Let's expand on this idea by exploring some statistics on the causes of death in this country. Statistics and numbers are not the be all and end all, but they can provide perspective, add to our knowledge, maybe even change the way we think or behave.

Ultimately, there is only one number we are concerned with. Our own. Rest assured it won't be found here.

MALNUTRITION SCORECARD: There is concern that those subsisting on a plant-based diet won't get the proper nutrition, and as a consequence will be malnourished. In 1999, 4,289 people died of malnutrition in the United States.[1] Most likely few, if any, were vegetarians. But let's assume they all were for the sake of argument.

There is concern that those subsisting on a meat-based diet won't get the proper nutrition, and as a consequence will be malnourished. It is estimated that 68 percent of deaths have their roots in the American meat-based diet.[2] Based on this percentage, the year 1999 saw 1,626,151 people die of a different kind of malnourishment.

That means for every vegetarian that died from his or her diet, 380 meat-eaters died from theirs.

LIFE EXPECTANCY: WHAT DO WE EXPECT? The assumption is that we are living longer and better. Good assumption?

An American male reaching 55 years old in 1990 could only expect to live 3 years longer than an American male from 1900.[3] Twenty-three countries rank ahead of the United States in Healthy Life Expectancy (HALE). According to the Division of Vital Statistics, in 1999, U.S. life expectancy was 76.7 years. According to program and damage theorists, humans have a genetically programmed maximum life expectancy of 120 years.[4]

We can expect more.

BYPASS SOMETHING ELSE: The risk of dying during heart bypass surgery is 5 to 12 percent. The risk of dying from angioplasty is 1 to 3 percent.[5] These would seem to be reasonable risks given the alternative. However, the risks may not be so reasonable, and the alternative misidentified.

Heart bypass surgery is estimated to prolong life in 2 percent of patients. Angioplasty is estimated to not extend life or prevent heart attacks at all.[6] A better alternative might be to bypass the SICK Diet.

GROWING CANCER—GROWING NOSE? "In the early 1900s there was no hope of survival, but today 49 percent will live 5 years after diagnosis of cancer."[7] (In 1900 cancer was the 10th leading cause of death. Today, cancer is the 2nd leading cause of death.)[8]

"Surgery, radiation, and chemotherapy are the only treatments that can combat cancer."[9] (Vegetarians have more than double the ability to destroy cancer cells by way of their immune systems.)[10]

The American Cancer Society announced in 1997, "There are no practical ways to prevent breast cancer, only early detection."[11] (According to Dr. Robert Hatherill, 90 percent of cancers are due to factors that have been identified and are within our control.)[12]

NEW KID IN TOWN: Alzheimer's disease, with all the earmarks of another degenerative disease connected to diet, was added as a cause of death classification in 1998. In 1999, it ranked 8th, causing 44,000 deaths.[13]

Nature designed the body to run its life expectancy course, then pass quietly away. When we see a cause of death classification for the occurrence, "Died Peacefully in Sleep," we will know that we are beginning to turn the corner.

STRIVE FOR PERFECTION: There were close to 2.4 million deaths in the United States in 1999; 1 death every 13 seconds. It's probably no surprise that circulatory diseases and cancer together made up a large share, 1.55 million deaths or 65 percent. With a very broad brush, here is a total breakdown of deaths in millions:[14]

- Heart / Stroke / Cancer: 1.55
- Diabetes / Kidney / Alzheimer's: 0.15
- Infectious / Respiratory / Pneumonia: 0.25
- Suicide / Liver Cirrhosis / HIV: 0.10
- Automobile / Accidents / Homicide: 0.10
- All Other: 0.25

Total: 2.4 Million

Let's suspend reality for a moment and as best we can erase the attitudes, assumptions, and perceptions we hold. We are going to generalize and exaggerate a bit in the hopes it will help us to envision a different way of looking at death, therefore a different way of looking at life. The theme is personal responsibility and taking control.

As it stands now there are 133 official causes of death. Yet not one of the causes accounts for a natural, peaceful, death. A cause that the body—a 100-trillion-cell machine, refined during 8 million years—is capable of, if not expected to achieve.

Let's assume for the moment that we ate the right diet, led exemplary lives, and always used good judgment. Many people already do. Theoretically then, why couldn't we strive to make a natural death the only cause of death?

Let's start from the premise that 68 percent of deaths are directly related to our flesh diets. The following independent assessment matches the 68 percent figure previously referenced. (1.55 million for Heart, Stroke, and Cancer, less 5 percent heredity for circulatory disease and 10 percent heredity, virus, and environment for cancer. Add 0.15 million for Diabetes, Kidney, and Alzheimer's. This comes to 1.62 million, or 68 percent of 2.4 million).

Infectious and respiratory diseases, and pneumonia would not appear to be affected by diet. However, the animal-based foods that degenerate our bodies take the place of plant-based foods that *regenerate* the immune system—the very system that is responsible for warding off invaders. So indirectly it is related to diet. Let's arbitrarily say we can prevent half of these deaths with an immune system operating at full power. (50 percent of 0.25 million is 0.13. That's an additional 5 percent affected by diet.)

Suicide, liver cirrhosis, and HIV. In varying degrees they are voluntary and self-imposed. We can argue extenuating circumstances that remove them from our control. But we can also argue that we are ultimately responsible for our actions. (100 percent of 0.10 adds another 4 percent of control.)

Automobile, accidents, and homicide. Foresight and good judgment could diminish all three. Even homicide. In 90 percent of homicides the parties are known to each other. Over time, the choices we make and lifestyle we lead can place us in the wrong place at the wrong time. We will arbitrarily assign a 75 percent factor. (75 percent of 0.10 contributes another 3 percent.)

We will conservatively apply a 50 percent factor to the "all other" category. (50 percent of 0.25 million is 0.13. Add another 5 percent of control.)

Now the 133 causes of death gets distilled down to a precise 6, which are:

- Within our control:

  - Diet (direct): 1.62 million (68 percent)
  - Diet (indirect): 0.13 million (5 percent)
  - Self-imposed: 0.10 million (4 percent)
  - Poor judgment: 0.08 million (3 percent)
  - Other: 0.13 million (5 percent)

  Total: 2.06 million (85 percent)

- Not within our control:

  - Unfortunate circumstances: 0.34 million (15 percent)

If we abate the 85 percent that are within our control, then the cause of death tally might someday look like this:

- Died Peacefully in Sleep: 2.06 million (85 percent)
- Unfortunate Circumstances: 0.34 million (15 percent)

Ultimately we would strive to identify and address the other 15 percent to bring them within our control.

There are two different ways to view this whole assessment, and both have validity.

The first way: An unrealistic, over-simplified picture of life that makes some questionable and perhaps offensive assumptions. It's too far-out to be taken seriously.

The second way: A lofty ideal suggesting that if we combine the potential of our bodies, with a change in our perspective, we could live longer, happier, and healthier lives. A perspective that suggests we do have a say on how we live and die by virtue of recognizing that diet, along with other factors, has a direct impact.

Both views can be true, yes, but the adoption of only one will advance us forward.

96: Doctors

DR. PHIL THEERICH AND DR. DEE SENT

We usually think of doctors as doctors, rather than as people. Maybe it's because when we visit doctors we are keenly focused on one objective only: getting well. The doctor's family life, fears and hopes, or opinions on the recent election are not important to us when we are sick. Nothing is for that matter. We never get to know the individual in the white coat, so we end up perceiving doctors as faceless healers cut from the same cloth. But they're not.

Medicine is like any other profession in that it attracts all types of people who have a diversity of biases, limitations, skills, and backgrounds. And people with a whole range of motives. Those who want to become doctors for selfless and altruistic reasons to give compassion and mercy, to those who want to become doctors for money and ego gratification to get power and prestige.

If we had a chance to interact with doctors when we weren't sick, we could see them as people and get a perspective we never had before. With this in mind, we have invited two doctors to join us, Dr. Phil Theerich and Dr. Dee Sent, with the hope that hearing them speak will help us to better provide for our own future health and illness-care.

First, we will hear from Dr. Dee Sent.

"Thank you for inviting me. I've wanted to be a doctor and make people well ever since I watched my mother waste away from cancer. I was just six. I stood by helplessly. Although I live with a passion to assist those who are ill, I still have that helpless feeling so much of the time.

"I received my training from the best medical school and graduated with honors. I can diagnose disease from a hundred yards away, prescribe from more than a thousand drugs by memory, and hook my patients up with any of the best 50 surgeons in town.

You think it would be enough, but it isn't even close.

"Most of my patients are suffering from chronic diseases for which I can only supply a crutch, not a cure. My medical schooling provided little nutritional education, so I've learned on my own about the power of plant-based foods and the equally powerful devastation of animal-based foods. I try to impart this knowledge to my patients, but most don't seem to want to hear it; most don't want to change their eating habits. I often lose their business as a result.

"They expect instead to get a prescription, to have a test run, to hear that surgery will solve their problem. And if I don't meet their expectations—even if I know diet changes will help them—I risk a malpractice suit. If I don't follow the recognized regimen—even if I know an alternative treatment, for say cancer, might be a better solution for them—I could lose my license. Then I am of no use to anyone.

"I know I'm a good healer, but I also know I can't hold a candle to the body's healing powers. It can perform magic if we would only recognize its potential and assist with its ability to do so.

"I don't know everything there is to know either. My continuing education consists of journal articles, scientific research, conferences, patient handouts, lectures, and publications that come from the pharmaceutical and meat and dairy industries. I know the information is biased, but I'm already logging 60 hours a week with patients, and don't have the time to do my own research.

"That's why I'm thrilled when I see patients who have utilized the Internet, or other resources, to research their own illnesses. They often find information I wasn't aware of. They come with questions. They want to be in charge of their own destiny. While most of my patients want me to tell them what to do, these patients rightfully want me to assist them.

"People must understand that we are not gods. People must understand we have limitations. People must understand that *they* hold the key to their health. Thank you."

Now we will hear from Dr. Phil Theerich.

"Thank you for inviting me. I must say I have never heard so much touchy-feely, bleeding heart malarkey in all my life from Alice in Wonderland over there. To suggest that something as simple as diet is the answer to the immense complexities of the diseases we are faced with today is utterly ridiculous. I never interfere with my patients' lifestyles and I know they respect that.

"This is war. A war we are losing, no doubt because of doctors like Ms. Sent. It's us against the evil side of Nature. We have to throw everything we have at it if we are to have a chance of winning. That means money, technology, drugs, and surgery. We doctors are the generals in this battle. We need every bit of cooperation from our patients if we are going to succeed—and that doesn't mean by having them help us by surfing the Internet.

"I don't have to worry about malpractice or losing my license because my patients know I will perform every test, try every drug, and then radiate it, laser it, or cut out the disease—whatever it takes.

"Sure, I make a lot of money, but can we put a price on health? Am I a God? Of course not. But to a patient I can cure, I bet I come pretty damn close.

"I love my work every bit as much as Ms. Sent. My chances of succeeding are only limited by the tools technology gives me and the patient's faith in my skills.

"I can make the difference between pain and pleasure, sickness and health, or life and death. And that is what I intend to keep on doing. Thank you."

We thank Dr. Phil Theerich and Dr. Dee Sent for talking with us and being so direct. It's hard to believe, given the extreme contrast in perspectives, these individuals share the same profession.

We hope their speeches were informative. We hope they helped us reach...some decent conclusions.

97: U.S. Rankings

TIME TO LOOK AT OURSELVES IN THE MIRROR

There is no doubt that America is the greatest country in the world. Few of us would want to live anywhere else. But we didn't get that way by denying reality, burying our heads in the sand, or accepting the status quo.

Most Americans consider our healthcare system, and health, second to none, and themselves reasonably well informed on health matters. But like the guy who never looks in the mirror can always believe he is a stud, Americans have done the same when it comes to looking at our collective health, and the factors that influence it.

Unfortunately, until we pick up the mirror and take an honest look at ourselves and our blemishes, we will never know the truth, and thus never be able to improve and progress. Let's place the mirror in front of our faces.

The United States has sophisticated technology, a temperate climate, and we rank number one in per capita healthcare expenditures.[1] So one might expect us to be pretty close to the top in the Healthy Life Expectancy (HALE), and Health System Performance categories published by the World Health Organization, right? We rank 24th and 37th, respectively.[2] Big powerhouses like Iceland and Malta have greater life expectancies, and Andorra and Columbia do better in overall health performance. Let's bring the mirror a little closer.

Less than 1 percent of our healthcare dollars go toward prevention.[3] We lead the world in malpractice suits.[4] Infant mortality is higher in New York City than in Shanghai.[5] We rank number one in hip fractures caused by osteoporosis.[6] We are the only nation in the industrialized world that doesn't guarantee minimum healthcare to every single citizen—42 million have no health coverage.[7] While this begins to explain our rank, there are more blemishes and wrinkles to see.

While European nations have access to alternative cancer care, the United States is the only country that actively denies alternative medicine.[8] While other countries are passing laws to make animal farming practices more humane, we are passing laws to unprotect animals.[9] While the industrialized world has banned antibiotics in animal feed, the United States still continues the practice.[10] Don't put the mirror down yet, we aren't finished.

One-half of adults, 100 million Americans, suffer from some form of a chronic disease, mostly due to diet.[11] Two-thirds of the world subsists on plant-based diets, while just 5 percent of Americans are vegetarians.[12] Where most worldwide diets get 75 percent of their calories from whole grains, the American animal-based diet gets 1 percent.[13] Food safety? Americans suffer from 76 million cases of food poisoning a year.[14] The United States incurs 50 times more cases of salmonella poisoning than say, Sweden.[15]

What did we think we were going to see in the mirror?

- Because milk is a staple in our diets, the average American believes that milk is a staple in 99 percent of the world's diets. The percentage of milk consumed by the rest of the world: 35 percent.[16]

- The percentage of Americans that believe that eating less meat reduces colon cancer risk: 2 percent.[17] Based on a study of 40 countries the correlation between animal fat and intestinal cancer is 82 percent.[18]

- The percentage of American women who believe there are dietary steps they can take to reduce their risk of breast cancer: 23 percent.[19] Based on a 40-country study the correlation between animal fat and breast cancer is 76 percent.[20]

- The percentage of men who believe there is a link between eating meat and prostate cancer: 2 percent.[21] Based on the study of 30 countries the correlation between animal fat and prostate cancer is 67 percent.[22]

Looking in the mirror can be painful, especially when what we see is not very attractive. However, the alternative is worse. Given what we know now, we can grow, make improvements, and move up in the standings. Then one day when we look in the mirror and say, "Mirror, mirror, on the wall who's the fairest of them all," the mirror will answer back, "You are, you healthy American stud."

98: Prevention

BENJAMIN FRANKLIN'S SEQUEL

"An ounce of prevention is worth a pound of cure." The adage put forth by Benjamin Franklin in *Poor Richard's Almanac* more than 250 years ago may have been his most profound and thoughtful insight.

Given that Mr. Franklin was a vegetarian, one might have thought he was referring to the health hazards of meat and the health benefits of vegetables in preventing disease when he created this adage. But he wasn't. He was alerting people to tips on preventing fires, and fire damage to their homes.

In America we have taken Mr. Franklin's advice to heart, becoming a nation voracious about not only fire safety, but about all aspects of prevention. From bicycle helmets to childproof safety caps, from air bags to warning labels, we do everything possible to try and prevent mishaps. In fact, many people would suggest we have gone overboard in the area of prevention.

If Ben Franklin had created his advice in reference to our health, and the consequences of a meat-based diet, would our obsessiveness about prevention have been focused toward diet, instead of general safety? Would, for example, seniors who are good about using a cane to prevent injuries, be equally focused about eating their leafy greens for the folic acid to help prevent Alzheimer's disease?[1]

Let's explore this concept with a list of parallel preventions like this one, and see if we can expand on Mr. Franklin's adage when it comes to what we eat.

- Men are pretty good about wearing an athletic cup to prevent groin injuries, but are they pretty good about eating tomatoes containing lycopene to help prevent testicular cancer?[2]

- We are pretty good about installing an antivirus protector on our computers to prevent data corruption, but are we pretty good about reducing the consumption of cured meats to help prevent brain cancer?[3]

• We are pretty good about using Travelers Cheques on vacation to prevent robbery, but are we pretty good about reducing the amount of animal protein in our diets to prevent the robbing of calcium, and the risk of osteoporosis?[4]

• We are pretty good about placing deadbolts on our doors to prevent break-ins, but are we pretty good about reducing iron-laden red meat in our diets to help prevent free radicals from breaking into our DNA, contributing to cancer, heart disease, and aging?[5]

• We are pretty good about wearing dark glasses to prevent damage to our eyes, but are we pretty good about eating carrots, sweet potatoes, and oranges to increase our consumption of beta-carotene and antioxidants to reduce the risk of cataracts?[6]

• We are pretty good about wearing our seat belts as protection against serious automobile injury, but are we pretty good about consuming fiber that's only found in plant-based foods as protection against diverticulitis, appendicitis, and colon cancer?[7]

• We are pretty good about using childproof safety caps to prevent drug and chemical poisoning, but are we pretty good about reducing our consumption of beef, chicken, and fish, to help prevent E. coli and salmonella poisoning?[8]

• We are pretty good about preventing our sinks and toilets from backing up by keeping our pipes clear, but are we pretty good about reducing our fat and cholesterol intake keeping our arteries clear to reduce the risk of hypertension?[9]

• We are pretty good about putting swim floats on our children to help prevent drowning, but are we pretty good about reducing their consumption of milk to help prevent asthma?[10]

- We are pretty good about painting our homes to keep the wood from being destroyed, but are we pretty good about reducing our consumption of beef to keep our forests from being destroyed?[11]

- We are pretty good about brushing our teeth to help prevent plaque buildup causing cavities and gum disease, but are we pretty good about reducing our consumption of fat and cholesterol-laden animal-based foods to help prevent plaque buildup causing atherosclerosis and heart attacks?[12]

- We are pretty good about purchasing enough automobile insurance to protect ourselves financially from property damage, personal liability, uninsured motorists, and medical costs, but are we pretty good about purchasing enough foods containing complex carbohydrates to protect ourselves from diabetes, hypoglycemia, weight gain, and fatigue?[13]

- We are pretty good about placing a screen in front of our fireplaces to prevent an uncontrolled fire from getting started, but are we pretty good about eating foods from the plant kingdom to maintain strong immune systems preventing an uncontrolled cancer from getting started?[14]

- We are pretty good about having an awareness that our children will suffer if we choose not to talk with them about sex and drugs, but are we pretty good about having an awareness that animals and starving people will suffer if we choose to eat meat?[15]

- We are pretty good about putting on sunscreen to decrease the risk of sun-dependent skin cancer, but are we pretty good about reducing our fat intake to decrease the risk of hormone-dependent prostate and breast cancers?[16]

If Mr. Franklin, being a vegetarian, was with us today, he would probably have a word or two to say about the diet practice. In fact, he might have many words to say. We would probably find them penned in a sequel to *Poor Richard's Almanac*, titled: *A Pound of Plant-based foods is Worth a Ton of Health.*

99: Celebrity

WORTHY OF IMITATION

If we're not vegetarians, then most likely it is not a topic we ponder often. In fact, the subject has crossed our minds maybe three times in the past year.

One time was when a vegetarian friend called—the one who wears no make-up, clothes that rarely match, and who we think is far too thin—inviting us to a potluck dinner party with the theme "Bean Fling."

The second time was at a party, where a person we didn't know cornered us by the buffet table and preached to us endlessly on the virtues of vegetarianism, while we tried to hide the fact we were holding a plate full of cocktail wieners and meatballs.

The third time was from television, when we witnessed an animal activist protesting the start of hunting season by running through a forest with an air horn in each hand warning the animals of impending danger.

Given our interesting encounters with vegetarianism, it's no wonder we give the diet as much thought—as we do to say—cleaning behind the refrigerator.

But what if our friend holding the Bean Fling was Kim Basinger or Dyan Cannon? What if the preaching party lecturer was Mel Gibson or Bo Derek? What if the animal activist was Paul McCartney or Mary Tyler Moore? Might we have a different view of vegetarianism given the celebrity of these vegetarians?

We all have people we admire and look up to. People whose qualities, principles, and accomplishments we hold in high regard. We call them role models. We find their habits, interests, and way of life worthy of imitation.

The following musicians, politicians, writers, movie stars, philosophers, spiritual leaders, social scientists, athletes, educators, inventors, artists, and activists are celebrities who have one thing in common: they are all vegetarians.[1] Might who they are make their principles and habits worthy of imitation? And is it conceivable that who they have become is due to one particular habit they have embraced?

- American writers Louisa May Alcott (*Little Women*), Henry David Thoreau (*Walden*), and Herman Melville (*Moby Dick*), who produced some of America's greatest literary works.

- Leonardo da Vinci and Benjamin Franklin who might best be called versatile geniuses for their prolific inventions and creativity.

- H. G. Wells who produced great science fiction and suspense, and Mark Twain who produced great humor and satire.

- British Playwrights William Shakespeare and George Bernard Shaw, two of the greatest dramatists ever.

- Songwriters and musicians Bob Dylan, Paul McCartney, Stevie Wonder, and James Taylor, who have few equals.

- Musicians and performers Tina Turner, Smokey Robinson, and Carlos Santana, whose energies and stage presences make them bigger than life.

- Plato and Socrates, Greek philosophers whose writings and teachings still hold meaning today.

- People with foresight like Charles Darwin (theory of evolution), Dr. Benjamin Spock (baby and child care), and Steven Jobs (co-founder of Apple computers), who broke new ground and cleared their own paths.

- Mathematical wizards, Pythagoras, Albert Einstein, and Isaac Newton, who helped make sense of the universe.

- People of courage who stood up and fought for the rights of others like Susan B. Anthony (women), Cesar Chavez (farm workers), Albert Schweitzer (the poor), and Ralph Nader (consumers).

- Spiritual leaders such as Gandhi, Buddha, and possibly Jesus.

- Movie stars with beauty and sex appeal like Candice Bergen, Brooke Shields, Bo Derek, Dyan Cannon, Kim Basinger, and Brigitte Bardot. Movie stars with machismo and sex appeal like Richard Gere, Mel Gibson, Tom Cruise, and Alec Baldwin.

- Icons of comedic genius, Milton Berle, Carol Burnett, and Bill Cosby. Icons of acting genius, Dustin Hoffman and Mary Tyler Moore.

- Television stars Jerry Seinfeld, Ted Danson, Meredith Baxter, and Ed Begley, Jr.

- Young, but already successful movie stars, Tobey Maguire and Drew Barrymore.

- Football coaches Marv Levy (Buffalo Bills and four consecutive Super Bowl appearances), and Tom Osborn (Nebraska and four national championships).

- Politicians Dennis J. Kucinich (Ohio congressman), and Andy Jacobs (Indiana congressman).

- Sports superstars and champions: The amazing endurance of Captain Alan Jones (17,003 consecutive pushups), and Dave Scott (six-time Ironman triathlon winner). The athletic achievements of female tennis champions Billie Jean King, Martina Navratilova, and Chris Evert. The Olympic feats of Carl Lewis and Edwin Moses. The bodybuilding accomplishments of Mr. America and Mr. Universe, Bill Pearl.

- A medley of talent, class, and integrity that includes Leo Tolstoy, Ralph Waldo Emerson, Margaret Mead, Vincent Van Gogh, Chubby Checker, Johnny Cash, Ringo Starr, Bill Walton, Barbara Feldon, Bob Barker, Henry Heimlich M.D., and Fred Rogers.

Did choosing to become vegetarians make a contribution to the success of these individuals?

Did choosing to become vegetarians remain consistent with the other intelligent choices these people made that contributed to their success?

Would these individuals have achieved at the level they had if they had not been vegetarians?

Would others who have achieved success that were not vegetarians have achieved even more if they had been?

All good questions that have no conclusive answers.

Most of us will never reach the accomplishments of these individuals. Most of us will never attain their status. But all of us can ponder the significance of their dietary choice, and all of us can give more thought to cleaning behind the refrigerator.

100: Quality of Life

THE IRONY OF THEIR SOLE COMPLAINT

The boy's mother and stepfather have lived a comfortable middle-class life. Both are in their mid-eighties. Both have exceeded their gender's life expectancy. Both have eaten the American SICK diet their entire lives.

It sounds like an argument *in support* of a meat-based diet. Then again, for the past 20 years or so they have together suffered from, and through, the following degenerative health problems:

Heart bypass surgery, gall bladder surgeries, osteoporosis, congestive heart failure, stenosis of the spinal column, prostate cancer, pacemaker implant, hypertension, mild stroke, phlebitis, hysterectomy due to endometriosis, rectal surgery due to harsh laxative, cataract surgery, right hip replacement, left hip replacement, skin cancer, obesity, diverticulitis, arthritis, double hernia, pinched nerve resulting in back surgery, hearing loss, diminishing mental function, and dental surgeries.

OK, so they have had some health problems. Most people in their later years have deteriorating health. It's an accepted reality. Having lived longer than the average American puts them ahead of the game, right? Yes, compared to everyone else who has lived on the same diet, they have done pretty well.

But if we combine the geneticists' hypothesis that humans have the potential to live 120 years, with the fact that those in other populations who subsist on the WELL diet live into their 90s with barely a scratch, then doing "pretty well" loses some of its luster. What looked like a pretty full life now looks like, at least in theory, a life that has been reduced by decades in both quantity and quality.

Quality of Life is a broad term, and without details the concept is rather impotent. Let's put some life into it.

For the past two decades, more than 20 percent of their lives, the boy's mother and stepfather have had more and more of their time taken up with the following activities:

Making doctors' appointments, driving to and waiting for the doctor, and being with doctors.

Confined in hospital beds, worrying about impending surgeries, and undergoing surgeries.

Going to physical therapy, purchasing equipment to assist in physical therapy, and doing physical therapy at home.

Taking medications, changing medications and dosages, and remembering to take medications.

Keeping track of medical bills, paying medical debts, and worrying about medical costs.

Reducing pain in the body, worrying about the future, and crying.

A long way from where—as their son recalls—their time used to go:

Playing golf, planting flowers, taking car trips, doing home repairs, playing bridge, flying cross-country on vacation, attending club meetings, going to plays, spending time at the beach, going to restaurants, doing home improvements, attending professional meetings, having friends for dinner, keeping up the yard, taking long walks, maintaining the cars, traveling to visit family, and relaxing, laughing, and smiling.

But today, the picture looks like this:

The golf clubs are now a home for spiders and the TV is the closest they get to a golf course.

Because the stepfather can't lift, bend over, climb a ladder, or stoop down, he has to stand by and watch home repairs and maintenance often done by people who do too little, charge too much, and care not the least.

Taking a walk is no longer a simple pleasure but a major production that is too tiring, too risky, and too painful.

Ditto for going to restaurants, meetings, and traveling cross-country.

Having friends over for bridge would be in the cards except many of them have passed away, are in retirement homes, or find traveling too tiring, too risky, and too painful also.

And relaxing, laughing, and smiling often take too much physical and mental energy to justify the effort.

The end of one's life—the last block of years—should not be lived like this. The last years of life should be the best years of life.

We should be rewarded for the years of going to a job, raising our children, following a schedule, and being responsible. It is time to sleep in, reminisce, keep a journal, paint, find joy with grandchildren, read, dole out wisdom, take up a new hobby, try a new sport, speak our minds, and visit all day.

It is a time for independence, not dependence. It is a time to look forward to tomorrow, not fear tomorrow.

What is amazing is that with all these two people have come up against and suffered through, they rarely complain. With one prominent exception.

We know it's an official complaint because it has been repeated more than once. One can tell by their tone of voice it really ticks them off. They complain about—and if we don't see the irony here, we will never know irony—the foods they have to eat now: Whole foods. Fruits and vegetables, pastas and potatoes, grains and beans, soups and salads. Less fat, less sugar, less sodium, less meat, less dairy—less of all the foods they have been eating their entire lives. It's not hard to understand their attitude. They are being told to undo habits, conditioning, and a way of life that has been with them forever.

The boy has three hopes for his mother and stepfather.

One: they will change their dietary habits. Two: the complaint about the foods they must now eat will be appreciated someday. Three: they will have many more somedays.

101: The Picture

284 PUZZLE PIECES — A CLEAR PICTURE

Last Christmas the dog got a hold of one of the presents—a jigsaw puzzle—then chewed up the box beyond recognition and scattered the pieces throughout the house. No one knew what the jigsaw puzzle picture was, so the family decided to find the pieces and try to solve the puzzle.

Now and then a piece was found and placed on a card table set up in the living room. Each piece by itself gave hardly a clue as to the nature of what the completed picture was. After about 100 pieces had been found, the puzzle began to take shape. A few educated guesses were made about the picture, but no one was 100 percent sure.

Finally, one day a member of the family fit a piece into the puzzle—piece number 284—and voila! The picture materialized. Not all the pieces had been found, but the ones that had, fit together perfectly to leave no doubt that the picture puzzle was solved.

Does everyone else see the picture, too?

1. EVOLUTION: Humankind and its ancestors evolved for most of 8 million years on a vegetarian diet.[1]

2. ICE AGE: Climatic changes of the Ice Age and drought, 3.5 million years ago, rendered plants scarce requiring hominids to eat animals in order to survive.[2]

3. ANATOMY: The human anatomy—grinding molars, no sharp claws, digestive system—is unlike a carnivores.[3]

4. SPEED: A study revealed that meat consumption is inversely related to body weight/speed: From a one-pound animal (dwarf galago) eating 70 percent dietary animal matter, to a 350-pound animal (gorilla) eating 1 to 2 percent animal matter.[4]

5. INSTINCT: How often do we see a human pouncing on a chicken, ripping it apart, salivating at the sight of its raw flesh, then sucking the warm blood from it?

6. BIOLOGICAL EVOLUTION: If we accept the Darwinian version of evolution, then we accept that we are primates descended from animals, and should therefore question the practical and philosophical justification for eating them.

7. CHOLESTEROL: The human body manufactures 500 milligrams of cholesterol a day—all that it needs. The Recommended Daily Allowance (RDA) for cholesterol is zero.[5]

8. CHOLESTEROL: The plant kingdom contains zero cholesterol.[6]

9. CHOLESTEROL: An American on the SICK diet ingests an additional 500 milligrams of cholesterol a day more than what the body manufactures.[7]

10. CHOLESTEROL: Chicken and fish contain twice the cholesterol as beef.[8]

11. CHOLESTEROL: A single egg contains 213 milligrams of cholesterol.[9]

12. CHOLESTEROL: The average American's cholesterol is 205 mg/dL.[10]

13. CHOLESTEROL: The average American vegan's cholesterol is 133 mg/dL.[11]

14. HEART DISEASE: After 35 years in the Framington Heart Study, those with cholesterol less than 150 mg/dL had no heart attacks.[12]

15. HEART DISEASE: An American dies every minute of a heart attack.[13]

16. HEART DISEASE: 25 men of the Hunzas of Kashmir, older than 90, who subsisted on a pure vegetarian were studied and found to have no trace of coronary artery disease.[14]

17. HEART DISEASE: Residents of rural China subsist primarily on grains, legumes, fruits, and vegetables. Cholesterol levels range from 90 to 150 mg/dL. As a result, coronary artery disease is virtually unknown.[15]

18. HEART DISEASE: When the Japanese, known for their predominately vegetarian diet, moved to other parts of the world and changed their eating habits a direct correlation developed between their diet and heart disease.[16]

19. HEART DISEASE: Coronary artery disease is 5 times lower for Greek men than American men; the Greek diet is plant-based.[17]

20. HEART DISEASE: In a 12-year Esselstyn study, severe heart disease was reversed in 95 percent of those going on a pure vegetarian diet.[18]

21. HEART DISEASE: The famous heart surgeon, Dr. Michael DeBakey, suggests that heredity accounts for about 5 percent of heart disease.[19]

22. ATHEROSCLEROSIS: During World War II Norway's supply of meat was virtually cut off. As a result the correlation between the reduction of fat consumption and circulatory disease in Norway from 1938 to 1948 was almost identical.[20]

23. ATHEROSCLEROSIS: Of American soldiers in their 20s who were autopsied during the Korean War, 35 percent had fibrous plaque in their coronary arteries, while the opposing forces subsisting on a predominately vegetarian diet showed no such damage.[21]

24. ATHEROSCLEROSIS: Russian physiologists fed egg yolks

to herbivore rabbits, and to carnivore dogs and cats. The rabbits produced atherosclerotic plaque similar to those occurring in humans. They couldn't produce atherosclerotic plaque in the dogs and cats.[22]

25. ATHEROSCLEROSIS: A study revealed that a low-fat vegetarian diet reduced cholesterol 24 percent (roughly 60 points) in 12 months, and caused 82 percent of the arterial plaque to shrink.[23]

26. ATHEROSCLEROSIS: Dr. Dean Ornish's program, based on a low-fat, whole-foods vegetarian diet, has shown to reverse atherosclerosis in 75 percent of people, with 80 percent being able to avoid surgery after 1 year on the program.[24]

27. ATHEROSCLEROSIS: Stress, lack of exercise, and heredity have little to do with the disease.[25]

28. HYPERTENSION: 50 million Americans have hypertension.[26]

29. HYPERTENSION: Hypertension is 13 times more likely in meat-eaters.[27]

30. HYPERTENSION: In the United States, 50 percent of the population older than 65 has hypertension with readings greater than 160 over 95.[28]

31. HYPERTENSION: In New Guinea and several African countries, blood pressures throughout life remain at a constant 110 over 70.[29]

32. HYPERTENSION: According to the *Journal of the American Medical Association* (1983), a study showed that for those with mild hypertension on drug therapy, the number of deaths was reduced by 1 percent.[30]

33. HYPERTENSION: A study revealed that after changing to a vegetarian diet 58 percent of people with hypertension came off their medication.[31]

34. HYPERTENSION: In African societies where hypertension is unknown their descendants in the United States experience hypertension that is epidemic.[32]

35. PROTEIN: An adult male puts out 4.32 grams of urinary nitrogen per day. Each gram represents 6.25 grams of broken down protein. Thus 27 grams of protein are required per day. 27 x 4 calories / gram = 108 calories / 2,400 calories = 4.5 percent protein / day.[33]

36. PROTEIN: Human breast milk, utilized at a time of critical growth and nutrition, contains 5.0 percent protein in calories.[34]

37. PROTEIN: The World Health Organization recommends 5.0 percent protein as a minimum requirement.[35]

38. PROTEIN: The U.S. RDA for protein is 10.0 percent.[36]

39. PROTEIN: The pure vegetarian (no meat, dairy, or eggs) eating only from the plant kingdom consumes 11.0 percent protein.[37]

40. PROTEIN: Experiments have shown that subjects eating only plant sources of protein have maintained nitrogen equilibrium.[38]

41. PROTEIN: According to the American Dietetic Association, if we get enough calories and eat a reasonable variety of plant-based foods, it is virtually impossible not to meet protein needs.[39]

42. PROTEIN: The primary disease of inadequate protein consumption is Kwashiorkor. There are virtually no cases of this disorder in the United States.[40]

43. PROTEIN: Research conducted on rats in 1914 to determine how to get livestock to grow faster is still used today as the basis of the claim that animal protein is superior for humans.[41]

44. PROTEIN: The average omnivore American consumes 16.5 percent protein—11.0 percent in animal protein.[42]

45. OSTEOPOROSIS: The average American ingests at least twice the protein the body requires of which 70 percent is animal protein, and it's acidic.[43] This increases the pH of the blood requiring the alkaline calcium from the bones to neutralize it.[44]

46. OSTEOPOROSIS: A study revealed that those on meat-based diets who ingested 1,400 milligrams of calcium daily had a negative calcium balance; those on low-protein diets ingesting 500 milligrams had a positive calcium balance.[45]

47. OSTEOPOROSIS: A study revealed that women who consumed a high ratio of animal to vegetable protein suffered 3 times the rate of bone loss, and 4 times the rate of hip fractures.[46]

48. OSTEOPOROSIS: A study revealed that the average bone loss of an omnivore woman is 35 percent at age 65; the average bone loss of an herbivore woman is 7 percent at age 65.[47]

49. OSTEOPOROSIS: Bantu women of Africa consume 240 to 450 milligrams of calcium on a predominately vegan diet. Osteoporosis is almost unknown amongst them.[48]

50. OSTEOPOROSIS: African Americans in this country, who ingest 1,000 milligrams of calcium a day, have 9 times the hip fracture rate of South African Blacks who ingest 196 milligrams of calcium a day.[49]

51. OSTEOPOROSIS: When African blacks move to affluent countries and change their diets and lifestyles, osteoporosis becomes common among them also.[50]

52. OSTEOPOROSIS: Eskimos routinely ingest 2,500 milligrams of calcium daily and maintain a negative calcium

balance. They have one of the highest number of osteo-porosis cases in the world.[51]

53. OSTEOPOROSIS: The four countries with the highest consumption of dairy products are the United States, Finland, Sweden, and England. They are also the four countries with the highest rates of osteoporosis.[52]

54. OSTEOPOROSIS: The United States ranks first in hip fractures caused by osteoporosis.[53]

55. OSTEOPOROSIS: 20 million American women suffer from osteoporosis.[54]

56. OSTEOPOROSIS: Calcium comes from the soil. Plants use it for varying needs, so vegetarians and vegans get their calcium from the plants.[55]

57. KIDNEY DISEASE: Excess protein in our diet makes the kidneys work harder by excreting more water, raising the fluid pressure that causes tissue damage and loss of kidney function.[56]

58. KIDNEY DISEASE: Animal protein from dairy products, cross-react with our body's protein-generating antibodies. These antigen-antibody complexes are trapped in the tiny blood vessels of the kidneys, causing inflammation and damage.[57]

59. KIDNEY DISEASE: A study from 1946 revealed that of 100 patients placed on a low-protein diet, 65 showed objective improvement in kidney function.[58]

60. KIDNEY DISEASE: Kidney stones form due to excess calcium from the bones being called on to neutralize the acidic animal protein in the blood, then ending up in high concentrations in the urine.[59]

61. KIDNEY DISEASE: 20 million Americans have kidney and urinary diseases.[60]

62. ULCERS: Animal protein foods—meats, cheese, eggs, milk—are acid forming. They upset the delicate balance between the protective mucus and stomach acid that can lead to ulcers.[61]

63. ULCERS: A study revealed that of 48,000 male health professionals, those that consumed 30 grams of fiber a day were half as likely to get ulcers as those who took in 13 grams a day.[62]

64. ULCERS: Most foods from the plant kingdom are base-forming (alkaline) and contain plenty of fiber.[63]

65. ULCERS: A study revealed that an internist changed the lives of his ulcer patients when he took them off dairy products for 2 weeks.[64]

66. ULCERS: 33 million Americans will sustain an ulcer at some point in their lives.[65]

67. AUTOIMMUNE DISEASE: Animal protein has shown to be implicated in autoimmune disease, as animal protein amino acid sequences cross react with human protein chains, confusing the immune system resulting in an attack on us.[66]

68. AUTOIMMUNE DISEASE: When free radicals—promoted by fats, oils, milk, and iron—attack immune cells, the immune system weakens, which diminishes the ability of the immune cells to distinguish between friend and foe.[67]

69. AUTOIMMUNE DISEASE: Animal fat has shown to greatly decrease natural killer cell activity and impact the clearing system that removes antigen-antibodies implicated in autoimmune disorders.[68]

70. AUTOIMMUNE DISEASE: More than 100 autoimmune diseases afflict 50 million Americans.[69]

71. ARTHRITIS: Theory says it is caused by an autoimmune response from animal proteins that has shared sequences of

amino acids with the collagen in our joints.[70]

72. ARTHRITIS: A study revealed that 6 subjects going on a pure vegetarian diet had complete disappearance of symptoms after 7 weeks.[71]

73. ARTHRITIS: Rheumatoid arthritis is rare in Africa, Japan, and China where the diets contain little fat, cholesterol, and animal protein.[72]

74. ARTHRITIS: When Blacks move from Africa to America and adopt a meat-based diet, their incidence of rheumatoid arthritis rises dramatically.[73]

75. ARTHRITIS: In the United States, 1 in 4 people suffers from osteoarthritis.[74]

76. MULTIPLE SCLEROSIS: Animal protein and animal fat are implicated in the autoimmune disease of the nervous system, multiple sclerosis.[75]

77. MULTIPLE SCLEROSIS: The nine countries with the highest rate of multiple sclerosis have a per capita fat consumption of 105 to 151 grams per day; the nine countries with the lowest incidence of multiple sclerosis have fat intakes of 24 to 60 grams per day.[76]

78. MULTIPLE SCLEROSIS: A long-term 34-year study tracked survival rates of multiple sclerosis patients. Symptoms of those that followed a diet restricting red meat and milk were slowed or stopped; the group had a 95 percent survival rate. Those that failed to follow the restricted diet had a 20 percent survival rate.[77]

79. MULTIPLE SCLEROSIS: The disease is rare in Asia, but common in Europe and North America.[78]

80. MULTIPLE SCLEROSIS: More than 250,000 Americans have multiple sclerosis.[79]

81. DIABETES (TYPE I CHILDHOOD): Strong evidence indicates a specific cows' milk protein sparks an autoimmune reaction, generating antibodies to bovine serum albumin and our own pancreatic cells. It is believed that this reaction destroys the insulin producing cells of the pancreas, causing insulin-dependent diabetes.[80]

82. DIABETES (TYPE I CHILDHOOD): One study found antibodies to cows' milk protein present in all 142 diabetic children at the time of disease diagnosis.[81]

83. ASTHMA: An autoimmune response is implicated in asthma for those with a hypersensitivity to animal protein, specifically cows' milk protein.[82]

84. ASTHMA: Asthmatics can find a marked improvement in their condition by eliminating cows' milk from their diets.[83]

85. ASTHMA: A long-term study utilized a vegan diet that resulted in significant improvement in 92 percent of the 25 patients.[84]

86. ASTHMA: A study showed that 20 of 38 patients receiving natural beta-carotene were protected against exercise-induced asthma.[85]

87. ASTHMA: It's predominately a disease of Western culture. Poorer nations see little of it.[86]

88. ASTHMA: The disease assails 17 million Americans, including 4.8 million children.[87]

89. CROHN'S DISEASE: Data suggests that animal protein and an autoimmune response in the intestine is the culprit.[88] Some suspect it may be caused by a microorganism present in cows' milk not killed by pasteurization.[89]

90. CROHN'S DISEASE: It appears that vegetable protein is associated with reduced incidence.[90]

91. CROHN'S DISEASE: The disease is mostly found in the United States, Scandinavia, and United Kingdom, where meat and dairy consumption is the highest.[91]

92. CROHN'S DISEASE: A half-million Americans suffer from it.[92]

93. FAT: The American SICK diet includes 40 percent of its calories in fat. The WELL diet includes 10 to 15 percent of its calories in fat.[93]

94. FAT: Humans do require fats in their diet, but only two—unsaturated linoleic and linolenic fatty acids—and they are only synthesized by plants.[94]

95. FAT: Dietary fat significantly increases the amount of hormones circulating in men and women—50 percent higher in some women—by over-production, by preventing excretion of hormones, or by both.[95]

96. FAT: Fiber is the mechanism that absorbs and excretes the hormones.[96] Herbivore women excrete 2 to 3 times more estrogen in the feces than their omnivore counterparts.[97] Fiber is only contained in the plant kingdom; there is no fiber in meat.[98]

97. BREAST CANCER: Breast cancer is a hormone-dependent cancer promoted by fat consumption: Omnivore women have 50 percent higher levels of estrogen—Herbivore women excrete 2 to 3 times more estrogen in the feces.[99]

98. BREAST CANCER: A study of 37 countries ranked in fat consumption / breast cancer rates revealed: Denmark (1st/1st), United States (7th/7th), Sri Lanka (37th/36th).[100]

99. BREAST CANCER: Affluent women in Japan who eat meat have an 8.5 times greater risk of breast cancer than the poorer Japanese women who can't afford meat.[101]

100. BREAST CANCER: The suspended consumption of cheese,

which contains roughly 70 percent fat, will reduce the risk of breast cancer up to 3 times.[102]

101. BREAST CANCER: A study of premenopausal women older than 40 found that the risk of postmenopausal breast cancer decreased by 54 percent with a vegetarian diet.[103]

102. BREAST CANCER: Women on estrogen therapy for more than 5 years will increase their risk of breast cancer by 30 to 40 percent.[104]

103. BREAST CANCER: Menstruation starts 4 years earlier and menopause begins 4 years later for women eating diets that are higher in fat. Eight years of higher levels of estrogen circulating in the body doubles the lifetime risk of getting breast cancer.[105]

104. BREAST CANCER: There is a peculiar discrepancy between the current age of menarche—a female's ability to bear children—of 12.5, and her level of maturity to be a mother. However, 175 years ago, when meat consumption and fat intake were significantly lower, menarche occurred at age 17.[106]

105. BREAST CANCER: The disease is diagnosed in 184,000 American women each year—one every 3 minutes—with 44,000 deaths attributed to the disease.[107]

106. OVARIAN CANCER: Ovarian cancer is a hormone-dependent cancer promoted by fat consumption: omnivore women have 50 percent higher levels of estrogen—herbivore women excrete 2 to 3 times more estrogen in the feces.[108]

107. OVARIAN CANCER: A study revealed that women who ate eggs three or more times a week, were 3 times more likely to get ovarian cancer than vegetarian women.[109]

108. OVARIAN CANCER: A study of 16,000 women in Norway revealed that those who drank two or more glasses of milk

a day had a substantially higher risk of ovarian cancer than women who drank less milk.[110]

109. OVARIAN CANCER: A study revealed that women who consume yogurt and cottage cheese have triple the risk of ovarian cancer as those who don't, as a result of the milk sugar, galactose, contained in the products.[111]

110. OVARIAN CANCER: In a 1989 study, Harvard University researchers noted that women with ovarian cancer had low blood levels of transferase, an enzyme involved in the metabolism of dairy foods.[112]

111. OVARIAN CANCER: *The Journal of the National Cancer Institute* reported that the higher a woman's cholesterol level, the greater her risk of ovarian cancer.[113]

112. OVARIAN CANCER: A study revealed that women on estrogen therapy for more than 5 years will increase her risk of ovarian cancer by 30 to 40 percent.[114]

113. OVARIAN CANCER: California Seventh-day Adventists—50 percent of whom are vegetarian—were found to have a lower risk of ovarian cancer than the general population.[115]

114. OVARIAN CANCER: 23,400 American women are diagnosed each year with ovarian cancer; 13,900 die from the disease.[116]

115. ENDOMETRIOSIS: Endometriosis is a hormone-dependent disease promoted by fat consumption: omnivore women have 50 percent higher levels of estrogen—herbivore women excrete 2 to 3 times more estrogen in the feces.[117]

116. ENDOMETRIOSIS: A study revealed that a 24-year-old woman who was treated with low-fat, purely vegetarian foods was noticeably better within 3 months, and at 6 months her pain was gone.[118]

117. ENDOMETRIOSIS: Women with high blood levels of

immune system weakening PCBs found in fish, have a higher prevalence of endometriosis.[119]

118. ENDOMETRIOSIS: The risk of endometriosis is typically reduced when menopause is handled without estrogen replacement therapy (ERT).[120]

119. ENDOMETRIOSIS: Heredity accounts for 4 to 5 percent of cases.[121]

120. ENDOMETRIOSIS: Endometriosis affects 12 million American women.[122]

121. PROSTATE CANCER: Prostate Cancer is a hormone-dependent cancer promoted by fat consumption; andros-terone and testosterone circulating in the bloodstream will produce a higher incidence of the cancer.[123]

122. PROSTATE CANCER: A Study of 6,500 men revealed that the risk of developing prostate cancer was increased by 3.6 times for those who ate eggs, cheese, and meat.[124]

123. PROSTATE CANCER: A study revealed that men who fill up with tomatoes (lycopene), carrots (beta-carotene), and cru-ciferous vegetables such as broccoli and cabbage, decrease their prostate risk by 41 percent.[125]

124. PROSTATE CANCER: In a study that reviewed 30 countries, the United States ranked 3rd in daily animal fat consump-tion, and 3rd in death rates due to prostate cancer.[126]

125. PROSTATE CANCER: The risk of prostate cancer for Seventh-day Adventist vegetarian men is one-third that of the general population.[127]

126. PROSTATE CANCER: For every 10 men who die of prostate cancer in Western Europe only 1 dies in Asia. Western Europeans consume 4 times more animal fat than Asians.[128]

127. PROSTATE CANCER: A man from Sweden will be 8 times

more likely to die from prostate cancer than a man from Hong Kong. A Swedish man's fat intake is twice that of a Hong Kong man's.[129]

128. PROSTATE CANCER: A case of prostate cancer is diagnosed every 3 minutes in the United States—198,000 a year. It causes 31,000 deaths a year.[130]

129. INFERTILITY: Infertility is hormone-dependent, promoted by fat consumption; testosterone circulating in the bloodstream will reduce sperm count in men.[131]

130. INFERTILITY: A study revealed that an injection of 200 milligrams of testosterone a day shut off sperm production in 70 percent of test subjects.[132]

131. INFERTILITY: In 1 out of every 3 cases, infertility is due to a problem with the man, specifically a deficient sperm count.[133]

132. INFERTILITY: In a study that reviewed 60 countries, a 77 percent inverse correlation existed between animal fat consumption and birth rates.[134]

133. HAIR LOSS: Heredity is the primary factor, but hair loss is also hormone-dependent, influenced by fat consumption.[135]

134. HAIR LOSS: First observed in 1942—and later studied— men who had their testicles removed for medical reasons, and therefore weren't producing testosterone, *also* weren't losing their hair. Little consolation. Later when they were given testosterone shots to compensate for their unfortunate operation, their hair fell out.[136]

135. HAIR LOSS: In Japan, where more people are changing to a more Western diet, more baldness is occurring.[137]

136. HAIR LOSS: A study revealed that hair falls out at twice the rate in the fall, when testosterone levels are higher, compared to the lower spring levels.[138]

137. FAT / FIBER: The SICK diet has half the complex carbohydrates and fiber, and nearly 4 times the fat as the WELL diet. Saturated fat is only found in the animal kingdom; complex carbohydrates and fiber are only found in the plant kingdom.[139]

138. DIABETES (TYPE II ADULT): A disease of too much fat, rather than too little insulin: Photomicrographs show that fat is hiding insulin receptor sites.[140] Complex carbohydrates cause insulin resistance to decrease, slowing absorption of sugars into the bloodstream, reducing the risk of diabetes.[141]

139. DIABETES (TYPE II ADULT): One study placed subjects on a low-fat vegan diet and saw their blood sugar levels drop 28 percent.[142] Fiber has shown to better synchronize with insulin.[143]

140. DIABETES (TYPE II ADULT): One study placed 10 patients on a 70 percent carbohydrate high-fiber diet. Sixteen days later, 9 of the patients were able to stop insulin.[144]

141. DIABETES (TYPE II ADULT): One study placed 80 patients on a low-fat diet, and 60 percent were off insulin in 6 weeks. Two more studies had 75 percent success rates.[145]

142. DIABETES (TYPE II ADULT): A study that reviewed 14 countries in fat consumption/diabetes rates revealed: Denmark (1st/1st), Japan (14th /14th).[146]

143. DIABETES (TYPE II ADULT): The people of Nauru, who live on a small Polynesian island and subsist on vegetables, grains, and fruits, had no diabetes prior to World War II. After the war, their country fell into riches, people began to include meat in their diets, and one-third of the population developed diabetes.[147]

144. DIABETES (TYPE II ADULT): Diabetes is rare among Africans, Asians, and Polynesians who subsist on plant-based diets.[148]

145. DIABETES (TYPE II ADULT): There are 15.7 million diabetics in the United States, with 798,000 new cases reported each year.[149] It takes 193,000 U.S. lives annually.[150]

146. COLON CANCER: Fiber binds with carcinogens, fats, and cholesterol, eliminating them from the body to reduce the risk of colon cancer.[151]

147. COLON CANCER: The muscle, fat, and ligaments of an animal diet can take 3 to 4 days—fat is solid at body temperature—to move sluggishly through the bowels, increasing the risk of colon cancer.[152]

148. COLON CANCER: A study reviewing 37 countries revealed an 82 percent correlation between the amount of daily fat consumed and the death rate from colon cancer. International studies suggest that fully 95 percent of colon cancer cases have a nutritional connection.[153]

149. COLON CANCER: According to the National Cancer Institute, when Japanese immigrants with low colon cancer rates moved to the United States and adopted the American meat-based diet, their rates rose to the level of the typical American.[154]

150. COLON CANCER: Every 4 minutes an American will be diagnosed with colon cancer—135,000 new cases annually. Every 10 minutes an American will die from colon cancer—56,000 deaths annually.[155]

151. DIVERTICULITIS: A disease of inflammation, and sometimes bleeding of the intestine, because of too much fat and too little fiber in the diet.[156]

152. DIVERTICULITIS: In a study, 70 diverticulitis patients were placed on a high-fiber diet. Before the diet they tallied 171 different symptoms. After a time on the diet, 88 percent of the symptoms disappeared, and the number of patients taking laxatives went from 49 to 7.[157]

153. DIVERTICULITIS: In the United States, 10 percent of those older than 40, and 35 percent older than 50, have evidence of this disease.[158]

154. IMPOTENCE: It is estimated that 85 percent of impotence cases are due to restricted artery blood flow to the penis as a result of a meat-based diet.[159]

155. IMPOTENCE: Roughly 10 percent of erectile dysfunction is considered to be emotional.[160]

156. IMPOTENCE: In the United States, 34 percent of middle age men suffer from impotence. By the age of 60, 1 in 4 men is impotent.[161]

157. IMPOTENCE: Men are capable of retaining their sexual vitality and activity well into their 80s and beyond.[162]

158. HEMORRHOIDS: Caused by straining in trying to evacuate hard, dry, underweight feces, courtesy of a meat-based diet.[163]

159. HEMORRHOIDS: Hemorrhoids are rare in Asia and Africa where the diets are predominately plant-based. In North America and Western Europe this is not the case.[164]

160. HERNIA: A hiatal hernia can occur from abdominal pressure of daily straining. In the United States, 1 out of 5 people has this problem.[165]

161. APPENDICITIS: A result of a small, hard, concentrated feces getting stuck in the appendix opening.[166]

162. APPENDICITIS: There are 250,000 cases each year of appendicitis in this country.[167]

163. APPENDICITIS: In rural Africa where the diet is plant-based many surgeons have never seen a single case.[168]

164. IRON: The body stores iron. Iron, especially the heme iron

resident in meat—but not contained in plants—creates excess iron storage that acts with oxygen, promoting free radical damage.[169]

165. IRON: The non-heme iron in plants keeps the body's stores lower. However, when the body is deficient in iron, non-heme iron in plant-based foods has the capability to increase its absorption rate by 10 times.[170] Plant-based foods have a much greater ability to maintain the correct balance of iron in the body.[171]

166. IRON: The average omnivore has 1,000 to 2,000 milligrams of stored iron, while the average herbivore has lower, safer amounts of stored iron in their bodies of 480 milligrams.[172]

167. CANCER: Excess iron encourages DNA damage that can lead to cancer.[173]

168. ATHEROSCLEROSIS: Iron makes atherosclerosis more likely to start.[174]

169. HEART DISEASE: During the childbearing years a woman's risk of heart disease is significantly less than a man's because her iron levels are held down by the natural loss of iron through menstruation. After menopause, her risk becomes the same as a man's.[175]

170. VISION LOSS: Oxidation, due to the bombardment of free radicals from excessive iron, light, or the environment, can lead to cataract development.[176]

171. VISION LOSS: Oxidation of the rods and cones, due to the bombardment of free radicals from excessive iron, light, or the environment, can lead to macular degeneration.[177]

172. ALZHEIMER'S DISEASE: A study revealed that free radicals interacting with iron, ever so present in the damage to other parts of the body, also play a role in the development of Alzheimer's.[178]

173. AGING: Overall tissue damage because of too much iron can accelerate the aging process.[179]

174. FREE RADICALS: Antioxidants are protective chemicals that neutralize free radicals and the tissue oxidation that they cause. Some examples are vitamin C, E, beta-carotene, and folic acid. All originate, and most come, from the plant kingdom.[180]

175. AGING: Beta-carotene, prevalent in carrots, has anti-aging properties.[181] It protects our skin from free radical damage caused by the sun.[182]

176. AGING: The Hunzas of Kashmir, who subsist on a 99 percent vegetarian diet, work and play at age 80 and beyond, have no cavities, father children, and have no heart disease into their 90s. They are active at age 100 and maintain 20/20 vision. Their broken bones heal in 3 weeks and they usually die of natural causes.[183]

177. ALZHEIMER'S DISEASE: A study revealed that Alzheimer's patients have low blood levels of the vitamin folic acid and high levels of the protein building block homocysteine.[184] (Homocysteine is converted from methionine—a protein 2 to 3 times more prevalent in meat.)[185]

178. ALZHEIMER'S DISEASE: Folic acid found in green leafy vegetables, and whole grains, prevents methionine from being converted to homocysteine.[186]

179. ALZHEIMER'S DISEASE: A study revealed that the homocysteine levels dropped 13 to 20 percent in just 1 week after the subjects switched to a vegan diet.[187]

180. ALZHEIMER'S DISEASE: A study revealed that reduced blood cholesterol levels (in this study, cholesterol was lowered by drugs) lowered the risk of developing Alzheimer's disease and other forms of dementia by 73 percent.[188]

181. ALZHEIMER'S DISEASE: A study revealed that people who remained free from any form of dementia had consumed higher amounts of beta-carotene, vitamin C, vitamin E, and vegetables than the people in the study who developed Alzheimer's disease.[189]

182. ALZHEIMER'S DISEASE: Alzheimer's disease has been diagnosed in 4 million Americans.[190]

183. VISION LOSS: Milk sugar, galactose, as we age is more difficult to break down and passes into the lens of the eye leading to cataracts.[191]

184. VISION LOSS: A study revealed that people who eat less than 3.5 servings of fruits and vegetables a day have 6 times the risk of developing cataracts.[192]

185. VISION LOSS: A survey revealed that people who ate the most beta-carotene and other carotenoids, particularly as supplied by spinach and collard greens, had almost half the risk of macular degeneration, as those eating fewer carotenoids.[193]

186. VISION LOSS: A study revealed that people who consumed higher intakes of two antioxidants found in green leafy vegetables, lutein and zeaxanthin, were 70 percent less likely to develop macular degeneration.[194]

187. VISION LOSS: People on fat-free intravenous fluids for reasons not related to glaucoma, improved their intraocular pressure, which reduces the risk of this disease.[195]

188. VISION LOSS: Research from the 1940s revealed a significant and continuous improvement in intraocular pressure, reducing the risk of glaucoma, when subjects were placed on a low-fat rice diet.[196]

189. HEARING LOSS: Evidence suggests that hearing loss could be caused by the immune system being compromised, since

ongoing repair is a must in maintaining the moving parts involved in hearing.[197]

190. HEARING LOSS: Hearing loss has been shown to improve after 4 months on a low-fat vegetarian diet.[198]

191. HEARING LOSS: A high homocysteine blood concentration could interfere with the blood flow to the inner ear.[199] (Homocysteine is converted from methionine, a protein 2 to 3 times more prevalent in meat.)[200]

192. HEARING LOSS: Folic acid found in green leafy vegetables, and whole grains, prevents methionine from being converted to homocysteine.[201]

193. HEARING LOSS: People in Third World countries eating their traditional diets that don't include meat have better hearing at the age of 70 than the average American has at 20.[202]

194. FATIGUE: Hypoglycemia, a condition of low blood sugar resulting in fatigue, can be caused by excess dietary fat consumption.[203]

195. FATIGUE: The remedy for hypoglycemia is to increase complex carbohydrates like rice, vegetables, or beans as they blunt the insulin response allowing a more gradual absorption of glucose.[204]

196. FATIGUE: Chronic fatigue syndrome (CFS) is basically a weakened immune system causing chronic weakness that can be made worse by animal protein, and strengthened by numerous plant-based foods including beta-carotene.[205]

197. BEHAVIOR: Dietary fat and lack of fiber increases testosterone levels in men making them more violent; daily animal fat consumption was plotted against sex offenses for 54 countries and a correlation of 50 percent was found.[206]

198. BEHAVIOR: Animal protein reduces tryptophane in the

brain, which in turn increases aggression. When daily animal protein consumption was plotted against the number of wars and civil wars for 58 countries, a correlation of 35 percent was found.[207]

199. BEHAVIOR: Whole grains, beans, and vegetables rich in complex carbohydrates increase the brain's supply of serotonin making people calm and even-tempered.[208]

200. BEHAVIOR: Omega-6 fatty acids from meat were found in significantly higher levels in 34 habitually violent criminals.[209]

201. BEHAVIOR: A vegetarian diet induces alpha waves, which indicate a state of neuromuscular relaxation, not just of the brain, but also of the whole body as shown by electroencephalograms (EEGs).[210]

202. CHILDREN: American children show fatty streaks in their arteries at 9 months, signs of atherosclerosis at 3 years, and scar tissue formation in the teen years.[211] Of 21 to 39-year-olds, 85 percent had fatty streaks, and 69 percent had fibrous plaque in the coronary arteries.[212]

203. CHILDREN: 17 percent of 6th to 8th graders have cholesterol levels greater than 180 mg/dL.[213]

204. CHILDREN: 1 in 8 American children has blood pressure that is too high.[214]

205. CHILDREN: 25 percent of children 6 to 17 years old are overweight.[215]

206. CHILDREN: Cancers in children were doubled with the consumption of hamburgers or hot dogs at least once a week.[216] Today, cancer is the second leading cause of death among children under 15; In 1950 it was a medical rarity when meat and dairy consumption was much lower.[217]

207. CHILDREN: The highest rates of leukemia are found in

children ages 3 to 13, who consume the most dairy products.[218]

208. CHILDREN: Childhood otitis media (ear infection) affects 10 million children and is linked to cows' milk allergy.[219]

209. CHILDREN: By the age of 19, Finnish children, who eat a high-fat diet, had a marked inability to hear high-frequency sounds.[220]

210. CHILDREN: Milk is suspected of triggering juvenile diabetes (Type I).[221]

211. CHILDREN: Increasing numbers of children, often as young as 10 years old, are being diagnosed with Type II diabetes.[222]

212. CHILDREN: A pediatrician recommended that all of his patients eliminate milk from their diets. The result? He did not have a single child with asthma.[223] In a study, 18,000 children showed a lower risk of asthma when they ate more vegetables and fiber that included vitamin E, calcium, and magnesium.[224]

213. CHILDREN: Clinical studies have shown that children on a diet of mostly vegetables, fruits, grains, and legumes, when consuming adequate calories, not only grow at normal rates, but also have been shown to attain greater height than omnivore children.[225]

214. CHILDREN: A study revealed that vegetarian children have higher I.Q.s.[226]

215. CHILDREN: The American Dietetic Association (ADA) approves a vegetarian diet for all ages, even those who are in a high-growth stage like infants and toddlers.[227]

216. FOOD POISONING: Every year 76 million people get sick and 5,000 people die from food poisoning.[228]

217. FOOD POISONING: 95 percent of food poisoning is to due

to meat, dairy, eggs, and fish.[229]

218. PLANTS: Experiments have shown that subjects eating only plant sources of protein have maintained nitrogen equilibrium.[230] According to the American Dietetic Association, if we get enough calories and eat a reasonable variety of plant-based foods, it is virtually impossible not to meet protein needs.[231]

219. PLANTS: Plant proteins' amino acid sequences are 100 percent different than human proteins. (Implicated in autoimmune disease are animal protein sequences similar to humans.)[232]

220. PLANTS: Phytochemicals, which include at least 1,000 active compounds, are found only in plants. They inhibit carcinogens, fight disease, and strengthen the immune system.[233]

221. PLANTS: The protective chemicals, antioxidants, all originated in the plant kingdom.[234]

222. PLANTS: Complex carbohydrates are only contained in plants.[235]

223. PLANTS: All minerals were manufactured in the earth at the same time it was formed. They are absorbed and delivered to us by way of plants.[236]

224. PLANTS: Fiber (cellulose) is found only in plants.[237]

225. PLANTS: All vitamins originate from plants. (Vitamin D is a hormone; vitamin B_{12} originates in the environment, but not in animals.)[238]

226. PLANTS: Plants contain only non-heme iron, which has the attributes to maintain the body's correct balance of iron.[239]

227. PLANTS: Plants are predominately alkaline—animals acidic.[240]

228. PLANTS: Unsaturated linoleic and linolenic fatty acids are the only fats required in the human diet—they are only synthesized by plants.[241]

229. PLANTS: Cholesterol is not found in plants.[242]

230. PLANTS: The ratio of proteins, carbohydrates, and fats in the aggregate from the plant kingdom matches up with human needs.[243]

231. PLANTS: Animals synthesize none of the nutrients essential to humans. Essential nutrients obtained from animal-based foods all originated in the plant kingdom.[244]

232. MENOPAUSE: Dr. Michael Klaper, MD, has watched many of his patients who eat a strictly plant-based diet go through menopause largely unfazed. (Menopause is not a disease.)[245]

233. DIETING: Americans are fatter than they were in 1990, with 50 percent currently overweight and 1 in 5 obese.[246]

234. DIETING: Our digestive system monitors both calories and nutrients by way of chemoreceptors.[247] It wants us to get enough to eat as well as get the proper nutrients. The SICK diet provides 40 percent of its calories from fat, which is weak in nutrients, consequently the body calls to be fed more.[248]

235. DIETING: Carbohydrates speed metabolism and are part of the cueing mechanism that alerts the body to fullness.[249] The WELL diet contains twice the calories of carbohydrates as the SICK diet.[250]

236. DIETING: Pure vegetarians weigh 10 to 20 pounds lighter, have 30 percent less body fat, and are 18 percent less (20 to 2 percent) obese than those consuming a meat-based diet.[251]

237. STRENGTH / STAMINA: Tests in strength and endurance at Yale University showed vegetarians had twice the stamina of meat-eaters.[252]

238. STRENGTH / STAMINA: A study in Paris found that vegetarians had 2 to 3 times more stamina than meat-eaters, and took only one-fifth the time to recover.[253]

239. STRENGTH / STAMINA: A test conducted with grip meters resulted in vegetarians having double the score of meat-eaters.[254]

240. STRENGTH / STAMINA: A test showed that immediately after subjects were fed a vegetarian diet they pedaled stationary bicycles almost 3 times longer than subjects who were fed a meat and dairy diet.[255]

241. STRENGTH / STAMINA: Carbohydrates should make up the largest portion of the athlete's diet; high-CHO diets optimize muscle and liver glycogen stores and have been shown to optimize performance during prolonged, and moderate intensity exercise.[256]

242. STRENGTH / STAMINA: Athletes who are winning are loading up on carbohydrates.[257]

243. STRENGTH / STAMINA: A Japanese baseball team went from last place to champions after every member was required to switch to a vegetarian diet.[258]

244. ENVIRONMENT: Animal agriculture depletes the amount of energy equal to running our automobiles.[259]

245. ENVIRONMENT: The production of all plant-based foods gives us more energy output than energy input. The production of all animal-based foods gives us less energy output than energy input.[260]

246. ENVIRONMENT: Animal agriculture consumes 50 percent of our water.[261]

247. ENVIRONMENT: Producing meat causes 17 times the water pollution as producing pasta.[262]

248. ENVIRONMENT: Livestock grazing has depleted 50 percent of the earth's forests.[263]

249. ENVIRONMENT: Soil erosion is occurring at 7 to 13 times the sustainable rate because of livestock grazing.[264]

250. ENVIRONMENT: One-third of the earth's land surface has been desertified to some degree by livestock grazing.[265]

251. ENVIRONMENT: Oil spills and sewer mishaps pollute the ocean less than livestock agriculture.[266]

252. ENVIRONMENT: One-half of endangered species, according to the Endangered Species Act, is due to cattle ranching.[267]

253. ENVIRONMENT: The extinction of species, and subsequent ecological breakdown, threatens human extinction.[268]

254. ANIMALS: Observing birds take flight gave our forefathers the knowledge, and provided the inspiration, to build the airplane. The ideas and prototypes for navigation, jet propulsion, and hydraulics came from the animal kingdom.[269]

255. ANIMALS: The water spider gave us the idea for the first diving bell. Hedgehog spines inspired space-station design. Bees, ants, and beavers gave us insights into advanced construction methods.[270]

256. ANIMALS: We can improve ourselves by studying, rather than consuming, animals for their qualities of character: the chicken for loyalty, the cow for patience, and the pig for friendliness.[271]

257. ANIMALS: We rely on the estimated 1.75 million species on earth to maintain hydrological cycles, regulate climate, contribute to the process of soil formation and maturation, store and cycle essential nutrients, absorb and break down pollutants, and more.[272]

258. RELIGION: The first page of the Bible suggests we are to *eat* plants ("herb-bearing seed / fruit of the tree") and *care* for the animals ("dominion"), not the other way around.[273]

259. RELIGION: Would God have placed our means of survival—food—in runaway animals, in another mammal's milk, and under a hen?

260. RELIGION: To eat meat—cause the death of an animal—would appear to encroach on most fundamental religious principles.

261. GLOBAL HUNGER: It takes 16 pounds of grain to produce 1 pound of feedlot beef; grain that produces 15 times the calories and 8 times the protein of beef.[274]

262. GLOBAL HUNGER: Feed the grain to human beings, instead of cattle for beef, and 2 to 3 times the current population could be fed.[275]

263. GLOBAL HUNGER: It is estimated that 1.2 billion on the planet are underfed and malnourished, and conservatively 15 million people a year die of starvation.[276]

264. IS IT POSSIBLE? Is it possible given that heredity is the culprit in but 5 percent of the cases of degenerative diseases, that what is believed to be our "family history" is more often "family habits"— children eating the same foods as their parents for 18 years, then carrying those learned habits on into adulthood?[277]

265. IS IT POSSIBLE? Is it possible that our enjoyment of meat is not the body telling us it nutritionally requires it, but instead, a desire that grows out of associations, reinforcement, and cultural conditioning?

266. IS IT POSSIBLE? Is it possible that Americans assume that because the majority—95 percent—in this country eat meat, that it must be proper? Or is this just a snapshot in

time—a snapshot that if taken of smoking at one time would have yielded the same assumption.[278]

267. IS IT POSSIBLE? Is it possible that the practice of vegetarianism contributed to the successes of Leonardo da Vinci, Benjamin Franklin, William Shakespeare, Plato and Socrates, Albert Einstein, Isaac Newton, Albert Schweitzer, and Vincent Van Gogh?[279]

268. IS IT POSSIBLE? Is it possible the following two numbers— 2 and 68—tell us a lot about the SICK diet habit? Medicines can lower our chances of dying of an infectious disease down to 2 percent, but despite the fact that we spend $1.5 *trillion* in healthcare costs, $141 *billion* on prescription drugs, including cholesterol lowering drugs, insulin therapy, hypertension medicines, estrogen therapy, and $8.6 *billion* in chemotherapy drugs, they haven't made a dent in our chances of dying of a degenerative disease directly influenced by diet of 68 percent.[280]

269. IS IT POSSIBLE? Is it possible that the USDA Food Pyramid Guidelines, which include meat and dairy foods—given that a large study showed that following it made little or no difference in the subjects' health compared to the average American—is biased by economic and political interests rather than being an unbiased nutrition model?[281]

270. IS IT POSSIBLE? Is it possible that the economic power of the meat and dairy industries influences the political machine to produce favorable laws and regulations that furthers the legitimacy and positive perception of their foods?[282]

271. IS IT POSSIBLE? Is it possible that the $2 billion spent on food ads, and the $5 billion spent on pharmaceutical ads, distorts our perception of nutrition and health?[283]

272. IS IT POSSIBLE? Is it possible that the media has a hard time reporting unbiased nutritional information if advertis-

ing revenue from the retail and wholesale animal-based food industries pay a portion of their bills?[284]

273. IS IT POSSIBLE? Is it possible that the educational materials and subsidized food provided to schools by the wholesale suppliers of meat and dairy products, and the government, creates early and deep psychological and physiological impressions, making it difficult to ever gain objectivity?

274. LONGEVITY: According to the *Journal of the American Medical Association* half of all adults—100 million Americans—suffer from one or more chronic diseases including heart disease, cancer, arthritis, diabetes, and kidney disease.[285]

275. LONGEVITY: Today, according to the National Cancer Institute, 80 percent of cancers are due to factors—diet and smoking—that are within our control.[286]

276. LONGEVITY: According to *The Surgeon General's Report on Nutrition and Health*, 68 percent of deaths in the United States are caused by diet-related diseases.[287]

277. LONGEVITY: According to the World Health Organization, 4,289 people died of malnutrition in the United States in 1999. Given that 68 percent of Americans died as a result of diet-related diseases, then 1.6 million died of a different kind of malnutrition. Although unlikely, assuming that all 4,289 were due to vegetarianism, then for every 1 vegetarian that died from his or her diet, 380 meat-eaters died from theirs.[288]

278. LONGEVITY: The United States has sophisticated technology, a temperate climate, and ranks number one in per capita healthcare expenditures, yet according to the World Health Organization (WHO), the U.S. ranks 24th in the world in Healthy Life Expectancy (HALE).[289] Could a factor be that Americans account for 4 percent of the earth's population but consume 23 percent of the world's beef?[290]

279. LONGEVITY: According to program and damage theorists, humans have a genetically programmed maximum life expectancy of 120 years.[291]

280. LONGEVITY: The cultures with the highest animal flesh consumption, the Laplanders, Greenlanders, and Eskimos, have a life expectancy of about 30 years.[292]

281. LONGEVITY: The Kirgese of Eastern Russia, who at one time lived chiefly on meat, rarely survived past the age of 40.[293]

282. LONGEVITY: According to the Division of Vital Statistics, in 1999, U.S. life expectancy was 76.7 years.

283. LONGEVITY: Vegetarian Seventh-day Adventist (SDA) men, on average, live 8.9 years longer than the typical North American male, while SDA women, on average, live 7.5 years longer than the typical North American female.[294]

284. LONGEVITY: According to world health statistics an unusually large number of the Yucatan Indians, Russian Caucasians, East Indian Todas, and Pakistan Hunzas, have a life expectancy of 90 to 100 years. Their diets are vegetarian.[295]

CONCLUSION

WE ONLY EVOLVE

By way of engineering and evolution every species, including humans, has a specific natural diet. If we were on a jury, and were now asked to reach a verdict on what the natural human diet was, what would be that judgment?

On one hand the science of food and its interaction with the human body appears to be the most complex issue we have ever had to unravel. On the other hand it may be the simplest. We of course don't know everything there is to know and we will add to our knowledge as time goes on. But at what point do we say we know enough to make a decision about our diet? As we stated previously, studies can go on forever but we don't.

This book is like a rope. Each piece of information, study result, and logical inference is a single strand of the rope. Every strand added to the rope makes the rope stronger. It's possible, even likely, that strands will break along the way—a figure will be proved wrong or a contrary fact will arise—but will a 1,000-strand rope with a handful of broken stands cause the rope to break?

Americans may not be alike when it comes to the issue of diet, but down deep we are alike when it comes to the following: We want to do the right thing. We want to be on the side of truth. We want to be aligned with God/Nature. And we want to live long and healthy lives. We must ask ourselves then: Is there a particular diet choice that is compatible with these principles?

Americans, on the whole, have something else in common—compassion and consideration for the rights of others. Can we reconcile our meat-eating habits with these qualities when an omnivore diet impacts the lives of animals and other human beings? And can we justify the diet if it profoundly impacts our family and children by way of our diminished health or reduced lifespan?

Will our next meal be a hamburger or a veggie burger? When there is so much riding on the answer are we willing to gamble with the choice?

History shows that we ultimately evolve. That is the nature of things. We learn, we adapt, we move forward. We seldom go backward. More people are becoming vegetarians. More vegetarian products can now be found in supermarkets. More people understand vegetarianism. More people are eating vegetarian meals. More people are eating less meat.

At future social gatherings most likely it won't be the vegetarians defending their diet choice, providing a sideshow attraction—the ones having their diet labeled. The term, vegetarian, will become as passé as "nerd," a label once applied to a person who fooled around with computers, that we now call *sir*, as in, "Sir, could I get you a cup of coffee or polish your Mercedes?" The focus instead will switch to the meat-eating "fleshetarians." *They* will be the ones asked to defend their habit, looked on with curiosity, and apologized to for not having meat at the social gathering.

Because we only evolve and because vegetarianism is growing, we know where we are headed. Therefore, there is no reason not to make our way there now.

BIBLIOGRAPHY

1. Abelow, B.J., et al. "Cross-cultural Association Between Dietary Animal Protein and Hip Fracture: A Hypothesis." *California Tissue Int.* 50, (1992): 14-8.
2. Ackerson, A. "Easing the Pain of Endometriosis." *Vegetarian Times*, (Summer, 2001): 8-10.
3. *Advertising Age Yearbook.* Crain Books, Chicago, (1984): 36.
4. Agence France-Presse. Sept. 3, 1997.
5. Akers, Keith. *A Vegetarian Sourcebook.* Vegetarian Press, 1993.
6. Akers, Keith. "Spiritual Traditions and Vegetarianism." www.compassionatespirit.com/spiritual-trads-and-veg.htm.
7. Aldercreutz H, Hämäläinen E, Gorbach, S.L., et al. "Diet and Plasma Androgens in Postmenopausal Vegetarian and Omnivorous Women and Postmenopausal Women with Breast Cancer." *American Journal of Clinical Nutrition.* 49, (1989): 433-42.
8. Allaby, Michael, Floyd Allen. *Robots Behind the Plow,* Rodale, 1974.
9. Allen, L. "Protein-Induced Hypercalciuria: A Longer Term Study." *Am J. Clin Nutr.,* 32 (1979): 741.
10. "Alliance for the Prudent Use of Antibiotics Publishes its FAAIR Report." *Journal of Clinical Infectious Diseases* 34, Supplement 3, (June 1, 2002). www.healthsci.tufts.edu/apua/Ecology/faair.html.
11. Altschuler, S. "Dietary Protein and Calcium Loss: A Review." *Nutr. Res.* 2 (1982):193.
12. *Alternative Medicine Cancer Therapies That Have Worked for Thousands.* Rideout Publishing Company. www.bonuspages.com/cancercuresinformation/breast.htm.
13. Altman, Nathan. "Revising the Basic Four." *Vegetarian Times* (1977): 9-14.
14. Altman, Nathaniel. "The Spiritual Side of Vegetarianism." *Vegetarian Times* (Nov-Dec 1977): 36-38.
15. Altschul, Aaron. *Proteins: Their Chemistry and Politics.* Basic Books (1965): 264.
16. "AMA Attacks Vegetarian Diet." *Vegetarian Times* (May-June 1979): 8-10.
17. "AMA Opposes Warning on Tobacco, Association Comes Under Sharp Criticism as It Takes Position Shared by Industry Against Mandatory Labeling of Cigarettes as a Health Hazard." *Medical World News* (Apr. 10, 1964): 51-53.
18. "AMA View Decried in Tobacco Dispute." *New York Times* (Mar 20, 1964): 23.
19. "America's Animal Factories: How States Fail to Prevent Pollution from Livestock Waste." Natural Resources Defense Council. www.nrdc.org/water/pollution/factor/cons.asp#note16.
20. American Academy of Allergy, Asthma, and Immunology Reports.... (Cited in: Thimian, Bernie. "16 Reasons Why People Avoid Dairy Products." 9, (1997) www.veggiepower.ca/16reason.htm.
21. American Association for the Advancement of Science. "Contraceptive Methods Go Back To Basics." *Science* 266 (Dec 1994): 1480.

22. American Cancer Society Cancer Response System, No. 8308, printed May 24, 1995.
23. American Cancer Society. "Statistics." www.cancure.org/statistics.htm.
24. "American Dietetic Association Position Paper on Vegetarianism." *Journal of Amer. Dietetic Assoc.* 97; 11. November 1997.
25. American Egg Board and National Dairy Council. Harrisburg, PA. Know-about Publications, 1975. (Cited in Robbins, *Diet.* 126-127).
26. American Heart Association (AHA). December 3, 2001. www.viahealth.org/disease/cardiac/stats.htm
27. *American Heart Journal.* 1964.
28. *American Heritage Dictionary of the English Language. Third Edition* (1996) Houghton Mifflin Company.
29. *American Journal of Cardiology* 69 (1992): 440.
30. *American Journal of Clinical Nutrition* 60 (1994).
31. *American Journal of Clinical Nutrition* 63 (1996).
32. *American Journal of Clinical Nutrition* 71 (2000).
33. *American Journal of Clinical Nutrition* 72 (2000).
34. *American Journal of Clinical Nutrition,* March 1983.
35. *American Journal of Epidemiology* 133 (1991).
36. *American Journal of Epidemiology* 145 (1997).
37. *American Journal Respir Crit Care Med* 151;5 (1995): 1401-8.
38. American Lung Association. Executive Summary: The American Lung Association Asthma Survey. 1998.
39. American Meat Institute. *The Meat Sourcebook.* Chicago, (1960): 43.
40. American Medical Association Council on Scientific Affairs. "Dietary Fiber and Health." *JAMA* 262 (1989): 542-46.
41. Amory, C. *Animail.* Windmill Books, 1976.
42. Analyst, The. "Asthma." www.digitalnaturopath.com/cond/C117993.html.
43. Analyst, The. "Multiple Sclerosis." www.digitalnaturopath.com/cond/C63825.html.
44. Anand, C. "Effect of Protein Intake on Calcium Balance of Young Men Given 500 Mg. Calcium Daily." *J. Nutr.* 104 (1974): 695.
45. Anderson J. "Update on HCF diet results." *HCF Diabetes Research Foundation Newsletter* 4, June 1982.
46. Anderson, J. "Health Implications of Wheat Fiber." *American Journal of Clinical Nutrition* 41 (1985): 1103.
47. Anderson, J. "Plant Fiber: Carbohydrate and Lipoprotein." *American Journal of Clinical Nutrition* 32 (1979): 346.
48. Anderson, J.W, K. Ward. "High-Carbohydrate, High-Fiber Diets for Insulin Treated men with Diabetes Mellitus," *American Journal of Clinical Nutrition* 32 (Nov. 1979): 2312.
49. Anderson, J.W. "Plant Fiber and Blood Pressure." *Ann Intern Med* 98 Part 2 (1983): 842.
50. Anderson, R.M. et al., "Transmission Dynamics and Epidemiology of BSA in British Cattle." *Nature* (Aug. 29, 1996): 779.
51. "Animal Mothers." www.geocities.com/Petsburgh/Haven/6979/mothers.html.
52. "Animal Waste Pollution in America: An Emerging National Problem." Minority Staff of the U.S. Senate Committee on Agriculture, Nutrition, and Forestry, Washington, D.C. (December 1997): 5.
53. *Animal World of Albert Schweitzer, The.* Joy, C. ed. Beacon Press (1950): 114-115.
54. *Ann Allergy* 49;3 (1982): 146-51.
55. *Ann NY Acad. Science* 889 (1999): 107-19.
56. "Antioxidants, Zinc, and Age-Related Macular Degeneration." *Archives of Ophthalmology* 119; 10, October 2001.

57. *Arch. Neurol.* 23 (1970): 460.
58. *Archives of Biochemistry and Biophysics* 336 (1996).
59. Armstrong, B. "Diet and Reproductive Hormones: A Study of Vegetarian and Non-Vegetarian Postmenopausal Women." *JNCI* 67 (1981): 761.
60. Armstrong, B., P. Doll. "Environmental Factors and Cancer Incidence and Mortality in Different Countries, With Special Reference to Dietary Practices." *International Journal of Cancer* 15 (April 1975): 617.
61. Ascherio, A., et al. "Dietary Intake of Marine N-3 Fatty Acids, Fish Intake, and the Risk of Coronary Disease Among Men." *New England Journal of Medicine* 332 (1995): 977-982.
62. Atassi, M.Z. *Immunochemistry of Proteins.* Plenum Press, New York (1977): 391.
63. Attributed to author Nicols Fox. (Cited by W. Andrews. "A Great Big Juicy Lie." 1998 www.hometown.aol.com/willster1/rant1.html).
64. Attributed to Cattlemen's Beef Board. (Cited in "US Faces Possible Mad Cow Risks." 12-15-00, www.rense.com/general6/faces.htm).
65. Attributed to Congressman Berkley Bedell, 1993 (Cited in Robbins, *Reclaim*, 220-221).
66. Attributed to Dr. J. Dan Baggert. (Cited in Oski, *Don' t Drink Your Milk*).
67. Attributed to Iowa Senator, Tom Harkin. (Cited in "Factory Farm Alarm." www.earth-save.org/news/factfarm.htm).
68. Attwood, Charles R., M.D. "Children Thrive on a Vegetarian Diet." www.newcenturynu-trition.com/public_html/webzine/archives/children_thrive.shtml.
69. Attwood, Charles R., M.D. "Complete" Proteins? www.vegsource.com/attwood/com-plete_protein.htm.
70. Attwood, Charles R., M.D. "The Case Against Dairy." (Interview with *Vegetarian Times*).
71. *Audubon.* December 1999.
72. Ausebel, K. *Hoxsey: How Healing Becomes a Crime* (A Documentary). Realidad Productions, Santa Fe.
73. Autoimmune Diseases Online. www.autoimmune-disease.com.
74. Avazim, Pitum. "Pate de Fois Gras." Amutah le-Ma'an Hayot Meshek (Assoc. for Farm Animals), Rishon le-Ziyyon, 1997.
75. Avocado, Professor Antonio. "Meat From Diseased Animals Approved for Consumers." July 17, 2000. www.vegsource.com/talk/science/messages/1180.html.
76. Ayres, Ed. "Will We Still Eat Meat? Maybe Not, If We Wake Up To What the Mass Production of Animal Flesh Is Doing to our Health, and the Planet's" *Time.* Nov. 8, 1999.
77. Ayres, Ed. *God's Last Offer.* New York/London, Four Walls Eight Windows (1999): 102-3.
78. Barnard R, "Response of Non-Insulin-Dependent Diabetic Patients to an Intensive Program of Diet and Exercise." *Diabetes Care* 5 (1982): 370.
79. Barnard, Christian. "Medicine Negated," Robert Lanza, ed, *One World: The Health and the Survival of the Human Species in the 21st Century.* Santa Fe: Health Press (1996): 105.
80. Barnard, Dr. Neal. "Beliefs About Dietary Factors In Breast Cancer Among Women, 1991-1995," *Preventive Medicine* 26 (1997): 109-13.
81. Barnard, Dr. Neal. *Food for Life.* Three Rivers Press, 1993.
82. Barnard, Dr. Neal. *The Power of Your Plate.* Book Publishing Co., 1990.
83. Barsotti, G., E. Morelli, et al. "A Special Supplemented Vegan Diet For Nephritic Patients." *American Journal of Nephrol.* 11; 5 (1991): 380-5.

84. Barzel, U. "The Effect of Excessive Acid Feeding on Bone." *Calc Tiss. Res.* 4 (1969): 94.

85. Batt, S. "Cancer, Inc." *Sierra Magazine.* (Sep-Oct 1999): 36.

86. Batt, S. *Patient No More.* Charlottetown, PEI, Canada. Gynergy Books (1994): 86.

87. Battaglia and Mayrose. *Handbook of Livestock Management Techniques.* Burgess Publishers, 1981.

88. Bauston, Gene and Lorri. Farm Sanctuary. "Brutality: Main Crop of Factory Farms." Special Report to EarthSave. www.earthsave.org/news/ff.htm.

89. Bazant, Nicolle., Nutrition Counselor. The Center for Well-Being of the Washington Hospital. Wilfred R. Cameron Wellness Center, Washington, Pa. www.wrcameronwellness.org/welladmin/healthy.html.

90. Beasley, R. "Low Prevalence of Rheumatoid Arthritis in Chinese: Prevalence survey in a rural community." *Journal Rheumatol.* 10 (Supplement 10) (1983):11.

91. "Beef Industry Going Bust." *Chicago Tribune.* June 18, 1998.

92. Begley, Sharon. "The End of Antibiotics." *Newsweek* (March 28, 1994): 47-51.

93. Behar, Richard and Michael Kramer. "Something Smells Fowl." *Time* (Oct 17, 1994): 42. and Jane Brody "Personal Health." *New York Times,* Oct 5, 1994.

94. Beighton, P. "Rheumatoid Arthritis in a Rural South African Negro Population." *Ann Rheum Dis.* 34 (1975): 136.

95. Bell, G. *Textbook of Physiology and Biochemistry,* 4th ed., Williams and Wilkins, Balentine (1954): 167-170. Cited in Table, "Comparison of Milk of Different Species." Robbins, *Diet.* 175.

96. Bell, J.C., S.R. Palmer, and J.M. Payne. *The Zoonoses: Infections Transmitted from Animals to Man.* Edward Arnold, London, 1988.

97. Bender, B. *Farming in Prehistory, From Hunter-Gatherer to Food Producer.* London, John Baker, 1975.

98. Bergstrom, J., L. Hermansen, E. Hultman, and B. Saltin. "Diet, Muscle Glycogen, and Physical Performance." *Acta Physiol Scand* 71 (1967): 140-150.

99. Berk, Lauren Elaine. "The American Cancer Society: Preventing Cancer or Protecting Big Business?" www.impactpress.com/articles/augsep00/cancer8900.html.

100. Berry, Rynn. *Food for the Gods*, Pythagorean Publishers (1998): 368.

101. Bertron, Patricia R., R.D., Carol M. Coughlin, R.D., Suzanne Havala, M.S., R.D., L.D.N., F.A.D.A., Virginia Messina, M.P.H., R.D., Neal D. Barnard, M.D., Nutrition Panel. Physicians Committee for Responsible Medicine (PCRM), "Vegetarian Diets: Advantages for Children." www.pcrm.org/health/Info_on_Veg_Diets/vegetarian_kids.html.

102. Best, Steve. "The Coming Crisis: Environmental Disaster, the Global Meat Culture, and Your Health," www2.utep.edu/~best/crisis.htm.

103. Bethea, Louise H. M.D., "Asthma: Destroying the Myths." 1998. www.allergyasthma.com/archives/asthma07.html.

104. Beyene, Y. *From Menarche to Menopause: Reproductive Lives of Peasant Women in Two Cultures.* Albany: State University of New York Press, 1989.

105. "Biases in the USDA," Press release issued by Physicians Committee for Responsible Medicine. www.nutrition.about.com/library/weekly/aa100400a.htm.

106. Bible. King James Version. *Genesis 1:26.*

107. Bible. King James Version. John 2:13-17, Note: The Greek word emporion has been translated as "meat market." (Cited in *Food for the Gods*, Rynn Berry, Pythagorean, New York, 1998).

108. Bjerklie, S. "Who Really Has the World's Safest Meat Supply?" *Meat and Poultry.* (August 1995): 97.

109. Black, A.H.S., J.I. Thornby, J.E. Wolf Jr., et al. "Evidence that a Low-Fat Diet Reduces the Occurrence of Non-Melanoma Skin Cancer." *Int J Cancer* 62 (1995): 165–9.

110. Blanchet, Trisha. "Autoimmune Disorders." *Vegetarian Times* (July, 2001): 20.

111. Blankenhorn, D.H., et al. "Beneficial Effects of Combined Colestipol-Niacin Therapy On Coronary Atherosclerosis and Coronary Venous Bypass Grafts." *JAMA* 257 (1987): 3233.

112. Bleifuss, Joel. "Killer Beef." *In These Times* (May 31, 1993): 12-15.

113. Blythman, Joanna. *The Food We Eat*. Michael Joseph: 154.

114. Borgstrom, Georg, (Cited in Lappé, Frances Moore. *Diet For a Small Planet*. 1975 edition: 22).

115. Borgstrom, Georg. "Impacts on Demand for the Quality of Land and Water." Presentation to the 1981 annual meeting of the American Association for the Advancement of Science.

116. Borgstrom, Georg. *Harvesting the Earth*. New York, Abelard-Schuman (1973): 64-65.

117. *Boston Globe,* July 7, 1996. (Cited in SATYA, "Welfare for Carnivores." Rice, Pamela. Oct. 1996. www.montelis.com/satya/backissues/oct96/welfare.html).

118. Bovard, J. "Farm Bill Follies of 1990." Cato Institute, Policy Analysis. Washington (Jul. 12, 1990): 4.

119. Bovard, J. "The Farm Fiasco." Institute for Contemporary Studies, San Francisco, 1989.

120. Boyd, G. "The Pressure to Treat." *Lancet* 2 (1980): 1134.

121. *Br J Rheumatol* 24 (1985): 321.

122. Brenner, B.M., T.W. Meyer and T.H. Hostetter. "Dietary Protein Intake and the Progressive Nature of Kidney Disease." *New Eng. J. of Med.* 307 (1982): 652-59.

123. Breslau, N. and G.C. Davis. "Migraine, Physical Health, and Psychiatric Disorder: A Prospective Epidemiologic Study In Young Adults." *J Psychiatr Res.*, Apr-Jun 1993.

124. Breslow, N., C.W. Chan, and G. Dhom, et al. "Latent Carcinoma of Prostate at Autopsy In Seven Areas." *Int Journal of Cancer* 20 (1977): 680-88.

125. Brewer, J., C. Williams, and A. Patton. "The Influence of High Carbohydrate Dets on Endurance Running Performance." *Eur J Appl Physiol* 57 (1988): 698-706.

126. Brody, J. "Health Toll for a Meat Diet Costs Billions." *New York Times, Santa Cruz Sentinel.* (Nov. 22, 1995): C-4.

127. Brower, Michael and Warren Leon. *The Consumer's Guide to Effective Environmental Choices: Practical Advice from the Union of Concerned Scientists.* New York: Three Rivers Press, Crown Publishers, 1999.

128. Brown, Lynda. "The Shoppers Guide to Organic Food." Fourth State (1998): 47.

129. Brown, Nancy Marie. "Sick Ice Cream." Research/Penn State 15; 1 (March 1994) www.rps.psu.edu/mar94/ice.html.

130. Brown, Sherrod, Rep. Sponsor H.R.1771, (introduced 5/9/2001); Latest Major Action: 5/22/2001 Referred to House subcommittee. www.house.gov/sherrodbrown.

131. "Browning of America, The." *Newsweek* (Feb. 22, 1981): 26.

132. Brubaker, David. "Planet on a Plate: Water Usage." Ph.D. Director, GRACE Project, Johns Hopkins University School of Public Health. www.vivausa.org/guides/planeton-aplate1.htm#waterusage.

133. Brune, William. State Conservationist, Soil Conservation Service. Des Moines, Iowa. Testimony before Senate Committee on Agriculture and Forestry, July 6, 1976.

134. Brunzell, J. "Improved Glucose Tolerance With High Carbohydrate Feeding in Mild Diabetes." *New England Journal of Medicine* 283 (1971): 521.

135. Budyko M.I., O.A. Drozdov, and M.I. Yudin. "The Impact of Economic Activity on Climate." *Soviet Geography* 12;10 (Dec. 1971): 666.

136. Burkholder, J.M. "Pfiesteria Piscicida and Other Toxic Pfiesteria-Like Dinoflagellates." North Carolina State University, 1997; and Chesapeake Bay Foundation, "Facts About Pfiesteria Piscicida."

137. Burkholder, J.M., et al. "Insidious Effects of Toxic Estuarine Dinoflagellate on Fish Survival and Human Health." *Journal of Toxicology and Environmental Health* 46 (1995): 501-22; and Chesapeake Bay Foundation, "Facts About Pfiesteria Piscicida in the Chesapeake Bay."

138. Burkitt, D.P. *Don't Forget Fiber in Your Diet.* New York, Arco, 1984.

139. Burkitt, D.P. *The Lancet* 2 (1972):1408. (Cited in Table 9. "Mean Weight of Stools and Transit Time in Different Populations." Akers, *Sourcebook*: 79).

140. Burkitt, D.P., "Headed in the Wrong Direction." *Lancet* 2 (1984):1475.

141. Burkitt, D.P., C. Latto, S.B. Janvrin, and B. Mayou. "Pelvic Phleboliths: Epidemiology and Postulated Etiology." *New England Journal of Medicine* 296 (1977): 1387-90.

142. Burkitt, D.P., H.C. Trowell, eds "Appendicitis." *Refined Carbohydrate Foods and Disease.* New York: Academic Press, 1978.

143. Burmeister, R. M.D. Describes case of a 24-year-old woman. www.pcrm.org/health/Preventive_Medicine/endometriosis.html.

144. Burros, Marian. "Health Concerns Mounting Over Bacteria in Chicken." *New York Times* (October 20, 1997): A1.

145. Burslem, J., G. Schonfeld, M.A. Howald, and S.W .Weidman. "Plasma Apoprotein and Lipoprotein Levels in Vegetarians." *Metabolism* 27 (1978): 711-719.

146. Butzer, K.W., "Accelerated Soil Erosion: A Problem of Man-Made Relationships." *Perspectives on Environment*, ed. I.R. Manners and M.W. Mikesell, Washington D.C.: Association of American Geographers, 1974.

147. Cairns, John. "The Treatment of Diseases and the War Against Cancer." *Scientific American*, November 1985.

148. Cairns, S. "Circulating Immune Complexes Following Food: Delayed Clearance in Idiopathic Glomerulonephritis." *Journal of Clinical Lab Immunol* 6 (1981): 121.

149. Calculation : $123 billion divided by 60 million American families.

150. Calculation: 550,000 deaths/year times $100,000/avg. expense per cancer case.

151. Calkins, B., et al. "Diet, Nutrition Intake, and Metabolism in Populations...." *Am J. Clin Nutr* 1 (1982):131.

152. Cameron, Ron. "The Gospel of the Ebonites." From, *The Other Gospels: Non-Canonical Gospel Texts.* Westminster Press (1982): 106.

153. "Campaign Update." *Humane Farming Association* XV. (Spring 2000): 1.

154. Campbell, T. Colon. "Still More Bull!" Editorial. www.earthsave.org/morebull.htm.

155. Campbell, T.C., B. Parpia, and J. Chen. "Diet, Lifestyle, and the Etiology of Coronary Artery Disease." The Cornell China Study, *American Journal of Cardiology* 82 suppl. (1998): 18T-21T.

156. Cantarow, A.C., and B.S. Schepartz. *Biochemistry.* W.B. Saunders, Philadelphia (1957): 152.

157. Caplan, Geoff. "Food & Mood: You Are What You Eat!" www.ediets.com/news/article.cfm/article_id,6074.

158. Carlson, E., et al. "A Comparative Evaluation of Vegan, Vegetarian, and Omnivore Diets." *Journal of Plant Foods* 6 (1985): 89-100.

159. "Carotenoids and Antioxidant Vitamins." *Am J Clin Nutr* 62; 6 Suppl (Dec 1995): 1448S-1461S.

160. Carper, Jean. *Food—Your Miracle Medicine.* HarperCollins Publishers, Inc. 1993.

161. Carr, R. "Antibodies to Bovine Gamma Globulin (BGG) and the Occurrence of a BGG-Like Substance in Systemic Lupus Erythematosus Sera." *Journal Allergy Clin Immunol* 50 (1972): 18.

162. Carroll, K. "Experimental Evidence of Dietary Factors and Hormone Dependent Cancers." *Cancer Research* 35 (1975): 3374.
163. "Carrot and Stick." *Vegetarian Times* (Dec. 1996): 14.
164. Carson, R.. *Silent Spring.* Crest Books, 1962.
165. Carter, B.S., H.B. Carter, and J.T. Isaacs "Epidemiologic Evidence Regarding Predisposing Factors to Prostate Cancer." *Prostate* 16 (1990): 187-197.
166. Case, R. "Type A Behavior and Survival after Acute Myocardial Infarction." *New England Journal of Medicine* 312 (1985): 737.
167. "Cattle Lose Battle for Species Protection." Environmental News Network, Oct. 9, 1997.
168. Center for Public Integrity, The. "Safety Last: The Politics of E. Coli and Other Food-Borne Killers." 1998.
169. Centers for Disease Control and Prevention reported in 1996. www.earthsave.org/news/19980901.htm.
170. Centers for Disease Control and Prevention. "How Livestock Antibiotics Threaten our Health." www.sierraclub.org/factoryfarms/antibiotics/health.asp.
171. Centers for Disease Control and Prevention. "Prostate Cancer Conference Report: Future Directions for Public Health Practice and Research in Prostate Cancer." www.cdc.gov/cancer/prostate/prosfuture/session1.htm.
172. Centers for Disease Control and Prevention. "Prostate Cancer Screening: A Decision Guide." www.cdc.gov/cancer/prostate/decisionguide/longdesc.htm.
173. Centers for Disease Control and Prevention. Asthma Prevention Program for Environmental Health. Center for Disease Control Asthma Prevention Program for Environmental Health, Center for Disease Control and Prevention, 1999.
174. Centers for Disease Control and Prevention: National Vital Statistics Reports, Deaths: Final Data for 1999. 49; 8 (September 21, 2001): 6.
175. Centers for Disease Control and Prevention: National Vital Statistics Reports, Deaths: Final Data for 1999. 49; 8 (September 21, 2001): Table 9 and Author's spreadsheet.
176. Centers for Disease Control: Potential Infectious Etiologies of Crohn's Disease 1999. www.crohns.org/research/cdc.htm.
177. Chan, J.M. et al. "Plasma Insulin-Like Growth Factor-I and Prostate Cancer Risk: A Prospective Study." *Science* 279 (1998): 563-6.
178. Chang, N. "Rheumatic Diseases in China." *Journal of Rheumatology* (suppl 10) 10 (1983): 41.
179. "Changes in the Growth in Health Care Spending: Implications for Consumers." April 1997. www.lightparty.com/Health/HealthCare2.html.
180. "Chemical Levels and Delinquent Behavior." *Journal of the American Medical Association,* February 1996.
181. Cheng, Beverly. "Is the United States Doing Enough to Prevent BSE?" January 19, 2001. www.meatingplace.com.
182. Chiodini, R.J. "Historical Overview and Current Approaches In Determining a Mycobacterial Etiology of Crohn's Disease." Mulder, C.J.J. and Tytgat G.N.J., editors. *Is Crohn's Disease a Mycobacterial Disease?* Dordrecht. The Netherlands: Kluwer Academic Publishers (1992): 1-15.
183. Chivers, Wood, and Bilsborough. *Food Acquisition and Processing in Primates.* Plenum Press, 1982.
184. Chopra, J.G., A.L. Forbes, J.P. Habicht. "Protein in the U.S. Diet." *The Journal of the American Dietetic Association.* 72 (March 1978): 253.
185. Chow, B.F. "The B_{12} Vitamins." *Nutrition: A Comprehensive Treatise* 2, G.H. Beaton and W.E. McHenry, eds. New York: Academic Press, 1964.

186. Chung, Hua Nei Ko Tsa Chih. 34 (1995): 79. *Arthritis Rheum* 34 (1991): 248.

187. *Clin Chim Acta* 203 (1991): 153.

188. *Clinical Science* 79 (1990): 331.

189. Cloudsley-Thompson, J.L. "Recent Expansion of the Sahara." *International Journal of Environmental Studies* 2;1 (June 1971): 35.

190. Cohen, P. "Serum Insulin-Like Growth Factor-I and Prostate Cancer Risk: Interpreting the Evidence." *Journal of the National Cancer Institute* 90 (1998): 876-9.

191. Cohen, Rabbi Alfred S. "Vegetarianism from a Jewish Perspective." *The Journal of Halacha and Contemporary Society.* 1:2 (Fall 1981): 50.

192. Cohen, Robert. "Consumer Reports Attacks Milk Critics." www.liferesearchuniversal.com/milkreport.html.

193. Cohen, Robert. "Milk - The Deadly Poison." www.notmilk.com/gotzits.html.

194. Colditz, G., et al. "The Use of Estrogens and Progestins and the Risk of Breast Cancer in Post-Menopausal Women." *New England Journal of Medicine* 332 (June 1995): 1589-93.

195. Collens, W. "Atherosclerotic Disease: An Anthropologic Theory." *Medical Counterpoint* (Dec. 1969): 54.

196. Collinge, John, et al. "Spongiform Encephalopathies: A Common Agent for BSE and vCJD." *Nature.* (Oct. 2, 1997): 449-50.

197. Collins, W.S. and G.B Dobkin. "Phylogenetic Aspects of the Cause of Human Atherosclerotic Disease." *Circulation.* Supplement 11; 32 (October 1965): 7.

198. Colon Cancer Alliance. White House Proclamation: National Colorectal Cancer Awareness Month, 2000, Washington, Feb. 29.

199. "Common Additives." The Big Carrot. www.thebigcarrot.ca/additives.htm.

200. Comparing pandas food consumption with humans. www.pandas.si.edu.

201. Connor, W.E. and S. Connor. "The Key Role of Nutritional Factors In the Prevention of Coronary Heart Disease. *Preventive Medicine* 1 (1972): 49-83.

202. Conservation International. September 2000. www.ecocities.net/Article16.html.

203. Contento, Dr. Isabel. "The Amino Acid Composition and Biological Value of Some Proteins, FAO, Rome." Dept of Nutrition Education, Columbia University.

204. Conversation with Brother Ron Pickarski, OFM (Cited in *Food for the Gods*, Berry: 226-227).

205. Conversation with Dr. Robert Kole (Cited in *Food for the Gods*, Berry: 186).

206. Conversation with Roshi Philip Kapleau (Cited in *Food for the Gods*, Berry: 75).

207. Cooke, H.B.S. "Pleistocene Mammal Faunas of Africa, with Particular Reference to Southern Africa." *African Ecology and Human Evolution.* eds. F.C. Howell and F. Bourliere, Chicago: Aldine Pub. Co., 1963.

208. Cornellussen, P.E. "Pesticide Residues in the Total Diet." *Pesticides Monitoring Journal* 2 (1969):140-152.

209. Couet, C., P. Jan, and G. Debry. "Lactose and Cataracts In Humans: A Review." *Journal of American Coll Nutrition* 10 (1) (1991): 79-86.

210. Cox, F.V., M.J Meynell and W.T Cooke. "Interrelation of Vitamin B_{12} and Iron." Abstract, *The American Journal of Clinical Nutrition* 9 (1961): 375.

211. Cramer, D.W., B.L. Harlow et al. "Galactose Consumption and Metabolism in the Relation to the Risk of Ovarian Cancer." *Lancet* 2; 8654 (1989): 66-71.

212. "Crisis Confronts 1.3 Billion." *Washington Post*, September 25, 1989, A1.

213. "Crohn's disease." Debate in the House of Lords. Lord Greenway, 2000 Jun 19:Column 82. www.veganoutreach.org/health/gotmilk.html#Crohn'sDisease.

214. Cummings, J.H., M.J., Hill, E.S. Bone, W.J Branch, and D.J.A Jenkins. "The Effect of Meat Protein and Dietary Fiber on Colonic Function and Metabolism. II. Bacterial Metabolites in Feces and Urine." *The American Journal of Clinical Nutrition* 32 (Oct. 1979): 2094.

215. Cunningham, A.S. "Lymphomas and Animal Protein Consumption." *Lancet* 1976 (Nov. 27): 1184-86.

216. Curb, J. "Long-Term Surveillance for Adverse Effects of Anti-Hypertensive Drugs." *JAMA* 253 (1985): 3263.

217. Cypress, B. "Medication Therapy in Office Visits for Hypertension: National Ambulatory Medical Care Survey, 1980." National Center for Health Statistics Advanced Data, No. 80. July, 22, 1982.

218. D'Elia, Armando. International Vegetarian Union, 6th European Vegetarian Congress. Bussolengo, Italy. September 21 - 26, 1997. "Consequences of Meat Protein on Human Behavior."

219. Darnton, John. "Britain Ties Deadly Brain Disease to Cow Ailment." *New York Times*, March 21, 1996, A-1.

220. Das Gupta, C.R., J.B. Chatterjea and P. Basu. "Vitamin B_{12} in Nutritional Macrocytic Anemia." *The British Medical Journal* 2 (Sep. 19, 1953): 645.

221. Davis, Brenda, R.D, et al. "The Rebuttal to the Dairy Farmer's of Canada Response to *Becoming Vegetarian.*" Fall 1996.

222. Davis, Brenda, R.D. "Plant Sources of Calcium." www.veggiepower.ca/caltable.htm.

223. Davis, Gail. *Vegetarian Food For Thought.* New Sage Press, 1999.

224. Davis, J.C., R. Finn, and L.J. Hipkin. St. Hill CA. "Do Plasma Glycoproteins Induce Lymphocyte Hypo-responsiveness and Insulin Resistance?" *The Lancet*, (Dec. 23, 30 1978): 1343-1345.

225. "Deadly E. coli Bug May Affect Half the Cattle." *Meat Industry Insight.* Nov. 15, 1999.

226. Decarli, A., et al. "Macronutrients, Energy Intake, and Breast Cancer Risk...." *Epidemiology* 8 (1997): 425-28.

227. Demarco, C. *Take Charge of Your Body: Woman's Health Advisor.* Winlaw, BC, Canada: Well Women Press (1994): 209.

228. Denslow, Julie, and Christine Padoch. *People of the Tropical Rainforest.* Berkeley, CA. *University of California Press* (1988) 169.

229. Deriaz, O., G. Theriault, N. Lavallee, G. Fournier, A. Nadeau, and C. Bouchard. "Human Resting Expenditure in Relation to Dietary Potassium." *American Journal of Clinical Nutrition* 54 (1991): 628-34.

230. Derrick, F. "Kidney Stone Disease: Evaluation and Medical Management." *Postgraduate Medical Journal* 66 (1979): 115.

231. Descartes, R. *Discourse on the Method of Rightly Conducting the Reason, and Seeking Truth in the Science.* John Veitch, Chicago (1920) iv.

232. Dewaal, Caroline Smith, and Louise Light. "Meat, Greed, and Deadly Microbes." *Vegetarian Times* (Nov. 1996) 89.

233. Dewalt, Billie. "The Cattle are Eating the Forest." *Bulletin of Atomic Scientists.*

234. "Diagnosis and Treatment of Alzheimer's Disease and Other Related Disorders." *JAMA* October 22 / 29, 1997.

235. "Diet and Stress in Vascular Disease." *JAMA* 176; 9 (June 3, 1961): 806.

236. "Diet and Urinary Calculi." *Nutrition Review* 38 (1980): 74.

237. "Diet, Nutrition Intake, and Metabolism in populations...." *Am J. Clin Nutr* 1 (1982): 131.

238. "Dietary Factors and Epithelial Ovarian Cancer." *British Journal of Cancer* 59; 1 (1989): 92-96.

239. Dietary Management of Blood Pressure, Howard University Medical Center, 1994.

240. *Dietitians Guide to Vegetarian Diets, The.* Appendix A, 1996.

241. Diplock, A.T. "Antioxidant Nutrients and Disease Prevention: An Overview." *Am J. Clin Nutr* 53 (1991): 189S-93S.

242. "Do You Get Enough Vitamin B_{12}?" Loma Linda University. *Vegetarian Nutrition & Health Letter* 3:5 (May 2000): 3.

243. Donahoe, Alanna. "America's Royalty: Burger King & Dairy Queen." www.lclark.edu/~soan221/96/foodtrend.html.

244. Donaldson, M.S., N. Speight, and S. Loomis. "Fibromyalgia Syndrome Improved Using a Mostly Raw Vegetarian Diet: An Observational Study." Oct. 24, 2001. www.immunesupport.com/library/showarticle.cfm/ID/3159/.

245. Dubey, J.P. "Toxoplasmosis." *Journal of the American Veterinary Medical Association* 189; 2 (1986): 168.

246. Duncan, I. "Can the Psychologist Measure Stress?" *New Scientist.* Oct 18, 1973.

247. Durning, Alan B. "Fat of the Land." Worldwatch Institute Report 4; 3 (May-June 1991) 12.

248. Durning, Alan B., and Holly Brough. "Taking Stock: Animal Farming and the Environment." Worldwatch Paper 103 (July 1991) 29.

249. Dwyer, J.T., et al. "Mental Age and I.Q. of Predominately Vegetarian Children." *Journal of the American Diet Association* 76 (1980) 142-7.

250. Dye, Michael. "Cow's Milk is the Perfect Food for Baby Calves, but Many Doctors Agree: It is Not Healthy for Humans." www.alphaomegafood.com/cowmilk.htm.

251. "E.R. Doctor Prescribes New Farm Policy for Congress." September 21, 1999. www.pcrm.org/news/health990921.html.

252. *Earth Island Journal.* "Food Slander laws." Fall 1995.

253. "Eat for Strength." (As told to Nicholas Senn by the hospital surgeons in Africa.) www.sdarm.org/pamphlet/strength.htm.

254. *Edenite Creed for Life, The.* Edenite Society, The. (1979): 19.

255. Edgson, Vicki and Ian Marber. "Nutrition Prescriptions and Supplements to Support a Health Immune System." co-authors of *The Food Doctor.* Collins and Brown, 1999. www.wrcameronwellness.org/welladmin/healthy.html.

256. Edwards M, and M. Waldorf. *Reclaiming Birth: History and Heroines of American Childbirth Reform.* Trumansburg, NY, Crossing Press (1984): 153.

257. Ellis, F. et al. "Incidence of Osteoporosis in Vegetarians and Omnivores." *American Journal of Clinical Nutrition* 25 (1972): 255.

258. Ellis, F.R. and T.A.B. Sanders. "Angina and the Vegan Diet." *The American Heart Journal* 93; 6 (June 1977): 803.

259. Ellis, F.R., and V.E.M.E. Montegriffo. "Veganism: Clinical Findings and Investigations." *American Journal of Clinical Nutrition* 23; 3 (March 1970): 249.

260. *Encarta 98 Desk Encyclopedia* & 1996-97 Microsoft Corporation.

261. Encyclopedia Britannica, Chicago, X (1974): 470.

262. Encyclopedia.com eLibrary. www.encyclopedia.com/html/b1/butter.asp.

263. Endometriosis Association Reports, The. www.pcrm.org/health/Preventive_Medicine/endometriosis.html.

264. Endometriosis Definition. Physicians Committee for Responsible Medicine. www.pcrm.org/health/Preventive_Medicine/endometriosis.html.

265. Enos, W. "Pathogenesis of Coronary Disease in American Soldiers Killed in Korea." *JAMA* 158 (1955): 912.

266. "Environmental and Health Consequences of Animal Factories." Natural Resources Defense Council Report, 1998.

267. "Environmental Quality—1979." *The Tenth Annual Report of the Council on Environmental Quality.* Washington, D.C. Dec. 1979.

268. "EPA Decides Carcinogen is OK for Eggs and Chicken." *Vegetarian Times.* July 1984.

269. *Epidemiologic Review.* 1996.

270. Epstein, F. "The Treatment of Reversible Uremia." *Yale Journal of Biological Medicine* 27 (1954): 53.

271. Epstein, Samuel E, M.D. "American Cancer Society: The World's Wealthiest 'Nonprofit' Institution." *International Journal of Health Services* 29; 3 (1999).

272. Epstein, Samuel E, M.D. *The Politics of Cancer.* East Ridge Press (1998): 539.

273. Esko, Edward. *Crime and Diet: The Macrobiotic Approach.* Japan Publications, Tokyo and New York, 1987.

274. Esselstyn, Jr., M.D., "Updating a 12-year Experience with Arrest and Reversal Therapy for Coronary Heart Disease." *American Journal of Cardiology* 84 (1999): 339-41.

275. Esselstyn, Jr., M.D., and B. Caldwell. "In Cholesterol Lowering, Moderation Kills." *EarthSave Magazine*, Summer 2001.

276. *Essene Gospel of Peace, The.* Translation of early Aramaic Texts, recounting the words of Jesus.

277. "European Scientists Say U.S. Beef Unsafe." *Santa Cruz Sentinel.* May 4, 1999, A-8.

278. "European Union Says Beef Hormone Can Cause Cancer." *Meat Industry Insights.* May 3, 1999.

279. Evans, P. "Relation of Longstanding Blood Pressure Levels to Atherosclerosis." *Lancet* 1 (1965): 516.

280. Exton-Smith, A. "Physiological Aspects of Aging: Relationship to Nutrition." *American Journal of Clinical Nutrition* 25 (1972): 853-59.

281. "Eye Disease Case-Control Study Group: Antioxidant Status and Neovascular Age-Related Macular Degeneration." *Arch Ophthalmol* 111 (1993): 104-9.

282. "Factory Farm Alarm: Animal Factories are Laying Waste to our Environment and to Public Health." EarthSave International. www.earthsave.org/news/factfarm.htm.

283. "Factory Farming Facts: In Defense of Animals." www.idausa.org/facts/factoryfarm-facts.html.

284. "Factory Farming: Mechanized Madness." PETA. www.peta-online.org/mc/facts/fsveg3.html.

285. "Facts of Fishing, The." *New Internationalist*, July 2000, p. 19.

286. *FAO Production Yearbook* 37 (1984): 263.

287. "Farm Animal Fun Facts." and "Animal Profiles." (courtesy Karen Graham, The Humane Society of the United States).

288. "Fatigue," Neuroscientists at the University of Virginia report. www.trans4mind.com/nutrition/fatigue.html

289. Fauber, John. "Recalls of Tainted Meat This Year are the Highest Ever." *Milwaukee Journal Sentinel*, Aug, 18, 2000.

290. FDA's "Bad Bug Book." www.ncagr.com/cyber/kidswrld/foodsafe/badbug/badbug.htm.

291. "Feeding The World - Seas Lose Bounty To Overfishing." *Philadelphia Inquirer.* Nov 15, 1996.

292. *Feedstuffs.* July 3, 1995.

293. Ferrer, J. "Milk of Dairy Cows Frequently Contains a Leukemogenic Virus." *Science* 213 (1981): 1014.

294. Feskanich, D., W.C. Willett, M.J. Stampfer, and G.A. Colditz. "Milk, Dietary Calcium, and Bone Fractures in Women: A 12-Year Prospective Study." *Am J Publ Health* 87 (1997): 992-7.

295. Fisher, Irving. "The Influence of Flesh-Eating on Endurance." *Yale Medical Journal* 13; 5 (1907): 205-221.

296. Fisher, Jeffery. *The Plague Makers*. New York: Simon and Schuster, (1994): 12.

297. Fisher, M., et al "The Effect of Vegetarian Diets on Plasma Lipid and Platelet Levels." *Archives of Internal Medicine* 146 (1986): 1193-7

298. Fitzgerald, B. *The Fitzgerald Report: A Report to the Senate Interstate Commerce Committee on the Need for Investigation of Cancer Research Organizations.* Congressional Record, Aug. 3, 1953.

299. Flynn, Meghan. M.S., R.D. "Colon Cancer: Diet May Hold Key to Prevention." *Environmental Nutrition*, July 1995.

300. Food and Agricultural Organization of the United Nations, *Production Yearbook* 29, 1975.

301. Food and Agricultural Organization of the United Nations. *FAO Production Yearbook* 1986. Rome, 1987. (Cited in Harris, *Scientific Basis*, Charts p. 52-63)

302. Food and Agricultural Organization, World health Organization Expert Group "Protein Requirements." United Nations Conf., Rome, 1965.

303. Food and Nutrition Board. *Recommended Daily Allowances*. Washington, DC, National Academy of Sciences.

304. Food Balance Sheets, 1979-1981 average. Food and Agriculture Organization of the United Nations. Rome, 1984.

305. Food Heritage, *Composition and Facts about Foods*, Mokelumme Hill, Cal. Health Research, 1971.

306. Food Safety and Inspection Service, United States Department of Agriculture, Consumer Information The Food Safety Educator 4; 1 (1999).

307. Food Safety Network, The. "Who's at Risk: Young Children." www.foodbiotech.org/pathogens/whorisk.htm#young.

308. Foster, G.D., T.A. Walden, I.D. Feurer. "Controlled Trial of the Metabolic Effects of a Very-Low-Calorie Diet: Short and Long Term Effects," *American Journal of Clinical Nutrition* 51 (1990): 167-72.

309. Fox, M. *Returning to Eden*. Viking Press, (1980): 3.

310. Fox, M. *Understanding Your Cat*. Coward, McGann & Geoghegan, New York (1974): 78.

311. Fox, Nicols. *Spoiled: The Dangerous Truth About a Food Chain Gone Haywire*. Basic Books, 1997.

312. Franklin Institute Online, The. "Tubular Circulation." www.sln.fi.edu/biosci/vessels/vessels.html.

313. Freeland-Graves, J., et al. "Zinc Status of Vegetarians." *Journal of American Dietetic Association* 77 (1980): S655-61.

314. Freeman, W.H. *Human Nutrition*. San Francisco (1978): 149.

315. Frei, B. "Ascorbic Acid Protects Lipids in Human Plasma and Low-Density Lipoprotein Against Oxidative Damage." *Am J. Clin Nutr* 54 (1991): 1113S-18S.

316. Freis, E. "Salt, Volume and the Prevention of Hypertension." *Circulation* 53 (1976): 589.

317. Frenkel, J.K. "Toxoplasmosis In Human Beings." *JAMA* 196 (1990): 240-8.

318. Friedland, R.P., T. Fritsch, K.A. Smyth, et al. "Patients With Alzheimer's Disease Have Reduced Activities in Mid-Life Compared With Healthy Control-Group Members." *Proc Natl Acad Science* 98 (2001): 3440-5.

319. Friend, P. "Dietary Restrictions Early and Late: Effects on the Nephropathy of the NZBxNZW Mouse." *Lab Invest* 38 (1978): 629.

320. Frommer, D. "Changing Age Of The Menopause." *Br Med Journal* 2 (1964): 349.

321. Frost and Sullivan Market Intelligence. Cited in Ralph Moss, *Questioning Chemotherapy*. New York, Equinox Press (1975): 75.
322. Fuhrman, Dr. Joel. "Autoimmune Disease Equals Digestive Dysfunction." *Fasting and Eating for Health*, 146-149.
323. Fukuzaki, H., R. Okamoto, and T. Matsuo. "Studies on Pathophysiological Effects of Postalimentary Lipemia in Patients With Ischemic Heart Disease." *Jpn Circ J.* 39; 3 (1975): 317-24.
324. Fulmer, Melinda. "Study: System for Seafood Safety Flawed," *LA Times*, Feb 14, 2001. (cited in Rice, *101 Reasons Why I'm a Vegetarian*, 2001, Fifth Edition).
325. Ganong, W.F. *Review of Medical Physiology*, Appleton and Lange, Norwalk (1991): 421.
326. Gardner, Gary, and Brian Halweil, "Underfed and Overfed: The Global Epidemic of Malnutrition." Worldwatch Paper 150, Worldwatch Institute, 2000.
327. Garland, C.F., et al. *Int J Oncol* 14; 5 (May 1999): 979-85.
328. Garland, D. "Role of Site-Specific, Metal-Catalyzed Oxidation in Lens Aging and Cataract: A Hypothesis." *Exp Eye Res* 50 (1990): 677-82.
329. Geil, P.B. and J.W. Anderson. "Nutrition and Health Implications of Dry Beans: A Review." *J. Am. Coll. Nutr.* 13 (1994): 549-558.
330. General Accounting Office report August 1992. "FDA Strategy Needed to Address Drug Residues in Milk." Cited in letter from Michael Hansen, Consumers Union, to Jerry Mande, Office of the Commissioner, FDA. May 24, 1993.
331. General Accounting Office. *Phosphates: A Case Study of a Valuable Depleting Mineral in America*, Report to Congress by the Comptroller General of the United States, EMD-80-21 (Nov. 30, 1979): 1.
332. Gerras, Charles. *The Complete Book of Vitamins*. Emmaus, PA: Rodale Press, 1977. Cited in Vegan 2000: Lifestyle of the Millennium. www.library.thinkquest.org/C004833/nutrients_en.shtml.
333. Getzendanner, Memorandum Opinion and Order: p. 5.
334. Gilda Radner Familial Ovarian Cancer Registry, The. "Risk Factors." www.ovarian-cancer.com/riskfactors.shtml.
335. Gilda Radner Familial Ovarian Cancer Registry, The. "Statistics." www.ovariancancer.com/statistics.shtml.
336. Gillespie, James R. *Modern Livestock and Poultry Production*. San Francisco, Delmar, 1997.
337. Gleason, S. "Menopause: It's Not a Disease." *Good Medicine*, Spring (1994): 9.
338. Global Biodiversity Assessment. UNEP. *Cambridge University Press*, 1995.
339. Glynn, K., et al. "Emergence of Multidrug-Resistant Salmonella Enterica Serotype Typhimurium DT104 Infections in the United States." *New England Journal of Medicine* 338 (1998): 1333-8.
340. Goff, Professor Douglas, Ph.D., "History of Ice Cream." Department of Food Science, University of Guelph. Guelph, Ontario. www.foodsci.uoguelph.ca/dairyedu/findsci.html.
341. Goldin, B. "Effect Of Diet on Excretion of Estrogens In Pre- and Postmenopausal Women." *Cancer Res.* 41 (1981): 3771.
342. Goldin, B.R., H. Adlercreutz, and S.L. Gorbach, et al. "Estrogen Excretion Patterns and Plasma Levels in Vegetarian and Omnivorous Women." *New England Journal of Medicine* 307 (1982): 1542-47.
343. Goldman, B.A. *The Truth about Where You Live*. New York: Random House, 1991.
344. Goldman, L. "The Decline in Ischemic Heart Disease Mortality Rates. An Analysis of Comparative Effects of Medical Interventions and Changes in Lifestyle." *Ann Intern Med* 101 (1984): 825.

345. Gonzales, Nicholas. *One Man Alone: An Investigation of Nutrition, Cancer, and William Donald Kelly*, unpublished Manuscript, 1987; cited in Richard Walters, *Options: The Alternative Cancer Book*, Garden City Park, NY: Avery, 1993.

346. *Good Medicine*, Autumn (1999): 7.

347. Goodhart, R. and M. Shils. *Modern Nutrition in Health and Disease."* Philadelphia: Lea and Febiger (1980): 91.

348. Goodman, D.C., T.A. Stukel, and Chiang-hua Chiang. "Trends in Pediatric Asthma Hospitalization Rates: Regional and Socioeconomic Differences." *Pediatrics* 101; 2 (Feb 1998): 208.

349. Goodwin and Mercer. *Introduction to Plant Biochemistry*. Pergamon Press, Oxford (1983): 118.

350. Gorbach, S. "Estrogens, Breast Cancer, and Intestinal Flora." *Rev. Infect Dis 6*; 1 (1984): S85.

351. Gorman, Christine. "The Low-Pressure Diet," *Time*. April 28, 1997.

352. Gover, Mike. "Study Shows Environmental Risk of Animal Waste." *Associated Press*, Dec. 28, 1997.

353. Government Accountability Project. "Fighting Filth on the Floor: A Matter of Life and Death for America's Families." (Nov. 9, 1995): 4.

354. Graboys, T. "Results of a Second-Opinion Trail Among Patients Recommended for Coronary Angioplasty." *Journal of the American Medical Association* 268 (1992): 2537.

355. Grady, D. "Scientists See Higher Use of Antibiotics on Farms." *New York Times*, January 28, 2001.

356. Gray, R. *The Colon Health Handbook*. Emerald Publishing Co., 1991.

357. Green, Patrice, M.D., and Allison Lee Solin. Commentary. "Deadly Dieting: The Truth behind the Atkins Plan." www.pcrm.org/health/Commentary/commentary9912.html.

358. Greene, Alan, M.D., F.A.A.P., and Khanh-Van Le-Bucklin, M.D. September 2001. www.drgreene.com/21_121.html.

359. Greene, Winston W, D.C., "Scientific Paper Abstracts on Vitamins." www.dcnutrition.com/vitamins/vitamin-abstracts.shtml.

360. Greenwood, S. *Menopause Naturally*. CA, Volcano Press (1992): 114.

361. Greer, G. *The Change: Women, Aging, and Menopause*. New York, Fawcett Columbine (1991): 118.

362. Griffiths, M., W.R. Sistrom, and R.Y. Stainer. "The Biology of Photo Synthetic Bacterium Which Lacks Colored Carotenoids." *Journal Cellular Comp. Physiology* 48 (1956): 473-515.

363. "Group's Surprising Beef with Meat Industry: Study Ranks Production of Beef, Poultry, and Pork as Second to Automobiles in Ecological Cost." *San Francisco Chronicle*, April 27, 1999.

364. "Growth Promoting Hormones Pose Health Risk to Consumers, Confirms EU Scientific Committee." The European Commission. Press Release: IP/02/604 Brussels. 23 April 2002. www.europa.eu.int/comm/food/fs/him/him_index_en.html.

365. Gruberg, E. and S. Raymond, *Beyond Cholesterol*. New York, St Martin's Press, 1981.

366. Guay, A.T., S. Bansal, and G.J. Heatley. "Effect of Raising Endogenous Testosterone Levels in Impotent Men With Secondary Hypogonadism: Double Blind Placebo-Controlled Trial With Clomiphene Citrate." *Journal of Clinical Endocrinology and Metabolism* 80; 12 (Dec 1995): 3546-3552.

367. Haapapuro, Eric R., et al. "Animal Waste Used as Livestock Feed: Dangers to Human Health." PCRM Review, 1997.

368. Haas, Elson M. M.D. *Staying Healthy with Nutrition: The Complete Guide to Diet and Nutritional Medicine*. Celestial Arts.

369. Haenszel, W. "Studies of Japanese Migrants, I. Mortality from Cancer...." *Journal of the National Cancer Institute* 40 (1968): 43.

370. Halpern, G.M. "Alimentary Allergy." *Journal of Asthma* 20; 4 (1993): 258.

371. Halweil, Brian. "United States Leads World Meat Stampede." Worldwatch Issues Paper. July 2, 1998.

372. Hamilton, J.B. "Male Hormone Stimulation Is Prerequisite and an Incitant In Common Baldness." *Am J. Anat* 71 (1942): 451-80.

373. Hammerly, Milt, M.D. "Take Charge & Let Go." www.healingpartner.com/articles/generalpublic/takecharge.html.

374. Hankinson, S.E., et al. "Circulating Concentrations of Insulin-Like Growth Factor-I and Risk of Breast Cancer." *Lancet* 351 (1998): 1393-6.

375. Hardinge, M. and F. State. "Nutritional Studies of Vegetarians. 1. Nutritional, Physical, and Laboratory Studies." *The American Journal of Clinical Nutrition* 2; 2 (Mar-Apr. 1954): 73.

376. Harris, J.P. "Autoimmunity of the Inner Ear." *Am J Otol* 10 (1989): 193-195.

377. Harris, R. *A Sacred Trust*. New York, New American Library (1966): 159.

378. Harris, S. "Organochlorine Contamination of Breast Milk." *Environmental Defense Fund*. Washington, D.C., Nov. 7, 1979.

379. Harris, William, M.D. The *Scientific Basis of Vegetarianism*. Hawaii Health Publishers, 1995.

380. Harty, S. *Hucksters in the Classroom*. Center for the Study of Responsive Law (1979): 23.

381. Harvard School of Public Health: Nurses' Health Study. *Journal of the National Cancer Institute* 91 (1999): 1751.

382. Hatherill, Dr. J. Robert, *Eat to Beat Cancer*. Renaissance Books, 1998.

383. Hatherill, Dr. J. Robert, Environmental Studies Department, University of California, Santa Barbara. "Vegetarianism Mental Benefits: The Correlation Between People Who Eat Meat and Violence." www.celestialhealing.net/mentalveg2.htm.

384. Haught, S.J. *Has Dr. Max Gerson a True Cancer Cure?* London Press 1962. Reprint ed., Canoga Park, California. Major Books, 1979.

385. Hauseman, P. *Jack Sprat's Legacy – The Science and Politics of Fat and Cholesterol*. Richard Mauk Publishers, NY, 1981.

386. Havala, Susan, M.S., R.D., F.A.D.A. "USDA School Meals Initiative for Healthy Children." *Vegetarian Journal*. Nov-Dec 1994.

387. Havala, Susan. *Being Vegetarian*, The American Dietetic Association, Chronimed Publishing (1996): 18.

388. Havala, Suzanne, M.S., R.D., "A Senior's Guide to Good Nutrition." Vegetarian Resource Group, 1998. www.vrg.org/nutrition/seniors.htm.

389. "He's Smarter Than You Think." *The Electronic Telegraph*. London, England. May 31, 1997.

390. Health Help: Digestive Problems and Conditions. www.innercleanse.com/healthinfoandnotes/digestiveproblems.html#diverticulitis.

391. Health Professionals Follow-up Study. Reported in "Dairy Products Linked to Prostate Cancer." *Associated Press*, April 5, 2000.

392. Health Research. *The Gospel of the Holy Twelve*. (1974): 8.

393. *Healthy Beginnings: A How To Guise to a Plant-Based Diet*. 2000.

394. "Healthy Food For Back to School." September 1998. EarthSave Press Release. www.earthsave.org/news/19980901.htm.

395. Healthy Life Expectancy (HALE) and Health Systems Performance Assessment. Health Systems Performance World Health Report 2000. World Health Organization. www3.who.int/whosis/menu.cfm.

396. Healthy Life Expectancy (HALE) and Health Systems Performance Assessment. World Health Organization. www3.who.int/whosis/menu.cfm.

397. Hegsted, D. "Minimum Protein Requirements of Adults." *American Journal of Clinical Nutrition* 21 (1968): 3520.

398. Hegsted, M. "Urinary Calcium and Calcium Balance In Young Men as Affected by the Level of Protein and Phosphorus Intake." *J. Nutr* 111 (1981): 553.

399. Heichelheim, FM. "Effects of Classical Antiquity on the Land." *Man's Role in the Changing Face of the Earth.*

400. Helsinki University Central Hospital Study. www.pponline.co.uk/encyc/0020.htm.

401. Hepner, G. "Altered Bile Acid Metabolism in Vegetarians." *American Journal of Digestive Diseases* 20 (1975): 935.

402. Hergenrather J., G. Hlady, B. Wallace, E. Savage. "Pollutants In Breast Milk of Vegetarians." *Lancet* 304 (1981): 792.

403. Hermon-Taylor, J. Presentation to Medical Journalists Association at the Royal Society of Medicine, London, January 24, 2000 (Cited in "Microorganisms In Milk Cause Crohn's Disease." *Environment News Service.* London, Jan 27, 2000.

404. Hertzler, A., and H. Anderson. "Food Guides in the United States," *Journal of Am Diet Assoc.* 64 (1974): 19-28.

405. Hibbeln J. R., J. Umhau, C. M. Linnoila, D. T. George, P. W. Ragan, S. E. Shoaf, M. R. Vaughhan, R. Rawlings, and N. Salem Jr. "A Replication Study of Violent and Nonviolent Subjects: Cerebrospinal Fluid Metabolites of Serotonin and Dopamine are Predicted by Plasma Essential Fatty Acids." *Biological Psychiatry* 44; 4 (August 15, 1998): 243-249.

406. Hill, M. "The Effect of Some Factors on the Fecal Concentration of...." *Journal of Pathology* 104 (1971): 239.

407. Hill, P. "Environmental Factors and Breast and Prostatic Cancer." *Cancer Res* 41 (1981): 3817.

408. Hindhede, M. "The Effect of Food Restrictions During War on Mortality in Copenhagen." *Journal of the American Medical Association,* 74; 6 (1920): 381.

409. Hirayama, T. "Epidemiology of Breast Cancer With Special Reference to the Role In Diet." *Preventative Medicine* 7 (1978): 173-95.

410. Hix, T. "Meat and Potatoes: Vegetarian Decisions in a Meat-Eating Society." 91; 9 (November 4, 1999). www.berry.edu/stulife/carrier/backissues/fall1999/11-4/life1.html.

411. Hoffer, A. and L. Pauling. "Hardin Jones Biostatistical Analysis of Mortality Data for Cohorts of Cancer Patients...." *Journal of Orthomolecular Medicine* 5 (1990): 143-54.

412. Hoffman, M. *The World Almanac and Book of Facts.* Pharos Books, New York (1992): 319.

413. Hoffman, Ronald, M.D. "Ulcers." *Conscious Choice.* November 1999. www.con-sciouschoice.com/holisticmd/hmd1211.html.

414. Holl, Adolph. *The Last Christian: A Biography of Francis of Assisi.* New York, Doubleday (1980): 209.

415. Holloway, M. "An Epidemic Ignored: Endometriosis Linked to Dioxin and Immunologic Dysfunction." *Sci Am* 270 (1994): 24-6.

416. Holman, R. "The Natural History of Atherosclerosis: The Early Aortic Lesions as Seen in New Orleans in the Middle of the 20th Century." *American Journal of Pathology* 34 (1958): 209.

417. Holmberg, Dr. Scott. "Hidden Danger in our Food," Channel 7 News (ABC). Nov. 7, 1984.

418. Homer, D. "The Growing Epidemic of Disease."
     www.innerlifewellness.com/disease.html.
419. "Hormonal Time Bomb?" *Time*. Aug. 2, 1971.
420. Houston, D.K., et al. "Age-Related Hearing Loss, Vitamin B_{12}, and Folate In Elderly
     Women." *Amer J Clin Nutr* 69 (1999): 564-71.
421. "How the Egg Industry Changed During the Last 20 Years." *Poultry Digest* (Jul
     1998): 232.
422. Hudson, N. *Soil Conservation*. London: B.T. Batsford, 1971.
423. Hudson, W.H. *The Book of a Naturalist*. George Duran Publishers (1919): 295-302
424. Hughes, G. "Molecular and Cellular Biology of the Inner Ear: The Next Frontier." *Am. J.
     Otol.* 10 (1989): 28-35.
425. Humphries, Bronwen. "History of Vegetarianism: The Diet of Early Humans."
     International Vegetarian Union. www.ivu.org/history/early/ancestors.html. (Hamilton
     and Busse. 1978.)
426. Huntington, G.S. *The Anatomy of Human Peritoneum and Abdominal Cavity*. Lea
     Brothers (1903): 189-199.
427. Hur, Robin, and Dr. David Fields. "America's Appetite for Meat is Ruining our Water."
     Vegetarian Times. Jan. 1985.
428. Hur, Robin, and Dr. David Fields. "Are High-Fat Diets Killing Our Forests?" *Vegetarian
     Times*. Feb. 1984.
429. Hur, Robin, and Dr. David Fields. "How Meat Robs America of its Energy." *Vegetarian
     Times*. April 1985.
430. Hur, Robin. "Food Reform: Our Desperate Need" Austin, Texas: Heidelberg Publishers.
     (1975): 151.
431. Hur, Robin. "Six Inches from Starvation; How and Why America's Topsoil is
     Disappearing." *Vegetarian Times*. (March 1985): 45-47.
432. Hur, Robin. "The Energy Cost of the Agri-food System." Unpublished manuscript,
     1981.
433. Hyde, R.M. and R.A. Patnode. *Immunology*. John Wiley and Sons, New York (1987):
     28.
434. "Impact of Market Concentration on Rising Food Prices." Subcommittee hearing on
     Antitrust. 96th Congress, April 1979. U.S. Government Printing Office: 13.
435. Imperato, P. and G. Mitchell. *Acceptable Risks*. Viking, New York (1985): 65-66.
436. Inaba, M. "Can Human Hair Grow Again?" Tokyo, Japan. Azabu Shokan, Inc., 1985.
437. "Induced Termination of Pregnancy Before and After Roe vs. Wade: Trends in
     Mortality and Morbidity of Women." American Medical Association Council on
     Scientific Affairs, Report H.
438. "Industry Forum." *Meat and Poultry*. (Mar. 1998). Per Delmer Jones, President, U.S.
     Meat Inspection Union.
439. Ingram, D.M., F.C. Bennett, D. Wilcox, N. de Klerk. "Effect of Low-Fat Diet on Female
     Sex Hormone Levels." *Journal of National Cancer Institute* 79; 6 (1987): 1225-29.
440. Institute for Planetary Renewal. "There Was No Slaughterhouse in the Garden of
     Eden." (Cited in Rice, *101 Reasons Why I'm a Vegetarian*, 2001, Fifth Edition).
441. *International Journal Vit Nutr Res* 69 (1999): 412.
442. "Invisible Menace: The, Agricultural Pollution Run-off in Our Nation's Streams." *Trout
     Unlimited*, Feb 1994.
443. Ioteyko, J., et al. *Enquete Scientifique Sur Les Vegetarians De Bruxelles*. Henri
     Lamertin, Brussels: 50.
444. Ippoliti, A. "The Effects of Various Forms of Milk on Gastric Acid Secretions, Studies
     In Patients With Duodenal Ulcers." *Annals of Internal Medicine* 84 (1976): 286.

445. "Iron Balancing Act, The." Loma Linda University. *Vegetarian Nutrition & Health Letter* 4:7 (Aug. 2001): 1.

446. "Iron Content of Foods." *Nutritive Value of Foods*. Consumer and Food Economics Institute, U.S. Dept of Agriculture, 1977.

447. "Is our Fish Fit to Eat?" *Consumer Reports*. (Feb 1992): 103-104.

448. Jacobs, D.R. Jr., L. Marquart, J. Salvin, and L.H. Kushi. "Whole-Grain Intake and Cancer: An Expanded Review and Meta-Analysis." *Nutr Cancer* 30 (1998): 85–96.

449. Jacobs, Lynn. *Waste of the West: Public Lands Ranching*. Tucson, Ariz.: Lynn Jacobs, 1991.

450. Jacobson, M.F., *The Complete Eater's Digest and Nutrition Scoreboard*. Anchor Press, New York (1985): 119.

451. Jacques, P.F. and L.T. Chylack Jr. "Epidemiologic Evidence of a Role For the Antioxidant Vitamins and Carotenoids In Cataract Prevention." *American Journal of Clinical Nutrition* 53 (1991): 352S-5S.

452. Janelle, K. et al., "Nutrient Intakes and Eating Behavior Scores of Vegetarian and Non-vegetarian Women." *Journal of American Dietetic Association* 95 (1995):180-5.

453. Johnson, N. "Effect of Level of Protein Intake on Urinary and Fecal Calcium and Calcium Retention of Young Adult Males." *J. Nutr.* 100 (1970): 1425.

454. Johnson, W.M., "What Has Been Happening to Land In America and What are the Projections." *Journal of Animal Science* 45; 6 (December 1977): 1469.

455. *Journal of Asthma* 22; 44 (1985): 13.

456. *Journal of Neuroepidemiology* 12 (1993): 28-36.

457. *Journal of Neurology* 57 (2000): 1439-1443.

458. *Journal of Nutrition* 129 (1999): 399.

459. *Journal of Nutrition* 74 (1961): 461.

460. *Journal of Photochem Photobiol* B 41 (Nov. 1997): 1-2,1-10.

461. *Journal of the American Medical Association* (June 29, 1979). One example.

462. *Journal of the American Medical Association* 164 (1972): 172.

463. *Journal of the American Medical Association* 276 (Nov 13, 1996): 1473.

464. *Journal of the American Medical Association* 282; 16 (1999): 1519-1522.

465. *Journal of the American Medical Association*. www.laleva.cc/petizione/english/ron-law_eng.html.

466. *Journal of the American Veterinary Medical Association*. (Stepaniak p. 38)

467. *Journal of the National Cancer Institute* (Sept 21, 1994).

468. *Journal of the National Cancer Institute* 88 (1996): 32-7.

469. *Journal of the National Cancer Institute* 88 (1996): 340-8.

470. *Journal of the National Cancer Institute* 88 (1996): 650. (*Nutrition Action Health Letter*, Oct 1996: 3).

471. *Journal of the National Cancer Institute* 92 (2000): 61-8. ("Vegetables Lower Prostate Cancer Risk." Loma Linda University. *Vegetarian Nutrition and Health Letter*. March, 2000.)

472. *Journal of the National Cancer Institute* 92 (Sept. 20, 2000): 1490.

473. Juskevich, J., et al. "Bovine Growth Hormone: Human Food Safety Evaluation." *Science* 249 (1990): 875-84.

474. Juvenal. (Quotation paraphrased.)

475. Kagawa, Y. "Impact of Westernization on the Nutrition of Japanese: Changes In Physique, Cancer, Longevity, and Centenarians." *Prev Med* 7 (1978): 205.

476. Kalechofsky, Roberta. *Haggadah for the Liberated Lamb*. Micah Pub (1985): 8.

477. Kannel, W. "Should All Mild Hypertension be Treated? Yes." *Controversies in Therapeutics*, L. Lasagna. ed., WB Saunders Co. (1980): 299.

478. Kaplan, N. "Mild Hypertension: When and How to Treat," *Arch Intern Med* 143 (255): 1983.
479. Kaplan, N. "Therapy for Mild Hypertension: Toward a More Balanced View." *JAMA* 249: (1983): 365.
480. Kapleau, Philip. *To Cherish All Life: A Buddhist Case for Becoming Vegetarian.* New York, Harper and Row (1981): 39-43.
481. Karjalainen, J., J. Martin, M. Knip, et al. "A Bovine Albumin Peptide as a Possible Trigger of Insulin-Dependent Diabetes Mellitus." *New Eng. J of Med.* 327; 5 (1992): 302-7.
482. Karleff, Ian. "Canadian Scientists Test E. coli Vaccine on Source." *Reuters News Service.* Aug. 10, 2000.
483. Kaur, Simran. "Eating Vegetarian to Save the Planet." www.simrankaur.com/eatingvegetariantosavetheplanet.
484. Kawate, R. "Diabetes Mellitus and Its Vascular Complications in Japanese Migrants on the Island of Hawaii." *Diabetes Care* 2; 161 (1979).
485. Keller, Bill. "Ties to Human Illness Revive Move to Ban Medicated Food." *New York Times* (Sept. 9, 1984): 1.
486. Kelley, V. "Enriched Lipid Diet Accelerates Lupus Nephritis In NZBxW Mice: Synergistic Action of Immune Complexes and Lipid In Glomerular Injury." *Am Journal of Pathology* 111 (1983): 288.
487. Kempner, W. "Some Effects of the Rice Diet: Treatment of Kidney Disease and Hypertension." *The Bulletin* 22 (1946): 358.
488. Kesteloot, H. Huang, and X.S. Yang, et al. "Serum lipids in the People's Republic of China: Comparison of Western and Eastern Populations." *Arteriosclerosis* 5 (1985): 427-433.
489. Kidd, David A., and Maribeth Abrams. "What Vegetarians Need to Know About Mad Cow Disease." *Vegetarian Voice* 25; 2 (Summer 2001): 8-13, 30.
490. King, Seth. "Iowa Rain and Wind Deplete Farmlands." *New York Times* (December 5, 1976): 61.
491. Kingma, J., and P. Roy. "Ultrastructural Study of Hypervitaminosis D Induced Arterial Calcification in Wistar Rats." *Artery* 16;1 (1988) 51-61.
492. Kirchner, M. "The Role of Hormones in the Etiology of Human Breast Cancer." *Cancer* 39 (1977): 2716.
493. Kivipelto, Miia. "High Blood Pressure and Cholesterol Levels Increase Risk." *British Medical Journal* (June 14, 2001).
494. Kjeldsen-Kragh, J., et al. "Controlled Trial of Fasting and One-Year Vegetarian Diet In Rheumatoid Arthritis." *Lancet* 338 (1991): 899-902.
495. Klein, R., B.E.K. Klein, T. Franke. "The Relationship of Cardiovascular Disease and Its Risk Factors to Age-Related Maculopathy: The Beaver Dam Eye Study." *Ophthalmology* 100 (1993): 406-14.
496. Klein, Richard. "Dieting Dangerously." *New York Times* (Jul. 14, 1997): A15.
497. Kradjian, Robert M., M.D., Breast Surgery Chief Division of General Surgery, Seton Medical Centre, Daly City, CA., "The Milk Letter: A Message To My Patients." www.afpafitness.com/milkdoc.htm.
498. Kristof, N. "China Sets Example in Health Care." *New York Times, Ann Arbor News.* (April 14, 1991): A-6.
499. Krohn, P. "Rapid Growth, Shot Life." *JAMA* 171 (1959): 461.
500. Kuller, L. "An Explanation for Variations in Distribution of Stroke and Arteriosclerotic Heart Disease Among Populations and Racial Groups." *American Journal of Epidemiology* 93;1 (1971).

501. Kuo, P. "The Effect of Lipemia Upon Coronary and Peripheral Circulation in Patients With Essential Hyperlipemia." *American Journal of Medicine* 26 (1959): 68.

502. Kurian, George Thomas. *The New Book of World Rankings.* Facts on File, Inc. New York (1991): 214.

503. Kushi Institute: Harvard University researchers noted. "Meat and Dairy Products." 1989. www.kushiinstitute.org/healing/meat-dairy.html.

504. Kushi, L.H. et al, *Am. J. Epidemiol* 149;1 (1999): 21-31. (Courtesy World Cancer Res. Fund).

505. Kyle, Dr. William L., ND, PhD. "Vegetarians Unlimited - 10 Reasons Why You Should Become a True Vegetarian!" Natural Health World. www.naturalhealthworld.com/articles/whyveg.html.

506. Lance, Gay. "Meat From Diseased Animals Approved for Consumers." *Scripps Howard News Service* (July 14, 2000).

507. *Lancet, The.* (Cited in "Meatless Menus for Prisons Make Dollars and Sense." Vlasak, Jerry, M.D., and Bernie Fischlowitz-Roberts.) www.pcrm.org/health/Commentary/commentary0012.html.

508. *Lancet, The.* (November 10, 2001).

509. *Lancet, The.* 355 (2000): 523.

510. Lang, John. "Environmentalists Rap Factory Farms for Manure Production." *Scripps Howard News Service* (June 9, 1998).

511. Lang, John. "U.S. Floating in Stinky Problem: Manure Pollution." *Desert News Archives* (April 29, 1998).

512. Langston, Peter. Fun People Archive. *WhiteBoard News* (May 7, 1997). www.langston.com/Fun_People/1997/1997AQD.html.

513. Lappé, Frances Moore, and Joseph Collins. *Food First: Beyond the Myth of Scarcity.* New York: Ballantine, (1977).

514. Lappé, Frances Moore, *Diet For a Small Planet.* New York, Ballantine Books (1991).

515. Lark, S. *The Estrogen Decision.* Los Altos, CA. Westchester Publishing (1994).

516. Larson, W.E. "Protecting the Soil Resource Base." *Journal of Soil and Water Conservation* 36;1 (Jan-Feb. 1981): 13.

517. Lauffer, R.B. *Iron Balance.* New York, St. Martin's Press (1991).

518. Lavine, Jay, M.D. "Nutrition and the Eye," The Vegetarian Resource Group. www.vrg.org/nutrition/eye.htm.

519. Law, M.R., N.J. Wald, T. Wu, et al. "Systematic Underestimation of Association Between Serum Cholesterol Concentration and Ischemic Heart Disease...," *British Medical Journal* 308 (1994): 363-6.

520. Lawrence, Jean. "High Fat, Low Carbs, What's the Harm." *CBS Healthwatch, Medscape,* Dec. 1999.

521. Lawrence, Ruth, M.D., University of Rochester School of Medicine (Spokeswoman for the American Academy of Pediatrics) *FDA Consumer* (June 1996).

522. LCA: Justice For Animals: Founder Chris DeRose. www.lcanimal.org/cmpgn/cmpgn_005.htm.

523. Leavenworth, Stuart. and Eli James Shiffer. "Airborne Menace." *Sunday Raleigh News and Observer,* July 5, 1998. (Quoting Viney Anaja, research professor; Department of Marine, Earth, and Atmospheric Sciences, North Carolina State University: 1A.)

524. Lempert, Phil. "Is Farmed Fish Really Healthier?" (August 27, 2001). www.supermarketguru.com/FoodSafety/arch_08-27-01.html.

525. Leonard, J.N., J.L. Hofer, and N. Pritikin. *Live Longer Now.* New York, Charter Books, (1974): 46.

526. Letson, David, and Noel Gjollehon. "Confined Animal Production and the Manure Problem." *Choices.* (3rd Quarter 1996): 18.

527. Lewinnek, G. "The Significance and a Comparative Analysis of the Epidemiology of Hip Fractures." *Clin Ortho Related Res* 152 (1980): 35.

528. Library of Congress: Committee On Environment and Public Works. U.S. Senate "A Brief Review of Selected Environmental Contamination Incidents With a Potential For Health Effects." (August 1980): 174-175.

529. Life Extension Foundation, *Life Extension Media, Disease Prevention, and Treatment.* Third Edition, Hollywood, FL. (2000): 21.

530. Lii, Jane. "China Booms, the World Holds Its Breath." *New York Times Magazine* (Feb. 18, 1996): 27.

531. Lindahl, O, L. Lindwall, et al. "Vegan Regimen With Reduced Medication in the Treatment of Bronchial Asthma." *Asthma* 22;1 (1985): 45-55.

532. Lindler, M. *Nutritional Biochemistry and Metabolism.* Elsevier Science Publishing Co., New York (1985): 70-71.

533. Linkswiler, H. "Calcium Retention of Young Adult Males as Affected by the Level of Protein and Calcium Intake." *Trans NY Acad Sci* 36 (1974): 333.

534. Lipsky, Joshua. "Study Claims BSE-Infected French Cows Entered Food Supply." (Dec. 18, 2000). www.meatingplace.com.

535. Lissner, L., D.A. Levitsky, B.J. Strupp, H.J. Kalkwarf, and D.A. Roe. "Dietary Fat and the Regulation of Energy Intake In Human Subjects." *American Journal of Clinical Nutrition* 46 (1987): 886-92.

536. Loggie, J. "Hypertension In the Pediatric Patient: A Reappraisal." *Journal of Pediatrics,* 94 (1979): 685.

537. Loma Linda University 20-year study (Cited in Robbins, *Diet,* p. 270).

538. Lommis, W. "Rickets." *Scientific American,* and *Human Nutrition* W.H. Freeman, San Francisco (1978): 193.

539. Lopez, Robert. *The Commercial Revolution of the Middle Ages, 950-1350.* Cambridge University Press (1982): 37.

540. Lovejoy, S.B. "Sources and Quantities of Nutrients Entering the Gulf of Mexico From Surface Waters of the U.S." EPA/800-R-92-002.

541. Lucas, P. "Dietary Fat Aggravates Active Rheumatoid Arthritis." *Clinical Research.* 29 (1981): 754A.

542. Lustgarden, Steve, and Debra Holton. "Women on the Verge of Health: The Vital Role of Food." www.earthsave.org/news/womenon.htm.

543. Lustgarden, Steve, and Debra Holton. Government Accountability Project (GAP), "What About Chicken?" (1996) www.earthsave.org/news/chicken.htm.

544. Lustgarden, Steve. "Bodyguards for the 21st century." www.earthsave.org/news/bodyguar.htm.

545. Luttrell, Clifton B. "The High Cost of Farm Welfare." Cato Institute, Washington, 1989.

546. Lyle, R.M., C.M. Weaver, D.A. Sedlock, S. Rajaram, B. Martin, and C.L. Melby. "Iron Status In Exercising Women: The Effect of Oral Iron Therapy vs. Increased Consumption of Muscle Foods." *Am. J. Clin. Nutr.* 56 (1992): 1049-1055.

547. Lyman, Howard F. *Mad Cowboy,* Scribner, 1998.

548. "Lymphoma." *Oncology.* May 22, 2000.

549. Mack, T. "Estrogens and Endometrial Cancer...." *New England Journal of Medicine* 294 (1976): 1262.

550. "Mad Cow Disease, Parts One and Two." *Rachel's Environment and Health Weekly.* (Jul. 9, 16, 1998).

551. *Mainstream.* (Summer 1983): 17.

552. "Making Food Safe" Oscar Mayer, (Cited in "The Business of Brainwashing: Corporations in the Classroom." www.compassionateliving.org/agenda2zw.htm).

553. Makinodan, T, J. Lubinski, and TC. Fong "Cellular, Biochemical, and Molecular Basis of T-Cell Senescence." *Arch Pathol Lab Med* 111 (1987): 910-14.

554. Malter, M, G. Schriever, U. Eilber. "Natural Killer Cells, Vitamins, and Other Blood Components of Vegetarian and Omnivorous Men." *Nutr Cancer* 12 (1989): 271-8.

555. "Mammograms: Is a Picture Worth a Thousand Words?" U.C.S.F. Breast Cancer Forum. March 14, 2001. www.breastcarecenter.ucsfmedicalcenter.org/forum/2001/march-minutes.html.

556. Managed Care Institute, Generic Pharmaceutical Association. www.gphaonline.org/news/facts.phtml.

557. Mandelman, Dobson, and Cox, Optometrists. "Vision News: Glaucoma." www.eye-docs.cc/content/visionnews.asp.

558. Mangels, Reed, Ph.D., R.D. "Calcium in the Vegan Diet." Vegetarian Resource Group www.vrg.org/nutrition/calcium.htm.

559. Mangels, Reed. "Protein in the Vegan Diet." Vegetarian Resource Group. www.vrg.org/nutrition/protein.htm.

560. Mangels, Reed. "Scientific Update." *Vegetarian Journal.* May-June, 2001.

561. Manuelidis, E.E., et al. "Suggested Links between different types of Dementias: Creutzfeld-Jacob Disease, Alzheimer Disease, and Retroviral CNS Infections." *Alzheimer's Disease and Associated Disorders* 3;1-2 (1989): 100-9.

562. Marcus, Erik. "The Meat Recall Sham: When is a Recall Not a Recall When it Involves Meat?" www.vegan.com/issues/1999/jan99/recalls.htm.

563. Marcus, Erik. *Vegan: The New Ethics of Eating.* McBooks Press, September 1997.

564. Marcus, R. "The Relationship of Dietary Calcium to the Maintenance of Skeletal Integrity In Man: An Interface of Endocrinology and Nutrition." *Metabolism* 31 (1982): 93.

565. Markarian, Michael. "Hunting For Dollars: Wildlife Mismanagement." *Vegetarian Voice* 25;2 (Summer 2001): 5-7.

566. Marmot, M. "Epidemiologic Studies of Coronary Heart Disease and Stroke in Japanese Men...." *American Journal of Epidemiology* 102 (1975): 511.

567. Marsh, A.G., T.V. Sanchez, O. Mickelsen, J. Keiser, and G. Mayor. "Cortical Bone Density of Adult Lacto-Ovo-Vegetarian and Omnivorous Women." *Journal of American Dietetic Association* 76 (1980): 148-51.

568. Martin, D.W., P.A. Mayes, V.W. Rodwell, and D.K Granner. *Harper's Review of Biochemistry.* Lange Medical Publications, Los Altos, CA. (1985): 673.

569. Mason, J. and P. Singer. *Animal Factories.* Avon Books, (1975): 117.

570. Mason, J. and P. Singer. *Animal Factories.* Crown Publishers (1980): 29-30, 48-49, 72.

571. Mason, Jim. "Assault and Battery." *Animals' Voice* 4;2 (Apr-May 1991): 33.

572. Mason, Jim. "Fowling the Waters." *E Magazine.* (Sep-Oct 1995): 33. (90 percent raised in factory farms).

573. "Massachusetts Male Aging Study." *Psychosomatic Medicine.* 1991 (Cited in "Meatless Menus for Prisons Make Dollars and Sense." Jerry Vlasak and Bernie Fischlowitz-Roberts, 2000. www.pcrm.org/health/Commentary/commentary0012.html).

574. Mathieson, R.A., J.L. Walberg, F.C. Gwazdauskas, D.E. Hinkle and J.M Gregg. "The Effect of Varying Carbohydrate Content of a Very-Low-Calorie Diet on Resting Metabolic Rate and Thyroid Hormones." *Metabolism* 35 (1986): 394-98.

575. Mayo Clinic Health Information, Nutrition Center: Diet and Disease, Handling Lactose Intolerance. www.walgreens.com/library/lifestyle/nutrition/diet/diet8.jhtml.

576. Mazess, R. "Bone Mineral Content of North Alaskan Eskimos." *Am J. Clin Nutr* 27 (1974): 916.

577. McAlister, N. "Should We Treat Mild Hypertension?" *JAMA* 249 (1983): 379.

578. McCance, R.A. and E.M. Widdowson. "The Composition of Foods." (1960): 22 and 124.

579. McCarthy, Coleman. "The Holes in the Deer-Hunting Defense." *Washington Post.* Nov. 24, 1992.

580. McClellan, W. "Prolonged Meat Diets With a Study of the Metabolism of Nitrogen, Calcium, and Phosphorus." *Journal of Biol Chem* 87 (1930): 669.

581. McClintock, Jack. "Twenty Species We May Lose in the Next 20 Years: And Then There Were None." *Discover* 21;10. October 2000. www.discover.com/oct_00/feat-species.html.

582. McCrea, F. "The Politics of Menopause: The Discovery of a Deficiency Disease." *Social Problems* (1983): 111-23.

583. McDougall, John, M.D. "Americans are Getting Fatter and Dying From It." Agora South Inc., 2000. www.earthsave.org/news/hiprotein.htm.

584. McDougall, John, M.D. "Anemia." The McDougall Program: Dietary and Lifestyle Implications. www.drmcdougall.com/science/anemia.html.

585. McDougall, John, M.D. "Natural Living" Radio Interview, WBAI, New York, March 1987.

586. McDougall, John, M.D. "Wellness Newsletter." (July-Aug. 99) www.drmcdougall.com/newsletter/july_aug.99.1.html.

587. McDougall, John, M.D. *McDougall's Medicine.* Piscataway NJ: New Century Publishers, 1985.

588. McDougall, John, M.D. *McDougall's Medicine: A Challenging Second Opinion*, New Win Publishing, 1985.

589. McDougall, John, M.D. *The McDougall Plan*, New Century Publications, Piscataway, 1983 p. 49-62.

590. McDougall, John, M.D. *The McDougall Program for a Healthy Heart.* (Cited in, "Does Aging Cause Hearing Loss?" www.hearinglossweb.com/Medical/Causes/aging.htm).

591. McDougall, John, M.D. *The McDougall Report: Lifesaving Facts Your Doctor Never Told* Trillium Health Products (1992): 32-38.

592. McDougall, Mary and John. *The McDougall Plan for Super Health and Life-Long Weight Loss*, New Jersey. New Century Publishers, 1983.

593. Mckdad, A., and et al. "The Spread of the Obesity Epidemic in the United States." *JAMA* 282 (1999): 1519-22. (Estimate of 2 percent by John Robbins, author and founder of EarthSave International.)

594. McKinlay, J. and S. McKinlay. "The Questionable Contribution of Medical Measures to Decline of Mortality of United States in the Twentieth Century." *Health and Society.* Milbank Memorial Fund. Summer, 1977.

595. McKnown, Thomas. *The Modern Rise of Populations.* Academic Press, Harcourt Brace, New York (1976): 152-163.

596. McNelly, J.A. "The Biodiversity Crisis: Challenges for Research and Management." Conservation of Biodiversity for Sustainable Development, O.T. Sandlund, et al, eds. *Scandinavian University Press,* 1992.

597. *Meat Industry Insights.* "CDC Says Deadly E. coli Cases Up Sharply In 1998." March 12, 1999.

598. *Meat Industry Insights.* "Deadly E. coli Bug May Affect Half the Cattle." Nov. 15, 1999.

599. *Meat Industry Insights.* "Microbiologists Battle E. coli," Oct. 26, 1999.

600. "Meat Inspection: A Rancid Rule Change." *St Louis Post-Dispatch* Editorial. Tuesday, July 18, 2000. www.commondreams.org/views/071800-104.htm.

601. "Meating of America, The." EarthSave Press Release, June 1998. www.earthsave.org/news/19980601.htm.

602. Med Web: "Atherosclerosis." medweb.bham.ac.uk/http/depts/path/Teaching/foundat/athero/Athero1.htm.

603. Medard, Gabel. Cornucopia Project, Preliminary Report. Rodale, Inc, Emmaus, Pa.: 33.

604. Mehl, Lewis., et al. "Outcomes of Elective Home Births: A Series of 1,146 Cases." *Journal of Reproductive Medicine* 19; 5 (1977): 281-90.

605. Melina, Davis, and Harrison, *Becoming Vegetarian*, Summertown, Tenn.: Book Publishing Co, 1995.

606. "Menopause." *Newsweek* (May 25, 1992): 39-44.

607. Mervyn, Len and Leonard. *Stomach Ulcers: Safe Alternatives Without Drugs.* Thorsons, May 1998.

608. Messina, V.K., and K.I. Burke. "Position of the American Dietetic Association: Vegetarian Diets." *J Am Diet Assoc* 97 (1997): 1317-1321.

609. Meyers, J., et al. "Six-Month Prevalence of Psychiatric Disorder in Three Communities." *Archives of General Psychiatry* 41 (1984): 959.

610. Microsoft Corporation. *Microsoft Small Business Consultant and Stat Pack.* Redmond, WA, 1988.

611. "Midwifery." *Los Angeles Times.* (April 28, 1992): E1.

612. Mikesell, M.W. "The Deforestation of Mount Lebanon." *Geographical Review* 59; 1 (Jan 1969): 1.

613. Miller, J.W. "Homocysteine and Alzheimer's Disease." *Nutr Rev* 57:4 (April 1999): 126-9.

614. Mills, P.K., et al. "Cancer Incidence Among California Seventh-Day Adventists, 1976-1982." *The American Journal of Clinical Nutrition* 59 (1994): 1136S-1142S. (suppl.).

615. Miranda, P "High-Fiber Diets in the Treatment of Diabetes Mellitus," *Ann Intern Medicine*, 88:482, 1978.

616. Mirkin, Gabe, M.D. "Folic Acid and Alzheimer's Disease." July 1, 2001. www.DrMirkin.com/nutrition/9218.htm.

617. Moen, M.H., and P. Magnus. "The Familial Risk of Endometriosis." *Acta Obstet Gynecol Scand* 72 (1993): 560-4.

618. Mohr, Paula. "More Milk Per Cow: Management and Genetics Boost Holstein Production Averages above 30,000 Pounds." *Farm Journal* (January 1996).

619. Mokhiber, H. *Corporate Crime and Violence: Big Business Power and the Abuse of the Public Trust.* San Francisco: Sierra Club Books (1989): 434.

620. Mondimore, Francis Mark. *Depression, The Mood Disorder.* The John Hopkins University Press. Baltimore, 1990.

621. Morrow, W. "Dietary Fat and Immune Disease." *Arthritis Rheum* 26 (1983):1532.

622. Moss, Ralph. *Questioning Chemotherapy.* New York, Equinox Press (1975): 21.

623. Moss, Ralph. *The Cancer Industry.* New York, Paragon House (1991): 116.

624. Multiple Vitamins, Minerals and Herbs. "The Function of Vitamins." www.a2zvita.com/MultipleVitamins.htm.

625. Murray, R.K., D.K. Granner, P.A Mayes. and V.W Rodwell. *Harper's Biochemistry.* Appleton and Lange, Norwalk, CT (1990): 576, 578.

626. Muwakkil, S. "Food Pyramid Scheme." *These Times.* (July 5, 2000).

627. Myers, N. *Conversion of Tropical Moist Forests.* Washington, D.C.,: National Academy of Sciences (1980): 3-4.

628. Myers, Norman. "Cheap Meat vs. Priceless Rainforests." *Vegetarian Times* (May 1982).

629. National Association of Biology Teachers. *The Responsible Use of Animals in Biology Classrooms.* Reston, Va.

630. National Cancer Institute. Bethesda, USA. (Cited in Barnard, *Food for Life*, 58).

631. National Cancer Institute. Bethesda, USA. (Cited in www.cancer2000.com/070199.html.)
632. National Cattleman's Beef Assoc. (NCBA) "Fact-Sheet—June 1998."
633. National Dairy Council, Nutrition Education Materials. (1985-1986 Catalog): 16-22 (0920N).
634. National Diabetes Information Clearing House. U.S. Department of Health and Human Services, 1 Information Way Bethesda, MD 20892-3560. National Diabetes Statistics: General Information and National Estimates On Diabetes In The United States, 2000. www.niddk.nih.gov/health/diabetes/pubs/dmover/dmover.htm.
635. National Eye Institute 15-Week Study, Bethesda, MD. "Seeing is Beleafing." *Vegetarian Times* (July 2001): 16.
636. National Geographic Channel, United Kingdom: "Animal Inventors." www.nationalgeo-graphic.co.in.
637. *National Geographic.* Feb. 1970.
638. National Institute of Allergy and Infectious Diseases. Fact Sheet: Asthma and Allergy Statistics. National Institute of Health.
639. National Institute of Health "Ratio of animal to vegetable protein." *Am J. Clin Nutr* (2001).
640. National Institute of Health: National Heart, Lung and Blood Institute. Data Fact Sheet: Asthma Statistics (1999).
641. National Kidney Foundation of Oregon and Washington, "Kidney and Urinary Tract Diseases." www.kidneywa.org/PublicInformation/UrinaryTractDisease.htm.
642. National Research Council (1982): 9-1, 9-2.
643. Natural Resources Defense Council: Testing the Waters. *A Guide to Water Quality at Vacation Beaches* (July 2002).
644. Naveh-Floman, N., and M. Belkin. "Prostaglandin Metabolism and Intraocular Pressure." *Br J Ophthalmol* 71 (1987): 254-6.
645. Nelson, Jeff. "Sorting through the Calcium Myths." www.vegsource.com/articles/cal-cium_update.htm.
646. Nelson, Jeff. The Man Willing to Take on Big Tobacco "Cow" Tows to Big Meat & Dairy." (1999). www.vegsource.com/articles/drkoop.htm.
647. Nelson, Sabrina. "How I Beat Relapsing Polychondritis." www.RelapsingPolychondritis.com.
648. Neuman, I., H. Nahum, and A. Ben-Amotz. "Prevention Of Exercise-Induced Asthma By a Natural Isomer Mixture of Beta-Carotene." *Ann Allergy Asthma Immunol* 82 (1999): 549–53.
649. *New England Journal of Medicine.* Mar. 26, 1981.
650. *New Scientist.* May 1994.
651. Nichols, Dr. Joe, M.D., www.nutritionref.com/main.html.
652. Niki, E., Y. Yamamoto, E. Komuro, and K. Sato. "Membrane Damage Due To Lipid Oxidation." *Am J. Clin Nutr* 53 (1991): 201S-5S.
653. Nilsson L.H, Hultman E. "Liver Glycogen In Man-the Effect of Total Starvation or a Carbohydrate-Poor Diet Followed By Carbo-Hydrate Refeeding." *Scand J Clin Lab Invest* 32 (1973): 325-330.
654. Noren, K. "Levels of Organochlorine Contaminants In Human Milk In Relation to the Dietary Habits of the Mothers." *Acta Pediatr Scand* 72 (1983): 811-6.
655. North Carolina Department of Health and Natural Resources. Correspondence from Dennis Ramsey to Karen Priest. (May 19, 1997).
656. North Carolina State University. 1995 Survey.
657. North, J. "Catching up on Smaller Profit Leaks." *Broiler Industry* (Jun. 1976): 41.
658. Northrup, Christiane. *Women's Bodies, Women's Wisdom.* New York, Bantam (1994).

659. Norvell, Candyce. "Why is Everyone Griping about School Lunches: Poor Nutrition in School Food Programs." *Current Health* 221; 5 (January 1995): 27.

660. NOVA WGBH Educational Foundation "A Plague on our Children." Boston, 1979.

661. Nsouli T., S. Nsouli, R, Linde, et al. "Role of Food Allergy in Serous Otitis Media." *Annals of Allergy* 73 (1994): 215-219.

662. N-Squared Computing, *Nutritionist III*. 4; 5, 1988. (Table "Protein: Percent of Calories." Harris, *Scientific Basis:* 41).

663. Null, Gary, Ph.D. "Medical Genocide Part 16," *Penthouse* (1987). Quoted in Barry Lynes, *The Healing of Cancer*. Queensville, Ontario: Marcus Books (1989): 10.

664. Null, Gary, Ph.D. *The Vegetarian Handbook*, St. Martin's Griffin, 1996.

665. Null, Steve and Gary. "How to Get Rid of the Poisons in Your Body." New York, Arco, 1977.

666. *Nutrition Action*. June 1999.

667. *Nutrition Cancer* 29 (1997): 29.

668. O'Connor, G.A. "A Regional Perspective Study of In-Hospital Mortality Associated with Coronary Artery Bypass Grafting." *Journal of American Medical Association* 266 (1991): 803.

669. Obituary Column (March 14, 1982): C-11, Riverside Herald. (Cited in Robbins, *Diet*: 262).

670. Ocean and Oceanography: "VIII resources." www.cosmiverse.com.

671. Ocean Facts: www.ovi.ca/fact_main.htm.

672. O'Connell, B. "Eating Right For Healthy Kidneys." *Diabetes Self-Management*. R.A. Rapaport Publishing, Inc. 2002.

673. Official Code Of Georgia Title 2. Agriculture Chapter 16. "Action For Disparagement of Perishable Food Products or Commodities." (Sample of state cited).

674. Ogunniyi, A., O. Baiyewu, O. Gureje, et al. "Epidemiology of Dementia In Nigeria: Results From the Indianapolis-Ibadan Study." *Eur Journal Neurol* 7 (2000): 485-90.

675. O'Keeffe K.A., R.E. Keith, G.D. Wilson, et al. "Dietary Carbo-Hydrate Intake and Endurance Exercise Performance of Trained Female Cyclists." *Nutr Res* 9 (1989): 819-830.

676. Ophir, O., et al. "Low Blood Pressure in Vegetarians...." *American Journal of Clinical Nutrition* 37 (1983): 755-62.

677. *Optimal Wellness Healthy News You Can Use*. "Deadly Pig Virus Returns" Issue 162 (July 16, 2000) www.mercola.com/2000/jul/16/pig_virus.htm.

678. Oregon Health Services, The. (April, 1997; June 2001) www.ohd.hr.state.or.us/acd/salmonella/facts.htm.

679. Ornish, Dean, M.D. "Can Lifestyle Changes Reverse Coronary Heart Disease?" *Lancet* 336 (1990): 129-33.

680. Ornish, Dean, M.D. "Effects Of Stress Management Training and Dietary Changes In Treating Ischemic Heart Disease." *JAMA* 54 (1983): 249.

681. Ornish, Dean, M.D. et al. "Intensive Lifestyle changes for Reversal of Coronary Heart Disease." *Journal of American Medical Association* 280 (1998): 2001-7.

682. Osborn, T. "Amino Acids in Nutrition and Growth." *Journal of Biological Chemistry* 17 (1914): 325.

683. Oski, Frank, M.D., *Don' t Drink Your Milk*. Teach Services, 1992.

684. Paganelli, R. "Detection Of Specific Antigen Within Circulating Immune Complexes: Validation of the Assay and Its Application to Food Antigen-Antibody Complexes Formed In Healthy and Food-Allergic Subjects." *Clin. Exp. Immunol.* 46 (1981): 44-53.

685. Page, Dr. Linda. "Secrets To Great Sex For Men Page: About Impotence." www.healthyhealing.com/SEX-Men-Impotence.html.

686. Page, I. "Prediction of Coronary Heart Disease Based on Clinical Suspicion, Age, Total Cholesterol, and Triglycerides." *Circulation* 42 (1970): 625.

687. Paik, D.C., D.V. Saborio, R. Oropeza, and H.P. Freeman. "The Epidemiological Enigma of Gastric Cancer Rates In the US: Was Grandmother's Sausage the Cause?" *Int J Epidemiol* 30 ; 1 (Feb 2001): 181-182.

688. Painter, NS. "Fiber Deficiency and Diverticular Disease of the Colon." eds. R.W. Reilly, and J.B. Kirsner. New York, Plenum, 1975.

689. Palmblad, J. "Lymphomas and Dietary Fat." *Lancet* 1 (1977): 142.

690. Parisi, A. "A Comparison of Angioplasty with Medical Treatment of Single Vessel Coronary Artery Disease." *New England Journal of Medicine* 326 (1992): 10.

691. Parsons, James. "Forest to Pasture: Development or Destruction?" *Revista de Biologia Tropical* 24 (1976): Supplement 1.

692. Passwater, R.A., Ph.D., *The Nutrition Superbook: Volume I*: "The Antioxidants, the Nutrients that Guard the Body Against Cancer, Heart Disease, Arthritis, and Allergies and Even Slow the Aging Process." New Canaan, CT: Keats Publishing (1995): 4-8, 184-186, 363.

693. Pate, R.R., B.J. Miller, J.M. Davis, C.A. Slentz, and L.A. Klingshirn. "Iron Status of Female Runners." *Int. J. Sport Nutr* 3 (1993): 222-231.

694. Paterson, C. "Calcium Requirements In Man: A Critical Review." *Postgrad Med. Journal* 54 (1978) 244.

695. Pearl, R. "Tobacco Smoking and Longevity." *Science.* Mar. 4, 1938.

696. Pearson, D., and , J. Anderson. *The Case Against Congress: A Compelling Indictment of Corruption on Capitol Hill.* New York, Simon and Schuster (1968): 329-330.

697. Peavy, William, and Warren Peary. *Super Nutrition Gardening.* www.geocities.com/vshouston/WhyOrganic.

698. Pelton, R., and T. Clarke. *How To Prevent Breast Cancer.* Fireside, 1995.

699. Pennington, J. *Food Values of Portions Commonly Used.* 14th ed., Harper & Row, New York, 1985.

700. Pennington, J., *Food Values of Portions Commonly Used*, Harper & Row, New York, 1989.

701. People for the Ethical Treatment of Animals. www.peta.org.

702. Perlman, D. "New Evidence Reported on Dioxin as Health Hazard." *San Francisco Chronicle.* (April 18, 1986): A-1, A-4.

703. "Pesticide Safety: Myths and Facts." National Coalition Against the Misuse of Pesticides.

704. Peters, J.M., S. Preston-Martin, S.J. London, et al. "Processed Meats and Risk of Childhood Leukemia." California, USA. *Cancer Causes Control* 5 (1994): 195–202.

705. Peterson, R. "Antibodies to Cow's Milk Proteins - Their Presence and Significance." *Pediatrics* 31 (1963): 209.

706. Phillips, R.L. "Role of Life-Style and Dietary Habits in Risk of Cancer Among Seventh-Day Adventists." *Cancer Research* 35 (1975): 3513-22.

707. "Physicians Committee for Responsible Medicine Cancer Awareness Survey." 1999. Reported in *Good Medicine* (Autumn 1999): 7.

708. Physicians Committee for Responsible Medicine Lawsuit Versus the U.S. Dept. of Agriculture and the U.S. Dept. of Health and Human Services." PCRM Website: 1999.

709. Pickering, T. "Treatment of Milk Hypertension and Reduction of Cardiovascular Mortality." *JAMA* 249 (1983): 399.

710. Pietila, H. "Deforestation is Turning Ethiopia into a Desert." *Baltimore Sun*, Dec 23, 1984.

711. Pimentel, D. and M. Pimentel. *Food, Energy, and Society.* New York: John Wiley and Sons (1979): 56, 59.

712. Pimentel, D., et al. "Conserving Biological Diversity in Agricultural/Forestry System." *Bioscience* 42 (1994): 354-62. Printed in Pimentel and Giampietro.
713. Pimentel, D., et al. "Energy and Land Constraints in Food Protein production." *Science*, Nov. 21, 1975.
714. Pimentel, D., et al. *Ecological Integrity: Integrating Environment, Conservation and Health.* Island Press, Washington DC, January 2001.
714a. Pimentel et al, "Land Degradation: Effects on Food and Energy Resources," *Science* 104 (Oct. 1976): 150.
715. *Plant Soil*, 167:305, 1994.
716. "Please Come In Time!" Dr. Helmut Keller. www.cancer2000.com/070199.html.
717. Plester, D., and A.M. Soliman. "Autoimmune Hearing Loss." *Am J Otol* 10 (1989): 188-192.
718. "Pork May Be the Source of Acute Hepatitis E Reported In US." *Mayo Clin Proc* 72 (December 1997): 1133-1136,1197-1198.
719. "Portrait of a Healer: Nicholas Gonzales, MD." *The Cancer Chronicles* (Summer 1990): 10.
720. Potter, John D. "Cancer Prevention: Food and Phytochemicals." Fred Hutchinson Cancer Research Center and University of Washington, Seattle, Washington. Brussels, Belgium. Second International Symposium. "The Role of Soy in Preventing and Treating Chronic Disease." September 15-18, 1996. www.soyfoods.com/symposium/oa1_1.html.
721. *Poultry Digest* (July 1978): 363.
722. *Poultry Tribune* (Feb, 1974).
723. Preston, Richard. *The Hot Zone*, New York: Anchor Books Doubleday (1994): 407-9.
724. *Preventive Medicine* 29 (1999): 87-91.
725. *Preventive Medicine* 30 (2000): 225-233.
726. Price, A.B., "Diverticular Disease (Pathology)." *Fiber Deficiency and Colonic Disorders*, ed. R.W Reilly and J.B Kirsner. New York, Plenum, 1975.
727. Pritikin, N. Quoted in *Vegetarian Times* 43:22.
728. Pronczuk, A., Y. Kipervarg, and K.C. Hayes. "Vegetarians Have Higher Plasma Alpha-Tocopherol Relative to Cholesterol than do Nonvegetarians," *J AM Coll Nutr* 11 (1992): 50-5.
729. "Pushing Drugs to Doctors." *Consumer Reports*. Consumers Union, Yonkers (Feb 1992): 87-94.
730. Putnam, Judy, and Shirley Gerber. "Trends in U.S. Food Supply 1970-97." *America's Eating Habits: Changes and Consequences* (n.d.), USDA, Economic Research Service, Food and Rural Economics Division, Agriculture Information Bulletin No. 750.
731. Quote on Vegetarianism. www.edu.pe.ca/sourishigh/Pages/Cmp6-03/Beth/Homepage/Quotes.htm.
732. Radio Interview w / Steven Rosen, 1987, (cited in: Rosen, Steven, *Diet For Transcendence*, Torchlight Publishing, 1997 p. 115.)
733. Randell, V.A., and F.J.G. Ebling. "Seasonal Changes in Human Hair Growth." *Br J Derm* 124 (1991): 146-51.
734. Rattigan, Patrick. *The Cancer Business.* www.harmonikireland.com/index.php?topic=cancerbusiness.
735. Ray, Carol and Wanda Koszewski. "Alzheimer's Disease and Nutrition." January 1998. www.ianr.unl.edu/pubs/foods/nf357.htm.
736. Raychoudhry, S.C. *Social, Cultural, and Economic History of India (Ancient Times)* Delhi: Surjeet Publications, 1978.
737. Recker, R. "The Effect of Milk Supplements on Calcium Metabolism, Bone Metabolism, and Calcium Balance." *American J. of Clinical Nutrition* 41(1985): 254.

738. Reddy, BS, et al, "Nutrition and its Relationship to Cancer," *Advances in Cancer Research*, 32:237, 1980.

739. Regenstein, Lewis. *How to Survive in America the Poisoned.* Acropolis Books (1982): 103.

740. Regenstein, Lewis. *The Politics of Extinction*, MacMillan Publishing Co., New York, (1975): 52-59.

741. Rennie, J. "Malignant Mimicry: False Estrogens May Cause Cancer and Lower Sperm Counts." *Scientific American* (Sept, 1993): 34-38.

742. Reported by Mike Hathorn as a candidate for Congress, and D.C. Amarasinghe, M.D., as a candidate for Congress websites.

743. Rice, Pamela. "101 Reasons Why I'm a Vegetarian." 1998 edition. www.vivavegie.org.

744. Rice, Pamela. "101 Reasons Why I'm a Vegetarian." 2001 edition. www.vivavegie.org.

745. Richards, E. "Vitamin C Suffers a Dose of Politics." *New Scientist.* Feb 27, 1986.

746. Ringrose, H. "Nutrient Intakes in an Urbanized Micronesian Population with a High Diabetes Prevalence." *American Journal of Clinical Nutrition* 32 (1979): 1334.

747. Risch, H., et al. "Dietary Fat Intake and Risk of Epithelial Ovarian Cancer." *Journal of the National Cancer Institute* 86 (1994): 1409-1415.

748. "Ritalin Maker Opens Drive to End Abuse." AP. *New York Times* (Mar. 28, 1996): A-13.

749. Rivellese, A. "Effect of Dietary Fibre on Glucose Control and Serum Lipoproteins In Diabetic Patients." *Lancet* 2 (1980): 447.

750. Robbins, John. *Diet for a New America.* Stillpoint, 1987.

751. Robbins, John. *Reclaiming Our Health.* H.J. Kramer, 1998.

752. Robbins, John. *The Food Revolution.* Conari, 2001.

753. Robbins, S.L., V. Kumar, and R.S. Cotran. *Pathlogic Basis of Disease*, W.B. Saunders Co., Philadelphia (1989): 163-237.

754. Roberts, J. "Blood Pressure Levels of Persons 6-74 years." United States, 1971-1974. *DHEW Pub. No.* (HRA) 203 (1977): 78-1648.

755. Roberts, W., R. MacRae, L. Stahlbrand. *Real Food for a Change.* Random House, Canada. 1999.

756. Robertson, W. "Should Recurrent Calcium Oxalate Stone Formers Become Vegetarians?" *British Journal of Urology* 51 (1979): 427.

757. Robertson, W. "The Role of Affluence and Diet In the Genesis of Calcium-Containing Stones." *Fortschritte der Urologie and Nephrologie* 11 (1979): 5.

758. Robinson, Ann, and Robbin Marks. "Restoring the Big River: A Clean Water Act Blueprint for Mississippi." Izaak Walton League, Minneapolis, MN, and the Natural Resources Defense Council, Washington D.C. (Feb. 1994): 13.

759. Roller, W.L., et al. "Energy Costs of Intensive Livestock Production." American Society of Agricultural Engineers. June 1975, St. Joseph, Michigan. Paper no. 75-4042, Table 7: 14.

760. Rose, D. "The Biochemical Epidemiology of Prostatic Carcinoma." *Dietary Fat and Cancer*, Alan Liss, Inc. New York, 1986.

761. Rose, D., et al, "International Comparisons of Mortality Rates For Cancer of the Breast, Ovary, Prostate, and Colon, and Per Capita Food Consumption." *Cancer* 58 (1986): 2363-2371.

762. Rose, D.P., A.P Boyar, C. Cohen, and L.E. Strong. "Effect of a Low-Fat Diet on Female Sex Hormone Levels in Women with Cystic Breast Disease." 1. Serum Steroids and Gonadotropins. *Journal of National Cancer Institute* 78; 4 (1987): 623-26.

763. Rose, William, Ph.D. "Comparative Growth of Diets...." *Journal of Biological Chemistry* 176 (1948): 753.

764. Rose, William, Ph.D., "The Amino Acid Requirements of Adult Man. XVI, The Role of the Nitrogen Intake." *Journal of Biological Chemistry* 217 (1955): 997.

765. Rosen, Steven. *Diet For Transcendence.* Torchlight Publishing, 1997.

766. Rosman, J. "Prospective Randomized Trial of Early Dietary Protein Restriction In Chronic Renal Failure." *Lancet* 2 (1984): 1291.

767. Ross, M.H. "Protein, Calories, and Life Expectancy." *Fed Proc* 18 (1959):1190-1207.

768. Rouse, I.L., B.K. Armstrong, and L.J. Beilin. "Vegetarian Diet, Lifestyle and Blood Pressure in Two Religious Populations." *Clinical Journal of Pharmacology and Physiology* 9 (1982): 327-30.

769. Rowen, Andrew, Loew Franklin, and Joan Weer. "The Animal Research Controversy: Protest, Process, and Public Policy—an Analysis of Strategic Issues." Boston: Center for Animals and Public Policy, 1995.

770. Rudd, G.L. *Why Kill for Food?* Indian Vegetarian Congress (1956).

771. Rudek, Joe, Ph.D. Senior Scientist, North Carolina Environmental Defense Fund in Hog Waste and Environmental Quality in North Carolina, Save Our State Forum. Raleigh, North Carolina (June 11, 1998): 47.

772. Ryan, Michael. "Emily the Cow." *Parade Magazine.* May 4, 1997. www.peaceabbey.org/sanctuary/emily1.htm.

773. Sacks, F.M. "Ingestion of Egg Raises Plasma Low Density Lipoproteins in Free-Living Subjects." *Lancet* 1 (1984): 647.

774. Sacks, F.M., W.P. Castellik, A. Donner, and F.H. Kass. "Plasma Lipids and Lipoproteins in Vegetarians and Controls." *The New England Journal of Medicine* 292; 22 (May 1975): 1148, 29. (Some of the "vegetarians" in the study ate fish although it was a small minority.)

775. "Safeguarding the Oceans." Environmental Defense. www.environmentaldefense.org/system/templates/page/focus.cfm?focus=2.

776. Safina, Carl. "The World's Imperiled Fish." *Scientific American,* Nov 1995.

777. Sagan, Carl. Quotation paraphrased.

778. Salonen, J.T., R. Salonen, K. Nyyssonen, H. Korpela. "Iron Sufficiency is Associated With Hypertension and Excess Risk of Myocardial Infarction: The Kuopio Ischemic Heart Disease Risk Factor (KIHD)." *Circulation* 85 (1992): 864.

779. Sancho, J. "Immune Complexes In Iga Nephropathy: Presence of Antibodies Against Diet Antigens and Delayed Clearance of Specific Polymeric Iga Immune Complexes." *Clin Exp Immunol* 54 (1983): 194.

780. Sanford, K.K., R. Parshad, R. Gantt. "Responses of Human Cells in Culture to Hydrogen Peroxide and Related Free Radicals Generated by Visible Light: Relationship to Cancer Susceptibility." J.E Johnson, R. Walford, D. Harman, J. Miquel eds. *Free Radicals, Aging, and Degenerative Disease.* New York, Alan R. Liss, 1986.

781. Sarasua, S. and D.A. Savitz. "Cured and Broiled Meat Consumption in Relation to Childhood Cancer." *Cancer Causes Control.* Denver, Colorado. 5 (1994): 141–8.

782. Satchell, Michael. "The American Hunter Under Fire." U.S. *News & World Report.* Feb. 5, 1990.

783. "Save Your Health - One Bite at a Time." EarthSave. www.earthsave.org/news/19980915.htm.

784. Schaefer, Dwight D. DC. Health Issues: Ask the Doctor. "The Shell Game." www.geocities.com/joerocam/ask_the_doctor.htm.

785. Schantz, Peter M. "Trichinosis in the United States, 1975: Increase in Cases Attributed to Numerous Common-Source Outbreaks." *The Journal of Infectious Diseases* 136; 5 (Nov. 1977): 712-715.

786. Scharffenberg, J.A., M.D., "Vegetarian Diets." *American Journal of Disabled Child* 133 (Nov. 1979): 1204.

787. Schell, O. *Modern Meat.* Vintage Books (1985): 59.
788. Schiel, K. "The War on Cancer Is a Fraud."
www.disinfo.com/pages/dossier/id336/pg1.
789. Schoeps, Hans-Joachim. *Jewish Christianity: Factual Disputes in the Early Church.*
D.R.A. Hare, Fortress Press (1969) 14.
790. "School Lunch Program Fails to Make the Grade." A Report by the Physicians
Committee for Responsible Medicine (PCRM), September, 2001.
791. Schouteden, A. *Ann de Soc. Des Sciences Med. Et Nat. de Bruxelles.* Henri Lamertin,
Brussels: 50.
792. Schulbach, Herb., et al. *Soil and Water* 38 (Fall 1978).
793. *Science News.* Jan 31, 1998.
794. *Scientific American.* January, 1892. (Cited in Barnard, *Food for Life*: 60.)
795. Scott, F.W. "Cow Milk and Insulin-Dependent Diabetes Mellitus: Is There a
Relationship?" *American Journal of Clinical Nutrition* 51 (1990): 489-91.
796. Seattle, Indian Chief. Paraphrased quotation.
797. Seddon, J.M., et al. "Smokers with Early Macular Degeneration." *J. Amer Med Assoc.*
1994.
798. Sedula, M. "Frequency of Systemic Lupus Erythematosus in Different Ethnic Groups in
Hawaii." *Arthritis Rheum* 22 (1979): 328.
799. Seidman, B.F. "Eating Lots of Vegetables May Help Prevent Non-Hodgkin's
Lymphoma." *Oncology.* May 22, 2000.
800. Semple, E.C. *The Geography of the Mediterranean Region, Its Relation to Ancient
History.* New York: AMS Press, 1971. (Reprinted from 1931 edition).
801. "Senate Grills Dietary Supplement Sellers." Senate Hearing Testimony, Sept. 11,
2001. www.usgovinfo.about.com.
802. Senate, Animal Agriculture, Information on Waste Management and Water Quality
Issues, GAO/RCED-95-200BR, Washington, D.C: 58-61.
803. Sever, P. "Blood Pressure and Its Correlation in Urban and Tribal Africa." *Lancet* 2
(1980): 60.
804. Severo, R. "Two Studies for the National Institute Link Herbicide to Cancer in
Animals." *New York Times.* June 27, 1980.
805. Shanmugasundarum, K.R., A. Visvanathan, et al. "Effect of High-Fat Diet on
Cholesterol Distribution In Plasma Lipoproteins, Cholesterol Esterifying Activity In
Leukocytes, and Erythrocyte Membrane Components Studied: Importance of Body
Weight." *American Journal Clinical Nutrition.* 44 (1988): 805-15.
806. Sherman, H. *Chemistry of Food and Nutrition.* MacMillan Co, N.Y. (1952,): 208.
807. Sherman, H. *The Science of Nutrition.* Columbia Univ. Press, N.Y. (1943): 177-198.
808. Shiver, Carl. *Die vergessenen Anfänge der Schöpfung und des Christentums.* Bad
Bellington, Germany: Order of the Nazarenes (1977) Section II, Part 3. English
Translation, *The Forgotten Beginnings of Creation and Christianity.*
809. Shu, X, et al. "Dietary Factors and Epithelial Ovarian Cancer." *British Journal of
Cancer* 59 (1989): 92-96.
810. Shukitt-Hale, Barbara, Marcelle Morrison-Bogorad. Agriculture Department's Human
Nutrition Research Center on Aging. Tufts University, Boston. *Journal of
Neuroscience.*
811. Sierakowski, R. "The Frequency of Urolithiasis in Hospital Discharge Diagnoses in the
United States." *Invest Urol* 15 (1978): 438.
812. Simon, C. "Soil and Land Biota Give, Not Take, CO_2." *Science News* 124;11 (Sept. 10,
1983): 166.
813. Simon, M, JD, MPH. "Dairy Industry Propaganda: A Tale of Two Mega-Campaigns."
www.vegan.com/issues/1999/apr99/dairyprop.htm.

814. Simon, M, JD, MPH. "Politics of Meat and Dairy." 1999.
      www.earthsave.org/news/polsmd.htm.
815. Simoons, F.J. "A Geographic Approach to Senile Cataracts: Possible Links With Milk
      Consumption, Lactase Activity, and Galactose Metabolism." *Digestive Diseases and
      Sciences* 27;3 (1982): 257-64.
816. Sims, L.S. *The Politics of Fat: Food and Nutrition Policy in America.* 1998.
817. Sinclair, A., and R. Gibson. "Essential Fatty Acids and Eicosanoids: Invited Papers
      From Third International Congress. The American Oil Chemists Society, Champaign
      (1992): 387.
818. Sinclair, W. "Block Warns of Crisis in Soil Erosion." The Washington Post, October 29,
      1981.
819. Singer, P. *Animal Liberation.* Avon Books (1975): 102.
820. Singh, I. "Low-Fat Diet and Therapeutic Doses of Insulin In Diabetes Mellitus." *Lancet*
      1 (1955): 422.
821. Slag, M. "Impotence in the Medical Clinic Outpatients." *JAMA* 249 (1983): 1736.
822. Smals, A.G.H., P.W.C. Kloppenborg, J. Benraad. Circannual Cycle In Plasma
      Testosterone Levels In Men." *Journal of Clinical Metabolism* 42 (1976): 979-82.
823. Smith P., and C. Daniel. *The Chicken Book.* Little, Brown, and Co: 51-124.
824. Smith, A.D.M. "Veganism: A Clinical Survey with Observations of Vitamin B_{12}
      Metabolism." *The British Medical Journal* 1 (June 16, 1962): 1655.
825. Smith, D. Howard. *Chinese Religions: from 1,000 B.C. to the Present Day.* New York:
      Holt, Rinehart, and Winston (1971): 11.
826. Smith, D.C. "Association of Exogenous Estrogen and Endometrial Carcinoma." *New
      England Journal of Medicine* 294 (1976): 1262.
827. Smith, D.M. "The Loss of Bone Mineral With Aging and Its Relationship to Hip
      Fracture." *Journal Clin Invest* 56 (1975): 311.
828. Smith, Dewaal Caroline. "Playing Chicken: The Human Cost of Inadequate Regulation
      of the Poultry Industry." Center for Science in the Public Interest (March 1996): 4.
829. Smith, Dr. Timothy J. *Renewal: The Anti-Aging Revolution.* "Defeating Free Radicals:
      The Key to Longevity." St Martins, November 1999.
830. Smith, Dr. Timothy, *Renewal: The Anti-Aging Revolution.* Chapter 1. Genetically
      Programmed Life Expectancy. St Martins Mass Market Paper. November 1999.
831. Smith, Gar. "Save the Tuna." *Earth Island Journal* (Fall 1994): 19.
832. Smith, Kirk, et al. "Quinolone-Resistent Campylobacter Jejuni Infections in Minnesota,
      1992-1998." *New England Journal of Medicine* 340 (1999): 1525-32.
833. Smith, M., and E. Elvove. "The Action of Irradiated Ergosterol in the Rabbit." *Public
      Health Reports* 44;21 (1929): 1248.
834. Smith, R. "Epidemiologic Studies of Osteoporosis In Women of Puerto Rico and
      Southeastern Michigan With Special Reference to Age, Race, National Origin and to
      Other Related or Associated Findings." *Clin Orthop* 45 (1966): 31.
835. Smith, R. Quoted in *Farm Journal* (Dec. 1973).
836. Smithsonian Institution. *Muse.* March '97. (Calculation: 12 million vegetarians of 280
      million Americans: 95 percent).
837. Snowdon, D. "Animal Product Consumption and Mortality Because of All Causes
      Combined: Coronary Heart Disease, Stroke, Diabetes, and Cancer in Seventh-Day
      Adventists." *American Journal of Clinical Nutrition* 48 (1988): 739-748.
838. Soler, M., C. Bosetti, S. Franceschi, et al. "Fiber Intake and the Risk of Oral,
      Pharyngeal and Esophageal Cancer." *Int J Cancer* 91 (2001): 283-7.
839. Solomon, L. "Osteoporosis and Fracture of the Femoral Neck in the South African
      Bantu. *J. Bone Joint Surg* 50B (1968): 2.

840. Solomon, L. "Rheumatic Disorders in the South African Negro. Part 1. Rheumatoid Arthritis and Ankylosing Spondylitis." *South Africa Medical Journal* 49 (1975): 1292.
841. *South Africa Medical Journal* 64 (1983): 552.
842. Spaulding, S.W., I.J. Chopra, R.S. Sherwin, S.S. Lyall. "Effect of Caloric Restriction and Dietary Composition on Serum T3 and Reverse T3 in Man." *Journal of Clinical Endocrinol Metabolism* 42 (1976): 197-200.
843. Spedding, C.R.W. "The Effect of Dietary Changes on Agriculture." B. Lewis and G. Assman, eds. *The Social and Economic Contexts of Coronary Prevention*. London: Current Medical Literature, 1990. (Cited in World Cancer Research Fund and American Institute for Cancer Research, *Food, Nutrition and the Prevention of Cancer: A Global Perspective* ,1997, p.557. Pimentel and Hall, *Food and Natural Resources*.)
844. Spence, J. "How We Use Plants." www.dur.ac.uk/~dbl0www/PUS/primuses.htm.
845. Spencer, Colin. "The Heretic's Feast, a History of Vegetarianism." 1996.
846. Spencer, J. "Hyperlipoproteinemias in the Etiology of Inner Ear Disease." *Laryngoscope* 85 (1973): 639.
847. Spencer, Vivian. *Raw Materials in the United States Economy 1900-1977*. Technical Paper 47, U.S. Dept. of Commerce, U.S. Dept of the Interior, Bureau of Mines: 3
848. Spock, Dr. Benjamin. *Dr. Spock's Baby and Child Care*. Pocket Books, June 1998.
849. Starch, Inra Hooper. *World Advertising Expenditures: A Survey of World Advertising Expenditures in 1985*. Mamaroneck, NY (1986): 5-10.
850. Stare, F. "Nutrition." *Annual Review of Biochemistry* 14 (1945): 431.
851. Stare, F. *Adventures in Nutrition*. Christopher Publishing, Hanover (1991): 23.
852. Starr, P. *The Social Transformation of American Medicine*. New York, Basic Books (1982): 98.
853. Staszewski, J. "Age at Menarche and Breast Cancer. *J. Natl Cancer Inst* 47 (1971): 935.
854. "State of the Planet, The." Climap. *Blue*. (April-May 2000): 67.
855. "State of the World." Worldwatch Institute, New York: Norton (1997): 105.
856. Stauffer, T. "Water: The Reason Israel Can't Give Up The West Bank." *Arlington Journal*. Jan. 27, 1982. Originally printed in Christian Science Monitor.
857. Stepaniak, Joanne, M.S.Ed. *The Vegan Sourcebook*. Lowell House, Los Angeles, 1998.
858. Stepaniak, Joanne, M.S.Ed., *Being Vegan*, Lowell House, Los Angeles, 2000.
859. Stocker, F.W., L.B. Holt, and J.W. Clower. "Clinical Experiments With New Ways of Influencing Intraocular Tension: I. Effect Of Rice Diet." *Arch Ophthalmol* 40 (1948): 46-55.
860. Strom, A. and R.A. Jensen. "Mortality from Circulatory Diseases in Norway, 1940-1945." *Lancet* 260 (1951): 126-129.
861. "Study Says Soil Erosion Could Cause Famine." *New York Times* (Sep 30, 1984): 20.
862. Supermarket Research. Nutrition Labels.
863. "Surveillance for Asthma: United States, 1960-1995." Morbidity and Mortality Weekly Report: CDC Surveillance Summaries 47 (1998).
864. Suzuki, David, and Holly Dressel. Quoted in *From Naked Ape to Super Species*. Toronto: Stoddart Publishing (1999): 59.
865. Suzuki, David. *The Sacred Balance: Rediscovering Our Place in Nature*. Vancouver, BC: Greystone Books (1997): 66.
866. Swank, R. "Changes in Blood Produced by a Fat Meal and by Intravenous Heparin." *American Journal of Physiology* 164;3 (1951): 798-811.
867. Swank, R. "Multiple Sclerosis: Twenty Years on a Low-Fat Diet." *Archives of Neurology*. 23 (1970): 460.
868. Swanson, D.R. "Migraine and Magnesium: Eleven Neglected Connections." *Perspectives in biology and medicine*. (Summer, 1988).

869. Swanson, Joy E., Cornell Cooperative extension (Q&A). "Antioxidant Nutrients." www.cce.cornell.edu/food/expfiles/topics/swanson/antioxidantsoverview.html.

870. Taik Lee, Kyu. "Chemicopathologic Studies...." *Archives of Internal Medicine* 109 (1962): 426.

871. Takacs, David. "Philosophies of Paradise." *The Johns Hopkins Univ. Press*. Baltimore, 1996.

872. Tannenbaum, A. and H. Silverstone. "The Genesis and Growth of Tumors. IV. Effects Of Varying the Proportion of Protein in the Diet." *Cancer Research* 9;3 (1949): 162.

873. Tanner, J.M. "Trend Towards Earlier Menarche in London, Oslo, Copenhagen, The Netherlands, and Hungary." *Nature* 243 (1973): 75-6.

874. Taylor, C.B. and S.K. Peng. "Vitamin D—Its excessive use in the USA." *Nutritional Elements and Clinical Biochemistry*. eds. M.A. Brewster and H.K. Naito, New York: Plenum (1980).

875. Teitel, Martin, and Kimberly Wilson. "Genetically Engineered Food: Changing the Nature of Nature." Rochester, V.T. *Park Street Press* (1999): 56.

876. *Tenth Annual Report of the Council on Environmental Quality, The*. "Environmental Quality—1979." Washington, D.C. (Dec. 1979).

877. "The Ugly Duckling Speaks Out About The Making Of Foie Gras." Eatveg.com. www.newveg.av.org/liverfat.htm.

878. Thimian, Bernie. "16 Reasons Why People Avoid Dairy Products." (1997). www.veg-giepower.ca/16reason.htm.

879. Thomson, G. "High Blood Pressure Diagnosis and Treatment: Consensus Recommendations Versus Actual Practice." *American Journal of Public Health* 71 (1981): 413.

880. *Thorax*. April 2000.

881. Thorogood, M., et al. "Plasma Lipids and Lipoprotein Cholesterol Concentrations in People With Different Diets in Britain." *British Medical Journal* 295 (1987): 351-353.

882. Thrash, A.M. and C.L. *Nutrition for Vegetarians*. Seale, Alabama: Tharsh Publications (1982): 68.

883. Tillman, DA. *Wood as an Energy Resource*. New York: Academic Press, 1978.

884. Tokuhata, G.K., W. Miller, E. Digon, T. Hartman. "Diabetes Mellitus: An Underestimated Public Health Problem." *Journal of Chronic Diseases* 28 (January 23, 1975).

885. Tolman, Jonathan. "Poisonous Runoff from Farm Subsidies." *Wall Street Journal* (Sept 8, 1995): A-10.

886. Topping, D.C. and W.J. Visek. "Nitrogen Intake and Tumorerigenesis in Rats Injected with 1,2-Dimethylhydrazine." *The Journal of Nutrition* 106 (1976): 1583.

887. Trentham, M.D., E. David, and H. Le Christine. "Relapsing Polychondritis Overview." *Ann Intern Med* 129 (1998): 114-122.

888. Tresl, Jacqueline, R.N., "High-Protein Diet Drawback: Stress —Too Much Protein Deprives You of Serotonin: The Body's Natural Chill Pill." www.theindychannel.com/sh/health/stressbusters/health-stressbusters-19991222-192048.html.

889. Trichopoulos, D. "Menopause and Breast Cancer Risk." *J. Natl Cancer Inst* 48 (1972): 605.

890. Triumph Prophetic Ministries (Church of God): "Did You Know?" www.hope-of-israel.org/thefirst.htm.

891. Trowell, H. "Dietary-Fiber Hypothesis of the Etiology of Diabetes Mellitus." *Diabetes* 24 (1975): 762.

892. Tuljapurkar, Shripad, Ph.D., Nan Li, Ph.D., and Carl Boe, Ph.D., at Mountain View Research, in Los Altos, California, Inc. Table 3: Fraction of total deaths attributable to selected causes, 1990. www.demko.com/m000801.htm.

893. U.S. Centers for Disease Control and Prevention.

894. U.S. Department of Agriculture 1994. (Cited in Vegan Orchard. www.essenes.cross-winds.net/vfacts.htm.)

894a. U.S. Department of Agriculture 1980. Appraisal: 50.

895. "U.S. Department of Agriculture Approves Rules for Meat Irradiation."

896. U.S. Department of Agriculture Economic Research Service. Provisions of the Food, Agriculture, Conservation, and Trade Act of 1990. *Agriculture Information Bulletin Number 624*, Washington (1991): vii.

897. U.S. Department of Agriculture Food Guide Pyramid. (Depicted in *Vegetarian Nutrition & Health Letter*, Loma Linda University, 4:3, March 2001.)

898. U.S. Department of Agriculture Handbook No. 456 "Nutritive Value of American Foods in Common Units." Protein Table, Seafood: 414.

899. U.S. Department of Agriculture History of Budgetary Expenditures of the Commodity Credit Corporation (FY 1990, 1991, Book 3): 2.

900. U.S. Department of Agriculture Statistics, 1989, United States Government Printing Office, Washington, DC, Table 623.

901. U.S. Department of Agriculture, Agricultural Handbook no. 8. Washington, D.C.: Government Printing Office, 1968.

902. U.S. Department of Agriculture, Economic Research Service. World Agricultural Supply and Demand Estimates, WASDE-256, Tables 256-6, -7, -16, -19. -23, World Bank, Poverty and Hunger. Washington DC: World Bank (1986): 24. Susan Oakie. "Health Crisis Confronts 1.3 Billion." *Washington Post* (September 25, 1989): A1.

903. U.S. Department of Agriculture, Economics and Statistics service. *Natural Resource Capital in U.S. Agriculture: Irrigation, Drainage and Conservation Investments Since 1900*. ESCS Staff Paper, March 1979.

904. U.S. Department of Agriculture. *Nutritive Value of American Foods*, Agricultural Handbook no. 456. Washington, D.C.: Government Printing Office, 1975.

905. U.S. Department of Health and Human Services, National Institute of Health "Surveillance, Epidemiology and End Results: Incidence and Mortality Data, 1973-1977." *National Cancer Institute*. Monograph 57, Bethesda, Maryland (June 1981): 4.

906. U.S. Department of Public Health and Human Services. "U.S. Surgeon General's Report on Nutrition and Health." Warner Books, 1989.

907. U.S. Environmental Protection Agency. (Cited in "Factory Farm Alarm," (2) www.earthsave.org/news/factfarm.htm).

908. U.S. Fish and Wildlife Service. "Survey on Hunting and Fishing." 1980.

909. U.S. General Accounting Office. Briefing Report to the Committee on Agriculture. "Animal Agriculture, Information on Waste Management and Water Quality Issues." GAO/RCED 95-200BR, Washington D.C., (1995): 58-61.

910. "U.S. Public Wrong About Dairy in Rest of the World." *The Dairy Express*. (Oct. 29, 1999): 6.

911. U.S. Renal Data System. USRDS 2001 Annual Data Report. Bethesda, MD: National Institute of Diabetes and Digestive and Kidney Diseases, National Institutes of Health (NIH), DHHS; 2001. www.kidneyetn.org/zframes-nkfetdisease.html.

912. U.S. Soil Conservation Services estimate. (Cited in Environmental Reasons for not Eating Animals www.pleasebekind.com/veg/enviro.htm).

913. U.S. Water Resources Council. "The Nation's Water Resources 1975-2000." Summary and Vol. 1. U.S. Govt. Print. Off., 1979. Washington, D.C.

914. Ullman, Dana. "Article on Homeopathy History." *Alternative Therapies*. (Sept. 1995): 13.

915. Ullman, Dana. "Chronic Fatigue Syndrome." *The One-Minute (or so) Healer*. www.innerself.com/Health/ullman_fatigue.htm.

916. Ullman, Dana. *Discovering Homeopathy*. Berkeley, CA, North Atlantic Books (1988): 40.

917. Ullman. Dana. *The One-Minute (or so) Healer*. Hay House, 2000.

918. Union of Concerned Scientists Press Release. "Seventy percent of all antibiotics given to healthy livestock." Jan, 8, 2001.

919. United Nations, International Year of the Ocean (YOTO). 1998 www.yoto98.noaa.gov/yoto/meeting/foreword.html.

920. United Press, "Food and Drug Administration: Meat Dye May Cause Cancer." *Washington Post*, Apr. 6, 1973.

921. Ursin, G., et al, "Milk Consumption And Cancer Incidence: A Norwegian Prospective Study." *British Journal of Cancer* 61 (1990): 454-459.

922. Useless Facts. www.geocities.com/gentryoraimo/uselessfacts.html.

923. Van, Z., and E.M. Bakker. "Paleobotanical Studies." *South African Journal of Science* 59 (1963) 332.

924. Vanderhaeghe, L.R., and J.D. Bouic. "The Immune System Cure." (1999): 194-195.

925. "Vegan From the Cradle: A Medical Doctor Explains Why an Animal-Free Diet for Babies Is His First Choice." *Vegetarian Times*, Sept. 1987.

926. Vegetarian Athletes: www.veggie.org/veggie/famous.veg.athletes.shtml. www.renewalresearch.com/book/the_case_against_a_carnivorous_diet.html. www.soystache.com/famousaz.htm. www.vegsource.com/articles/lewis_intro.htm. www.ivu.org/people/sports/index.html. www.efn.org/~goveg/articles.html.

927. Vegetarian Celebrities: www.soystache.com/famousaz.htm. www.ivu.org/people/sports/index.html. www.renewalresearch.com/book/the_case_against_a_carnivorous_diet.html.

928. "Vegetarian Diets for Children: Right from the Start." Physicians Committee for Responsible Medicine. www.pcrm.org/health/Info_on_Veg_Diets/veg_diets_for_children.html.

929. Vegetarian Society Information Sheet. Vitamin B12. www.vegsoc.org/info/b12.html.

930. Vegetarian Society: "Cheese & Rennet." www.vegsoc.org/info/cheese.html.

931. Vegetarian Society: "Vegetarian Nutrition for Children."_www.vegsoc.org/info/childre1.html.

932. *Vegetarian Times*. April 1998.

933. *Vegetarian Times*. July 1998.

934. Veldman, J.E. "The Immune System In Hearing Disorders." *Acta Otolaryngol Supple* 458 (1988): 67-75.

935. Vernia, P., M.R., Ricciardi, C. Frandina T. Bilotta, and G. Frieri. "Lactose Malabsorption and Irritable Bowel Syndrome. Effect of a Long-Term Lactose-Free Diet." *Ital J Gastroenterol* 27; 3 (Apr 1995): 117-121.

936. Virag, R. P. Bouilly, and D. Fryman. "Is Impotence an Arterial Disorder? A Study of Arterial Risk Factors In 440 Impotent Men." *Lancet* 1 (1985): 181-84.

937. Virato, "Reverence For Life," Sunday, June 24, 2001. www.veggieplace.com.

938. Vitamin and Mineral Complex Ingredients. www.herbshop.com/thy_vits.htm.

939. Vorherr, B. *Breast Cancer*. Baltimore: Urban & Schwarzenberg. 1980.

940. Vorman, Julie. "Feces, Vomit, On Raw Meat a Growing Risk." *Reuters News Service*. Sept. 6, 2000.

941. W.S.P.A. UK Advocates for Animals. www.advocatesforanimals.org.uk/foie_gras.htm.

942. Wachman, A. "Diet and Osteoporosis." *Lancet* 1 (1968): 958.

943. Walden, T.A., G.D. Foster, K.A. Letizzia, J.L. Mullin. "Long Term Effects of Dieting on Resting Metabolic Rate in Obese Outpatients." *JAMA* 190;264 (1990): 707-11.

944. Walker, A. "The human Requirement of Calcium: Should Low Intakes Be Supplemented?" *Am J. Clin Nutr* 25 (1972): 518.

945. Walker, A. "The Influence of Numerous Pregnancies and Lactations on Bone Dimensions in South African Bantu Women and Caucasian Mothers." *Clin Science* 42 (1972): 189.

946. Walker, R. "Calcium Retention in Adult Human Male as Affected by Protein Intake." *J. Nutr.* 102 (1972): 1297.

947. Walser, M. "Does Dietary Therapy Have a Role in the Predialysis Patient?" *American Journal of Clinical Nutrition* 33 (1980): 1629.

948. Walton, Eve Shatto, R.D., L.D.N. "Are You Getting Enough Iron, or Perhaps Too Much?" Vegetarian Resource Group, 1994. www.vrg.org/journal/iron.htm.

949. Warner, K. *Selling Smoke: Cigarette Advertising and Public Health.* Washington, DC: American Public Health Association (1986): 19.

950. *Water Quality at Vacation Beaches, A Guide to.* July 2002. www.nrdc.org/water/oceans/nttw.asp.

951. Watson, E.L.G. *Animals in Splendor.* Horizon Press (1967): 43-47.

952. Watson, R.R., R.H. Prabhala, D.E. Randall, M.Z. Nichaman, L.W. Pickle, and T.J. Mason. "The Effect Of Beta-Carotene On Lymphocyte Subpopulations In Elderly Humans: Evidence For A Dose-Response Relationship." *American Journal of Clinical Nutrition* 53 (1991): 90-94.

953. Weaver C.M., et al. "Dietary Calcium: Adequacy of a Vegetarian Diet." *American Journal of Clinical Nutrition* 59 (1994): 1238S-41S (suppl).

954. Weber, Gary. Statement made on *Oprah*: "What is fed to cattle...has been cooked at temperatures high enough to sterilize it." (Cited in Robbins, *Food Rev.*:149).

955. Weber, Peter. "Oceans in Peril." *E Magazine.* May-June 1994.

956. Wei, W.S., et al. *J Clin Epidemiol.* 47;8 (Aug 1994): 829-36.

957. Weiss, N., et al. "Increasing Incidence of Endometrial Cancer in the United States." *New England Journal of Medicine* 294;23 (1976): 1259.

958. Welch, C. "Cinecoronary Arteriography in Young Men." *Circulation* 42 (1970): 647.

959. West, K. *Epidemiology of Diabetes and Its Vascular Lesions.* New York: Elsevier (1978): 353-402.

960. "What Humans Owe to Animals." *Economist.* Aug. 19, 1995.

961. "What's Wrong With Fish?" *Vegetarian Times.* August 1995.

962. Whitaker, Julian. *Reversing Heart Disease.* New York, Warner Books (1985): 3-4.

963. "Why Be A Vegetarian?" Essene Nazarene Church of Mount Carmel. www.essene.com/Essene%20Teachings/Vegetarian.html.

964. Willeberg, P. "An International Perspective on Bovine Sommatotropin and Clinical Mastitis." *Journal of the American Veterinary Medical Assoc* 205;4 (1994): 538-41.

965. Willett, W., D. Hunter, et al. "Dietary Fat and Fiber in Relation to Risk of Breast Cancer: An Eight Year Follow-Up." *JAMA* 268;15 (1992): 2037-44.

966. Willett, Walter. Chairman of Nutrition Department—Harvard School of Public Health. Co-author of study (Cited in Robbins, *Food Revolution.*: 112).

967. Williams, G.M., B.S. Reddy, and J.H. Weisburger. "The Role of Metabolic Epidemiology and Laboratory Studies in the Etiology of Colon Cancer." *Advances in Medical Oncology, Research and Education* 3, *Epidemiology.* New York: Pergamon Press, 1979.

968. Williams, R. "The Trophic Value of Foods." Proceedings of the National Academy of Science 70; 3 (March, 1973): 710-713.

969. Williams, Ted. "Assembly Line Swine." *Audubon.* (March-April 1998): 27.

970. Wilson, E.O. "The Insect Societies." *Harvard University Press.* 1974.

971. Wilson, Edward O. "The Diversity of Life." Cambridge, MA: *Harvard University Press,* 1992.

972. Wilson, J. *Journal of Pediatrics* 84 (1974): 335.

973. Wilson, Robert. *Feminine Forever.* New York, David McKay, 1966.

974. Wokes, F., J. Badenoch, and H.M. Sinclair. "Human Dietary Deficiency of Vitamin B_{12}." *American Journal of Clinical Nutrition.* 3;5 (Sept-Oct. 1955): 375.

975. Wolfbauer, C.A. "Mineral Resources for Agricultural Use." *Agriculture and Energy,* William Lockeretz, ed., New York: Academic Press (1977): 301-14.

976. Wolfson, D. *Beyond the Law: Agribusiness and Systemic Abuse of Animals Raised for Food or Food production.* Farm Sanctuary (1999): 48, 51.

977. Wolinsky, H. and T. Brune. *The Serpent on the Staff: The Unhealthy Politics of the American Medical Association.* New York: Tarcher/Putnam (1994).

978. "Women With Hearing Loss May Benefit By Boning Up on Calcium." *Environmental Nutr* (Oct. 1998): 8.

979. "Women's Information About Menopause is Limited." North American Menopause Society. Sept 4, 1993.

980. Woolf, Jim. "Have Hogs Caused Milford Maladies?" *Salt Lake Tribune.* Jan 26, 2000.

981. World Alzheimer's Congress, July 2000. (Studies from 1993 and 1999 cited in www.vegsource.com/articles/alzheimers_homocysteine.htm. "Alzheimers: Losing Your Mind for the Sake of a Burger." Jeff Nelson).

982. World Cancer Research Fund and American Institute for Cancer Research. *Food, Nutrition and the Prevention of Cancer: A Global Perspective* (1997): 509.

983. World Conservation Union, The: Conservation International. "Red List of Threatened Species." September 8, 2000. www.ecocities.net/Article16.html.

984. World Conservation Union, The: List of Threatened Species.

985. World Health Organization Press Release. "World Health Organization Meeting on the Medical Impact of the Use of Anti-microbial Drugs in Food Animals. Berlin, Germany, Oct. 4, 1997," (October 20, 1997).

986. World Health Organization, Press Release. "WHO Issues New Healthy Life Expectancy Rankings." Washington, D.C., and Geneva, Switzerland. June 4, 2000.

987. World Health Organization. *World Health Statistics Annual.* Geneva 1989.

988. *World Health Statistics Annual,* FAO Production Yearbook. (Tables: Harris, *Scientific Basis:* 52-65).

989. *World News Tonight* Segment, May 31, 1999. www.vegan.com/issues/1999/sep99/pcrm.htm.

990. World Resources Institute, The. "World Resources, 1990-91: A Guide to the Global Environment." *Oxford University Press* (1990): 268.

991. Worldwatch Institute. *Vital Signs.* New York: Norton (1996): 108.

992. Worldwatch Institute's *State of the World* 1997 (Chapter Four): 64.

993. Wynder, E. "The Dietary Environment and Cancer." *Journal of American Dietetic Assoc* 71 (1977): 385-92.

994. Wynder, E., et al. "Breast Cancer Weighing the Evidence for a Promoting Role of Dietary Fat." *Journal of the National Cancer Institute* 89 (1997): 766-75.

995. Wynder, E., et al. "Tobacco Smoking as a Possible Etiologic Factor in Bronchogenic Carcinoma." *Journal of the American Medical Association* (May 1950): 329-338.

996. Yasugi, T., T. Tochihara, T. Fujioka, et al. "Eicosopentanoic Acid, Docosahexanoic Acid and Cerebral Hemorrhage: EPA and DHA Loading Study in Spontaneously Hyperactive Rats." *Am. J. of Cardio* 71;11 (1993): 916-20.

997. Young, Don., and Kerry O'Banion. University of Rochester. (Cited in Age Venture News Service. www.demko.com/m981116.htm#two).

998. YourDoctor, Inc. 1998. www.breastdoctor.com/breast/mammogram/cancer.htm.

999. Zahradnik, F. "EPA Suppresses Rural Water Study." *The New Farm.* Jan. 1984.

1000. Zeil, H. "Increased Risk of Endometrial Carcinoma..." *New England Journal of Medicine* 293 (1975): 1167.

1001. Zemel, M.B. "Calcium Utilization: Effect of Varying Level and Source of Dietary Protein." *Am J. Clin Nutr* 48 (1988): 880-83.

REFERENCES

(BRACKETED NUMBERS CORRESPOND TO BIBLIOGRAPHY)

Introduction, "The Diet Has Chosen Us." 1[836], 2[836], 3[463, 547 p.154], 4[425], 5[326].

Chapter 1 Introduction, "Evidence." 1[379 p.26], 2[892].

1. Scientific Evidence: 1[425].

2. Evolution: 1[425], 2[425], 3[425, 845, 379 p.18], 4[379 p.12], 5[425, 379 p.16], 6[425, 183], 7[425], 8[650].

3. Anatomy: 1[82 p.170], 2[426], 3[197], 4[750 pp.258-259], 5[664 p.144], 6[139].

4. Dieting: 1[464, 379 p.26], 2[379 p.98], 3[662, 588 p.219, 81 p.61], 4[81p.61, 301], 5[81 p.95], 6[496], 7[943, 308], 8[588 p.219], 9[259, 774, 375, 258, 593].

5. Studies: 1[81 p.60], 2[295], 3[443], 4[966], 5[156], 6[274], 7[820, 78, 45], 8[541], 9[373], 10[369], 11[240, 462, 459, 188], 12[81 p.44], 13[33 p.1223], 14[33 p.1214], 15[162, 965], 16[836].

6. Countries and Cultures: 1[987, 988], 2[409], 3[488, 155], 4[992], 5[746], 6[1], 7[587], 8[840, 94, 90], 9[754], 10[316], 11[750 p.280], 12[31 p.741-745], 13[750 p.154].

7. Degenerative and Infectious Disease: 1[892], 2[906], 3[666], 4[631], 5[217, 709], 6[194], 7[986], 8[418].

8. Nature: 1[662, 588 p.219, 81 p.61, 305, 904, 532, 662], 2[943, 308], 3[95, 301, 662, 727], 4[379 p.12], 5[463, 547], 6[425], 7[326], 8[428], 9[81 pp.29-30, 830], 10[249, 295, 443], 11[588 p.185-187], 12[751 pp.238-240], 13[873, 762, 439, 342], 14[751 pp.136-155], 15[796], 16[777], 17[474].

Chapter 2 Introduction, "Plants." 1[664], 2[359, 379 p.12], 3[554], 4[544], 5[443, 394].

9. Carbohydrates: 1[588 p.219], 2[662, 588 p.219, 81 p.86, 95, 301, 727], 3[81 pp.110-111, 842, 574, 583], 4[583, 588 p.219, 134, 351, 29], 5[583], 6[574, 229], 7[81 pp.110-111], 8[81 p.71, 750 p.256, 688], 9[134], 10[535], 11[662, 588 p.219, 81 p.61 p.86, 305, 904, 532], 12[664].

10. Vitamins: 1[568], 2[624], 3[624], 4[359], 5[538], 6[349, 625, 538], 7[844], 8[379 p.12], 9[430], 10[450, 752 p.83], 11[752 p.91], 12[784, 874].

11. Calcium: 1[737], 2[576], 3[294], 4[944, 527, 304, 286], 5[1001], 6[398, 44, 946, 453, 533], 7[375, 313, 151, 158, 452], 8[839, 944, 945, 840], 9[567], 10[558], 11[639], 12[9], 13[811], 14[1], 15[81 p.144], 16[28], 17[662, 588 p.219, 81 p.61 p.86, 305, 904, 532].

12. Iron: 1[517], 2[778], 3[517], 4[780], 5[305, 904], 6[305, 904, 857], 7[857], 8[517, 445], 9[517, 445], 10[841, 30(51:1990)], 11[30(49:1989, 30(53:1991)], 12[517], 13[445], 14[445].

13. Immune System: 1[783], 2[905], 3[750 p.329], 4[630], 5[544], 6[255], 7[553], 8[89], 9[89], 10[89], 11[89], 12[89], 13[89], 14[89], 15[667, 458], 16[938], 17[938], 18[938], 19[938], 20[554], 21[505], 22[433, 62], 23[753, 481, 43, 867], 24[689, 621], 25[517, 778, 780], 26[160].

14. Antioxidants and Phytochemicals: 1[544], 2[544], 3[544], 4[81 p.5], 5[544], 6[652, 315, 241], 7[869].

15. Athletes: 1[664 p.19], 2[98, 653, 675, 125], 3[329], 4[904], 5[546, 693], 6[24], 7[295, 443], 8[443], 9[791], 10[926, 750 p.158-163, 752 pp. 78-79].

16. Children: 1[904], 2[30(51:1990), 841], 3[81 p.60], 4[567], 5[387], 6[387], 7[430], 8[81 p.159], 9[394], 10[394], 11[786], 12[394], 13[433], 14[925], 15[307], 16[208, 918], 17[68], 18[873], 19[11, 517, 778, 872], 20[608], 21[101], 22[192], 23[848], 24[931].

17. Vitamin B_{12}: 1[929], 2[242], 3[857 p.216], 4[752 p.91], 5[242], 6[242 p.1], 7[715], 8[32], 9[441], 10[242], 11[242], 12[220, 210, 185], 13[30], 14[882, 509], 15[5 p.35, 81 pp.156], 16[242], 17[242 p.3], 18[242 p.1], 19[332], 20[664 p.151], 21[259, 974, 824].

18. Varieties and Flavors: (None).

Chapter 3 Introduction, "Meat and Dairy." (None).

19. Beef: 1[514 pp.69 p.445-6, 843, 904], 2[513], 3[902], 4[379 p.98, 371], 5[821], 6[366], 7[295], 8[547 p.136].

20. Pork: 1[423, 53], 2[571], 3[14], 4[898], 5[699], 6[514 p.435, 262], 7[199], 8[368], 9[687], 10[739], 11[876, 660, 804], 12[96], 13[522], 14[677], 15[718].

21. Chicken and Fish: 1[662, 588 p.219, 81 p.61 p.86], 2[700], 3[700], 4[700], 5[145], 6[156], 7[662], 8[898], 9[886, 939, 122, 567, 433, 62], 10[828, 144, 367], 11[93], 12[447, 961], 13[961], 14[961, 569], 15[996], 16[221, 961], 17[81 p.100], 18[93, 14].

22. Milk: 1[857], 2[972], 3[661], 4[878 No.12], 5[878 No.9], 6[293], 7[481], 8[370], 9[66, 433, 62], 10[589], 11[737], 12[944, 527, 304, 286], 13[966], 14[211], 15[177, 190, 374], 16[757], 17[391], 18[224], 19[221], 20[319], 21[815, 209], 22[444], 23[878 No.3], 24[567], 25[898], 26[92], 27[92, 374], 28[833, 857 p.223], 29[521], 30[752p.100], 31[81 p.104], 32[222, 898].

23. Dairy Products: 1[894], 2[930], 3[898], 4[193], 5[193], 6[226, 994], 7[340], 8[898], 9[575], 10[935], 11[930], 12[70], 13[586], 14[898], 15[211], 16[922], 17[898], 18[262], 19[129], 20[81 p.159, 397, 588 p.219], 21[964], 22[737], 23[430].

24. Eggs: 1[664 p.48], 2[901, 203], 3[203], 4[898], 5[81 p.37, 145, 625], 6[773], 7[661], 8[857 p.191-193].

25. Cholesterol and Fat: 1[588 p.102] 2[625, 145], 3[625, 532], 4[662, 588 p.219, 81 p.61 p.86, 305, 904, 532], 5[753, 625, 145, 662, 588 p.219, 81 p.61], 6[81 p.104], 7[590 pp.66-7, 297, 774], 8[81 pp.34-5, 26], 9[275, 81 p.64], 10[898], 11[699], 12[583], 13[464, 379 p.26, 730], 14[379 p.26], 15[488, 155], 16[82 p.15], 17[519], 18[195], 19[111, 201].

Chapter 4 Introduction, "Contaminants." 1[355], 2[465, 832, 296].

26. Antibiotics: 1[355], 2[355], 3[514 p.135], 4[92], 5[296], 6[296], 7[832], 8[170], 9[339], 10[296], 11[918, 465, 832, 296], 12[417, 752 p.140], 13[485], 14[985], 15[170], 16[10], 17[130].

27. Hormones: 1[787], 2[632], 3[875, 618], 4[177, 190], 5[374], 6[330], 7[473], 8[497], 9[430, 874, 491], 10[277], 11[664 p.35], 12[664 p.35], 13[664 p.35], 14[665], 15[364], 16[419], 17[278].

28. Pesticides: 1[164], 2[991], 3[703], 4[419], 5[739], 6[415], 7[180], 8[208, 918, 343, 654], 9[268], 10[702], 11[876, 660, 804], 12[750 p.329], 13[508, 128], 14[651], 15[268], 16[649, 528], 17[654, 402], 18[649, 528], 19[741], 20[551], 21[378], 22[739].

29. Food Poisoning: 1[893], 2[311], 3[92, 339], 4[828, 144, 367], 5[306], 6[81 p.135], 7[678], 8[93, 81 p,135], 9[378], 10[598, 482], 11[895, 599], 12[307], 13[311], 14[169, 170], 15[169, 170], 16[282], 17[785], 18[290], 19[290], 20[597].

30. Mad Cow Disease: 1[547 p.84], 2[547 p.84], 3[196], 4[50], 5[489, 547 p.96], 6[547 p.84], 7[547 p.97], 8[489], 9[489], 10[489], 11[550], 12[489], 13[489], 14[489, 181], 15[814], 16[489], 17[489, 219], 18[954, 489 p.9], 19[547 p.96, 489 p.13], 20[752 p.145-6], 21[534], 22[561, 547 p.87], 23[489 p.9, 547 p.94].

31. Meat Inspection: 1[174, 378], 2[828, 144, 367], 3[828 p.2, 93], 4[543], 5[752 p.118], 6[752 p.118], 7[752 p.118], 8[311 p.258], 9[752 p.136], 10[324], 11[232], 12[940], 13[600, 75], 14[289, 562], 15[562], 16[600], 17[438], 18[353], 19[353], 20[75], 21[920].

Chapter 5 Introduction, "Animals." (None).

32. The Cow: 1[466], 2[466, 88], 3[857 p.37], 4[835], 5[87, 787, 570], 6[960], 7[379 p.12], 8[309, 41 pp.34-35], 9[231], 10[750 p.40], 11[750 p.108], 12[937].

33. The Pig : 1[571], 2[423], 3[389], 4[750 p.29], 5[951], 6[787], 7[752 p.199].

34. The Chicken: 1[572], 2[951], 3[823], 4[287], 5[287], 6[287], 7[287], 8[287], 9[287], 10[287], 11[287], 12[951], 13[951, 474, 823 p.160], 14[287, 246], 15[287], 16[287], 17[287], 18[421], 19[637], 20[819], 21[722], 22[819 p.97 p.112, 570 pp.56-58], 23[657], 24[287, 750 p.54], 25[960].

35. Animal Intelligence: 1[287], 2[701], 3[51], 4[740], 5[287], 6[287], 7[41 p.18], 8[512], 9[772], 10[750 p.43], 11[750 p.37, 970], 12[310], 13[41 p.12], 14[750 p.39].

36. Vegan: 1[629], 2[769].

37. Factory Farms: 1[283], 2[283], 3[284, 570 p.29-30 p.48-49 p.72, 721, 245], 4[245], 5[269, 311, 8], 6[63], 7[289, 562], 8[174], 9[67], 10[76], 11[136, 137, 758, 540], 12[909], 13[570 p.5 p.6-8 p.76, 721], 14[968].

38. Veal and Foie Gras: 1[752 p.183], 2[153], 3[750 pp.114-117], 4[750 pp.114-117], 5[74], 6[74, 941], 7[877].

39. Hunting: 1[565], 2[97], 3[565], 4[857 p.77], 5[857 p.78], 6[565], 7[782], 8[908, 579], 9[565], 10[857 p.74], 11[857 p.74-75], 12[106], 13[857 p.80].

Chapter 6 Introduction, "The Environment." 1[76], 2[664 pp.78-9], 3[4], 4[919], 5[428], 6[114].

40. Water Depletion: 1[132], 2[856], 3[77], 4[902, 894a], 5[76], 6[15], 7[131], 8[514 p.69, 71], 9[71], 10[865], 11[865], 12[865], 13[131, 752 p.238, 913], 14[664 p.78, 743], 15[115, 792], 16[76], 17[116, 752 p.240].

41. Energy Depletion: 1[664 pp.78-9, 432], 2[514, 664 p.78], 3[429], 4[759, 547 p.125], 5[336], 6[752 p.214], 7[711, 904], 8[904, 713], 9[847], 10[429], 11[664 pp.78-9].

42. Soil Depletion: 1[697], 2[28], 3[422], 4[133, 490, 431], 5[247], 6[912, 516], 7[431], 8[514 p.81], 9[855], 10[818, 714a], 11[861], 12[28], 13[28], 14[603, 975, 331], 15[5 p.121], 16[207, 923, 189].

43. The Land: 1[990], 2[5 p.92], 3[5 p.92], 4[300], 5[326, 5 p.125], 6[5 p.84], 7[428, 454, 894a], 8[449], 9[513], 10[449], 11[627], 12[712], 13[4], 14[449], 15[752 p.283, 894a], 16[146], 17[843], 18[5 p.89], 19[5 p.89], 20[5 p.94, 513, 247], 21[5 p.86], 22[736], 23[612, 800], 24[399], 25[710], 26[371].

44. The Oceans: 1[919], 2[671], 3[919], 4[671], 5[955], 6[643], 7[885], 8[919, 775], 9[919], 10[442, 524], 11[442], 12[285], 13[955], 14[776], 15[524], 16[524, 755], 17[776], 18[831], 19[755], 20[919], 21[919], 22[670], 23[919], 24[919], 25[919], 26[919], 27[919, 483].

45. The Forests: 1[691, 628, 233, 428, 454], 2[627], 3[750 pp.363-4], 4[228], 5[135, 812], 6[752 p.255], 7[883], 8[428].

46. Animal Waste: 1[336], 2[510], 3[282], 4[655], 5[771], 6[523], 7[656], 8[743 No.2], 9[266], 10[352, 52], 11[52], 12[907], 13[247], 14[114], 15[547 p.129, 292, 969, 19], 16[52], 17[76], 18[526], 19[909], 20[909], 21[980], 22[511, 999], 23[854], 24[127, 363], 25[114].

47. Species Extinction: 1[338, 971], 2[871], 3[77 p.57], 4[752 p.234 p.270], 5[167], 6[363], 7[983], 8[864], 9[596, 983], 10[723, 871], 11[77 p.27], 12[77 p.27], 13[871], 14[581], 15[581], 16[864].

Chapter 7 Introduction, "Disease: Killers." 1[274, 679, 681], 2[520], 3[165], 4[299, 346], 5[641].

48. Heart Disease: 1[26], 2[408], 3[860], 4[265, 195], 5[750 p.215], 6[488], 7[870, 385], 8[566], 9[82 p.33-4], 10[82 p.15], 11[590 p.66-7, 297, 774], 12[274, 679, 681], 13[274], 14[235].

49. Atherosclerosis: 1[312], 2[602], 3[588 p.101], 4[416], 5[881], 6[881], 7[265], 8[958, 686], 9[591], 10[588 pp.115–118], 11[61], 12[680, 501, 846], 13[588 p.119], 14[525, 5 p.63, 81 p.48, 82 pp.33-4, 588 p.106, 166].

50. Hypertension: 1[477, 587 pp.203-230, 279], 2[559, 520], 3[536], 4[217, 709], 5[239], 6[590], 7[49], 8[478, 577, 709, 120, 479, 879], 9[216], 10[774], 11[768], 12[676], 13[351], 14[500], 15[590 p.213], 16[803], 17[316], 18[588 p.174].

51. Prostate Cancer: 1[23], 2[760], 3[81 p.71], 4[81 p.71], 5[537], 6[706], 7[391, 471], 8[738], 9[987, 301], 10[124], 11[124], 12[707], 13[587 p.6], 14[171], 15[172], 16[165].

52. Colon Cancer: 1[987, 988], 2[299, 346], 3[198], 4[967, 401, 406], 5[750 p.256], 6[139, 664 p.xix], 7[993, 214], 8[346], 9[669].

53. Breast Cancer: 1[698], 2[23], 3[998, 555, 588 p.32], 4[588 pp.31-33], 5[588 pp.31-33], 6[472], 7[663, 147], 8[272], 9[492, 162, 965], 10[350, 342], 11[341], 12[475, 320, 59, 407, 853, 889], 13[470], 14[987, 988], 15[409], 16[469].

54. Ovarian Cancer: 1[335], 2[335], 3[341, 504], 4[341], 5[837, 747, 809], 6[921], 7[211], 8[503], 9[503], 10[809], 11[761], 12[468], 13[467], 14[837], 15[334], 16[475, 320, 59, 407, 853, 889], 17[987, 988], 18[502].

55. Cancers: 1[23], 2[630], 3[382], 4[642, 468, 504], 5[614, 939, 60], 6[614, 60], 7[60], 8[381, 799], 9[215], 10[327], 11[460], 12[956], 13[109], 14[549, 1000, 826], 15[838], 16[781], 17[704], 18[58], 19[448], 20[720], 21[794], 22[384], 23[345, 719].

56. Diabetes: 1[884], 2[634], 3[866], 4[224, 323, 805], 5[724], 6[47, 615, 749], 7[48], 8[820, 78, 45], 9[959, 484, 746, 891], 10[481], 11[634], 12[634], 13[634], 14[634], 15[634].

57. Kidney Disease: 1[672], 2[270], 3[641], 4[811], 5[641], 6[911], 7[911], 8[911], 9[95, 301, 662, 727], 10[122], 11[122], 12[811], 13[230, 756], 14[236], 15[148, 779], 16[486], 17[947], 18[884, 588 p.255], 19[487], 20[766], 21[83].

58. Aging: 1[829], 2[894, 200], 3[830], 4[463], 5[81 p.9], 6[617], 7[544], 8[544], 9[362], 10[815, 209], 11[451], 12[829], 13[810], 14[829], 15[829], 16[829], 17[829], 18[100, 27], 19[765 p.11].

59. Alzheimer's disease: 1[616], 2[613], 3[616], 4[725], 5[981], 6[456], 7[997], 8[616], 9[457], 10[493], 11[674, 318], 12[829], 13[735], 14[735], 15[234].

Chapter 8 Introduction, "Disease: Hardships." (None).

60. Osteoporosis: 1[588 p.64], 2[542], 3[827], 4[564], 5[588 p.64, 639, 9, 453], 6[304, 286, 578], 7[578, 942, 84], 8[580], 9[737], 10[588 p.74], 11[588 p.74], 12[587 p.67], 13[576], 14[944, 945], 15[834], 16[34], 17[694, 224, 953, 375, 313, 151, 158,452], 18[588 p.69], 19[801], 20[257, 910].

61. Endometriosis: 1[264], 2[2], 3[263, 658], 4[658 p.166], 5[2], 6[617], 7[143], 8[341], 9[341], 10[2], 11[415], 12[81 p.129, 288, 184, 915, 692, 529], 13[81 p.128, 924, 952, 89, 544, 553], 14[263], 15[143].

62. Hearing Loss: 1[424], 2[424], 3[420], 4[978], 5[34], 6[420], 7[613], 8[616], 9[616], 10[717, 376, 934], 11[590], 12[590], 13[590], 14[424].

63. Vision Loss: 1[891], 2[209], 3[328, 56], 4[517], 5[451], 6[518], 7[281, 495], 8[728, 554], 9[56], 10[797, 159], 11[635], 12[557], 13[644], 14[859].

64. Impotence, Infertility, Hair Loss: 1[366], 2[936], 3[685], 4[821, 366, 936], 5[685], 6[325], 7[21], 8[7], 9[987, 301 p.127], 10[372], 11[733, 822], 12[436].

65. Hemorrhoids, Hernia, Appendicitis: 1[139], 2[139], 3[967, 401, 406], 4[81p.131], 5[141], 6[138], 7[138, 793, 932], 8[142], 9[253],10[81 p.131].

66. Ulcers, Crohn's, Diverticulitis: 1[917], 2[304, 286, 578, 444], 3[607, 413], 4[36], 5[176], 6[213], 7[182], 8[403], 9[31], 10[390, 40], 11[390], 12[726], 13[688].

67. Autoimmune Diseases: 1[110], 2[110, 753, 481, 531, 494, 840, 94, 90, 28, 73, 187], 3[260], 4[379 p.45-50], 5[322], 6[187], 7[121, 186], 8[161], 9[178, 798], 10[57], 11[455], 12[887].

68. Asthma: 1[863, 38, 173, 638, 640], 2[42], 3[348], 4[103], 5[910], 6[683], 7[66, 433, 62], 8[66], 9[880], 10[455], 11[54], 12[37], 13[648], 14[544, 81 p.5, 554], 15[322], 16[705, 684], 17[379 p.45-50], 18[110].

69. Childhood Illnesses: 1[661, 817], 2[293], 3[781, 704], 4[536], 5[433, 62, 795], 6[750 p.329], 7[750 p.329], 8[249], 9[880], 10[68], 11[928], 12[307], 13[416, 881], 14[962], 15[317], 16[20], 17[169], 18[786], 19[358], 20[320, 59, 407, 853, 889], 21[101, 931].

70. Fatigued: 1[357], 2[81 p.129], 3[81 p.129, 288], 4[81 p.128], 5[917], 6[750 p.297, 446], 7[584], 8[139, 356], 9[184, 915], 10[924, 288, 952], 11[244], 12[692, 529], 13[739], 14[584 p.222-3, 676].

71. Food and Behavior: 1[894, 200], 2[987, 301 pp.124-127], 3[987, 301pp.124-127], 4[987, 301 pp.124-127], 5[218], 6[620, 868], 7[888], 8[400], 9[383], 10[383, 180], 11[507], 12[273], 13[405], 14[157], 15[573], 16[218], 17[81 p.158], 18[218].

Chapter 9 Introduction, "Religion." (None).

72. Dominion: 1[636], 2[636], 3[890], 4[202].

73. The Bible: 1[770 p.87], 2[770 p.92], 3[770 pp.89-90], 4[789], 5[392, 254].

74. God: (None)

75. Jesus: 1[732], 2[789], 3[107], 4[276], 5[770 p.87], 6[539], 7[770 p.87].

76. Religions: 1[808 2[789], 3[732], 4[152], 5[206 p.75], 6[392, 254], 7[204 pp.226-227], 8[191], 9[480], 10[414], 11[205], 12[6], 13[6], 14[6], 15[6], 16[6], 17[476], 18[765 p.2, 5 p.178], 19[825].

77. Global Hunger: 1[326], 2[514 p.69 pp.445-6], 3[513, 247], 4[5 p.136].

Chapter 10 Introduction, "Manipulation." 1[64], 2[734].

78. Protein: 1[850], 2[397], 3[585], 4[764], 5[302], 6[95], 7[303], 8[314 p.165], 9[301], 10[240], 11[240], 12[662, 904], 13[69], 14[589 p.99], 15[592, 379 p.43], 16[387 p.16], 17[886, 939, 122, 567, 433, 62, 753, 481, 43, 867, 365, 31], 18[664 pp.47-48, 894], 19[752 p.71], 20[682], 21[763], 22[95, 767, 280, 499, 806, 807], 23[664 p.36], 24[347], 25[314].

79. Food Guide Pyramid: 1[897], 2[33], 3[906, 463], 4[626, 814], 5[814], 6[13, 404], 7[404, 851], 8[857 p.56, 626], 9[626], 10[626], 11[816], 12[816], 13[897], 14[708], 15[105], 16[897].

80. Beef Trade Associations: 1[91], 2[112], 3[163], 4[39], 5[601], 6[601], 7[461], 8[682], 9[168, 601], 10[252, 673], 11[547 p.16], 12[646], 13[933], 14[731].

81. Dairy Council: 1[989], 2[813], 3[701], 4[966, 706, 391], 5[435], 6[857 p.222, 661, 481, 66, 422, 62, 878], 7[989], 8[386, 250], 9[925, 589], 10[563, 989], 11[737], 12[645], 13[563], 14[645], 15[1001, 397, 44, 946, 453, 533, 375, 151, 158, 452, 839, 944, 945, 840].

82. School Donations: 1[243, 750 pp.129-130], 2[380], 3[750 p.131], 4[25], 5[25], 6[633], 7[552, 904], 8[385 p.207], 9[899], 10[552], 11[790], 12[386], 13[659], 14[790], 15[790], 16[790], 17[433, 62, 925], 18[786], 19[790].

83. Government Subsidies: 1[427], 2[410, 896], 3[545], 4[118], 5[903, 714, 102], 6[440,251], 7[900, 899], 8[291], 9[118], 10[117], 11[814], 12[261], 13[379 p.66, 906].

84. Advertising: 1[28], 2[38], 3[849], 4[412, 729], 5[434], 6[39], 7[814], 8[752 p.83], 9[752 p.83], 10[305, 898], 11[862], 12[3], 13[849], 14[610], 15[588 pp. 8-9], 16[588 pp. 8-9, 81 p.86].

85. Illness-Care: 1[544], 2[666, 584 pp.223-4], 3[631], 4[217, 709], 5[472], 6[194], 7[418], 8[986], 9[892].

86. Pharmaceutical Industry: 1[595, 79, 594], 2[918, 832, 296], 3[556], 4[588 p.5, 65], 5[742], 6[217, 709], 7[590 pp. 222-3], 8[316], 9[48, 820, 78, 45], 10[959], 11[748, 751 p.161], 12[321], 13[631, 716], 14[345], 15[554], 16[630], 17[337], 18[337], 19[488].

87. Medical profession: 1[179, 154], 2[345], 3[977, 437], 4[256 p.153], 5[256 p.154, 611], 6[72, 298, 22], 7[914, 916], 8[852], 9[977 pp.128-129], 10[333], 11[589 p.7], 12[588 p.254], 13[274, 344], 14[16], 15[81p.145], 16[949], 17[695], 18[977 p.145], 19[995], 20[977 pp.148-150], 21[619], 22[377], 23[696, 977 p.158], 24[17, 18], 25[126].

88. Cancer Business: 1[751 p.229], 2[99], 3[751 p.229], 4[150], 5[734], 6[321], 7[788], 8[588 pp.6-7], 9[588 pp.6-7, 998, 555, 588 p.32], 10[622], 11[588 p.6], 12[86], 13[345], 14[411, 745], 15[623], 16[321], 17[982, 382], 18[99], 19[12], 20[99], 21[85], 22[751 p.270], 23[271].

89. Menopause: 1[337, 81 p.44, 227, 582, 973, 658 p.434], 2[337], 3[979], 4[194], 5[360, 194], 6[751 p.151], 7[957, 227 p.214], 8[104, 606], 9[743 No.93], 10[337], 11[227], 12[751 p.147], 13[361, 609], 14[658 p.434].

Chapter 11 Introduction, "Insight." (None).

90. Our Children: (None).

91. Freedom: 1[903, 714, 102, 440, 251, 900, 899, 291, 119, 117, 814, 261, 379 p.66, 906], 2[903], 3[127], 4[379 p.98, 371], 5[149], 6[912, 516], 7[627].

92. Psychology: (None).

93. Society: (None).

94. Meat and Tobacco: 1[995, 385 p.28 p.196], 2[750 p.218, 836], 3[949], 4[408], 5[750 p.150], 6[995], 7[385 p.28 p.196], 8[750 p.218, 836].

95. Death Statistics: 1[174], 2[906], 3[418], 4[830], 5[668, 590 p.211], 6[666, 690, 354], 7[588 pp.6-7], 8[905], 9[751 p.270], 10[554], 11[272], 12[382], 13[174], 14[175].

96. Doctors: (None).

97. U.S. Rankings: 1[751 p.3], 2[395, 396], 3[140], 4[751 p.3], 5[498, 530], 6[587 p.67], 7[751 p.3], 8[751 p.370], 9[976], 10[832], 11[463], 12[836], 13[450], 14[93], 15[108], 16[910], 17[346], 18[988], 19[80], 20[988], 21[707], 22[987, 301].

243[662, 588 p.219, 81 p.61, 305, 904, 532, 662], 244[379 p.12], 245[337], 246[464, 379 p.26], 247[379 p.98], 248[662, 588 p.219, 81 p.61], 249[81 p.95], 250[662, 588 p.219, 81 p.86, 95, 301, 727], 251[259, 774, 375, 258, 593], 252[295], 253[443], 254[791], 255[443], 256[98, 653, 675, 125], 257[664], 258[750 p.158-163], 259[664 pp.78-9], 260[752 p.214, 711, 904], 261[514 p.69, 71], 262[127, 363], 263[691, 628, 233, 428, 454], 264[912, 516], 265[449], 266[919], 267[167], 268[871], 269[636], 270[636, 890], 271[287], 272[596, 983], 273[106], 274[514 pp.69 p.445-6, 843, 904], 275[513, 247], 276[326, 5 p.136], 277[82 p.33-4, 299, 346, 382, 617], 278[836], 279[927], 280[906, 892, 179, 154, 556, 321], 281[33 p.1223 p.1214], 282[266, 168, 601, 252, 673, 488, 386, 250, 742], 283[412, 729], 284[547 p.16, 610], 285[463], 286[630], 287[906], 288[174], 289[986, 751 p.3], 290[371], 291[830], 292[750 p.154], 293[765 p.11], 294[373], 295[750 p.154].

INDEX

505

carbohydrates, 75
endurance tests, 76
world-class vegetarian athletes, 76
Autoimmune Diseases, 273-276
a story, 274
Americans affected, 273
animal proteins, 275
cause unknown, 273
Colonel Otto M. Yune, 274
examples of, 275
number of autoimmune diseases, 273

Beef, 94-97
economics, 96
environment, 96
global hunger, 96
health, 95
image, 97
properties, 95
three definitions, 94
Beef Trade Associations, 333-336
annual beef revenue, 333
educational aids, 333
food slander laws, 334
media police, 335
medical print advertising, 334
nutrition labels, 333
plugging the holes, 333
political contributions, 334
TV media, 335
Bible, the, 302-305
creation of animals, 303
front-page news, 302
Genesis 1:28, 303
Genesis 1:29, 302
guideline for the human diet, 302
vegetarian diet arguments, 305
Breast Milk
diabetes, 235
in vegans, 128
omnivore mothers, 128, 284
percent of protein, 51
pesticides in, 128, 284
rats (percent of protein), 327

Calcium
adequate (vegetarians), 252
African Bantu, 252
amino acids, 63

baked into the planet, 65
Dairy Council, 337-340
dairy products, 64, 226, 251
deficiency (cows' milk), 106
Eskimos, 62, 252
fractures, 42
Harvard study, 62
immune system roles, 70
kidney stones, 238
negative balance, 62, 251
neutralize protein, 251
nutrients (one acre of land) , 186
organic soil, 181
RDA, 64
supplements, 251
Tooth Fairy, 62
true / false quiz, 62
vegans and vegetarians, 63, 252
WELL diet, 63
Cancer
cancers - not random and mysterious, 229-232
diet and 17 cancers, 230-232
perception of other diseases, 229
within our control, 230
of the breast, 222-224
chemotherapy, 223
losing the war, 222
mammograms, 222
prevention, 224
WELL vs. SICK diet, 223
of the colon, 219-221
new cases, 219
percent correlation, 219
protein, 220
snail in molasses, 220
soup can under sink, 220
witches' brew, 220
of the ovaries, 225-228
causes of, 225
dairy products, 226
diet - eggs in one basket, 228
diet given secondary status, 227
estrogen, 227
Mother Nature tried, 225
of the prostate, 216-218
cancer awareness survey, 217
cases per year, 216
fiber in the diet, 216

animal, 63, 64, 95
athletes, 75
autoimmune disease, 275
   asthma, 276, 280
   lupus, 276
   multiple sclerosis, 276
   relapsing polychondritis, 276
   rheumatoid arthritis, 275
calcium balance, 63, 111
casein, 108
children's needs, 79
cows' milk, 105, 235
Crohn's disease, 47, 271
fatigue, 290
fossil fuel, 179
hearing loss, 259
human requirement, 42, 101, 111, 326
in an egg, 112
in breast milk, 51
in chicken and fish, 101
in pork, 99
in SICK diet, 238
kidney disease, 239
kidney stones, 238
killer T-cells, 290
Kwashiorkor, 327
nutrient ratio, 39
Osborne and Mendel, 327
osteoporosis, 251
percent in foods, 326
plant kingdom - human needs, 51
produced on acre of land, 186
proportions, 326
protein - tiger in our closet, 324-328
risk of heart disease, 106
SIDS, 285
too much - the harm, 326
tumor promotion, 220, 230, 231
utilization, 328
war (correlation), 293
Psychology, 386-390
   aversion therapy, 389
   behavior modification, 389
   classical conditioning, 386
   desensitization, 389
   dog and pigeons, 386
   instrumental learning, 387
   makes us human, 390

Quality of Life, 417-419
   last years of life, 419
   mother and stepfather, 417
   not ahead of the game, 417
   the details, 417
   the irony, 419
   three hopes, 419
   twenty years, 417
   where time used to go, 418

Religions, 313-316
   all-exclusive, 313
   Buddhism, 315
   Christianity, 316
   early vegetarian sects, 313
   fundamental principles, 313
   Hindu, 315
   Islam, 315
   Jainism, 316
   Judaism, 316
   reason or rationalize, 316
   spinning the laws, 314
   Taoism, 316
Reversing Disease with Diet
   arterial plaque, 117
   arthritis, 42
   atherosclerosis - Dr. Dean Ornish, 208
   cancer, 73
   diabetes, 42
   12-year Esselstyn study - heart disease, 42

School Donations, 341-345
   "educational" materials, 342
   government commodities, 343
   health problems, 344
   icon of childhood, 344
   prescription required, 345
   two points of view, 341
Scientific Evidence - Overview, 28-31
   categories of evidence, 29
   confirmation or revelation, 31
   definition, 28
   Doctor's Sy and Ince, 28
   Rose Garden, the, 31
   University of Utopia, 28
Society, 391-393
   assumptions, 392